Oxford American Handbook of
Sports Medicine

W0091892

Published and Forthcoming Oxford American Handbooks

Oxford American Handbook of Clinical Medicine
Oxford American Handbook of Anesthesiology
Oxford American Handbook of Clinical Dentistry
Oxford American Handbook of Clinical Diagnosis
Oxford American Handbook of Clinical Pharmacy
Oxford American Handbook of Critical Care
Oxford American Handbook of Emergency Medicine
Oxford American Handbook of Geriatric Medicine
Oxford American Handbook of Nephrology and Hypertension
Oxford American Handbook of Obstetrics and Gynecology
Oxford American Handbook of Oncology
Oxford American Handbook of Otolaryngology
Oxford American Handbook of Pediatrics
Oxford American Handbook of Physical Medicine and Rehabilitation
Oxford American Handbook of Psychiatry
Oxford American Handbook of Pulmonary Medicine
Oxford American Handbook of Rheumatology
Oxford American Handbook of Surgery

Oxford American Handbook of Sports Medicine

Edited by

Jeffrey R. Bytomski

Head Medical Team Physician
Associate Professor and Director
Primary Care Sports Medicine Fellowship
Duke University Medical Center
Durham, North Carolina

Claude T. Moorman, III

Associate Professor
Head Team Physician and Director
Duke Sports Medicine
Duke University Medical Center
Durham, North Carolina

with

Domhnall MacAuley

School of Life and Health Science
University of Ulster
Department of Epidemiology
The Queen's University of Belfast
Northern Ireland

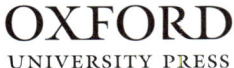
OXFORD
UNIVERSITY PRESS

OXFORD
UNIVERSITY PRESS

Oxford University Press, Inc. publishes works that further
Oxford University's objective of excellence
in research, scholarship and education.

Oxford New York

Auckland Cape Town Dar es Salaam Hong Kong Karachi
Kuala Lumpur Madrid Melbourne Mexico City Nairobi
New Delhi Shanghai Taipei Toronto

With offices in

Argentina Austria Brazil Chile Czech Republic France Greece
Guatemala Hungary Italy Japan Poland Portugal
Singapore South Korea Switzerland Thailand Turkey Ukraine Vietnam

Copyright © 2010 by Oxford University Press, Inc.

Published by Oxford University Press Inc.
198 Madison Avenue, New York, New York 10016

www.oup.com

Oxford is a registered trade mark of Oxford University Press

First published 2010

Library of Congress Cataloging-in-Publication Data

Oxford American handbook of sports medicine / edited by Jeffrey R. Bytomski,
Claude T. Moorman with Domhnall MacAuley.

    p. ; cm. — (Oxford American handbooks)

Adapted from: Oxford handbook of sport and exercise medicine / edited by
Domhnall MacAuley. 2007.

Includes bibliographical references and index.

ISBN 978–0–19–537219–9

1. Sports medicine—Handbooks, manuals, etc. I. Bytomski, Jeffrey R. II. Moorman,
Claude T. III. MacAuley, Domhnall. IV. Title: Handbook of sports medicine.
V. Series: Oxford American handbooks. [DNLM: 1. Sports Medicine—Handbooks.
2. Athletic Injuries—Handbooks. QT 29 O97 2010]

RC1211.O938 2010

613.71—dc22   2009023186

9 8 7 6 5 4 3 2 1

Printed in China
on acid-free paper

Preface

The world of sports medicine is becoming more complex as athletes receive care from a multi-faceted team including physicians, athletic trainers, physical therapists, and sports psychologists, to name a few. Many other professions assist in the care of athletes as well. Sports medicine is unique in balancing a safe return to sports while aggressively treating the problem in the least amount of time. With extensive media coverage of elite athletes, every athlete from children to the average "weekend warrior" expect the same level of care given to their sports elite figures. The sports medicine team is stretched on a daily basis to provide cutting-edge care while maintaining a full schedule.

The purpose of this Handbook is to have a reliable source readily available to those who are on the frontlines of sports medicine care. It is meant to be a reference as care providers travel from the office, to the training room, to the sideline, and around the world. Our aim for this text is to bridge the gap between comprehensive knowledge and quick access at the point of care by multiple levels of providers. This book is adapted from the original British version and has the advantage of knowledge collected from many experts around the globe. We have provided some practical chapters on procedures and radiology as well as exposure to many of the techniques used in the evolving world of sports psychology. The scope of the text ranges from discussion of event coverage and prepartication exams to both acute and chronic treatment of common medical and orthopedic problems in athletes.

We hope you gain the knowledge and insight needed to take care of your athletes at the highest level, wherever your travels take you.

Acknowledgments

This Handbook has only come together through the time, effort, and sacrifice of many individuals, not unlike the sports medicine team caring for its athletes at the highest level. The authors did a wonderful job of reviewing the previous text while updating and molding the new chapters to their current version. The clinical experience and knowledge of Dr. Moorman was without equal in assuring a quality text in the orthopedic chapters. Also, Andrea Seils at Oxford University Press has been instrumental in making this publication a high-quality Handbook. I would also like to thank all of the families of the contributors for their sacrifice in allowing the contributors to take time away from their schedules to make this a fine Handbook.

And finally, I would like to thank Shanda, Jarek, Trevor, and Alexandra for their patience and sacrifice as I spent time away from them in preparing the Handbook you have in front of you.

Jeffrey R. Bytomski

Contents

Detailed contents

List of color plates

Contributors

Kenton L. Anderson, MD
Resident Physician
Division of Emergency Medicine
Duke University Medical Center
Durham, North Carolina

David Berkoff, MD
Assistant Professor of Surgery
Division of Emergency Medicine
Duke University Medical Center
Durham, North Carolina

Blake Boggess, DO
Assistant Professor
Department of Family Medicine
Division of Sports Medicine
Duke University Medical Center
Durham, North Carolina

Jeffrey R. Bytomski, DO
Head Medical Team Physician
Associate Clinical Professor and
Director
Primary Care Sports Medicine
Fellowship
Duke University Medical Center
Durham, North Carolina

Albert Cook, MD
Sports Medicine Fellow
Duke University Medical Center
Durham, North Carolina

Greg Dale, PhD
Associate Professor of the Practice
of Health,
Physical Education and Recreation
Duke University
Durham, North Carolina

Husam Darwish, MD
Foot and Ankle Fellow
Duke University
Durham, North Carolina

Marc DeJong, MD
Primary Care Sports Medicine
Southern Illinois Sports Medicine
Belleville, Illinois

Stephanie Diamantis, MD
Resident
Department of Dermatology
University of North Carolina at
Chapel Hill
Chapel Hill, North Carolina

Mark Easley, MD
Assistant Professor
Department of Surgery
Division of Orthopedic Surgery
Duke University Medical Center
Durham, North Carolina

Brett Fritsch, MD
Sports Medicine Fellow
Duke University Medical Center
Durham, North Carolina

William Garrett, MD, PhD
Professor, Department of Surgery
Division of Orthopedic Surgery
Duke University Medical Center
Durham, North Carolina

John Hedge, DO
Primary Care Sports Medicine
Piedmont Family Practice
at Tega Cay
Fort Mill, South Carolina

Luke Hoagland, MD
Resident Physician
Department of Radiology
Harvard University
Boston, Massachusetts

Stacy Kennedy, MD
Rheumatology Fellow
Duke University Medical Center
Durham, North Carolina

Kevin Krasinski, MD
Sports Medicine Fellow
Duke Sports Medicine
Durham, North Carolina

Nancy Major, MD
Associate Professor
Department of Radiology
Division of Musculoskeletal
Radiology
Duke University Medical Center
Durham, North Carolina

Joe T. Minchew, MD
Orthopedic Spine Surgery
North Carolina Orthopedic
Associates
Durham, North Carolina

Claude T. Moorman, III, MD
Associate Professor
Head Team Physician
and Director
Duke Sports Medicine
Duke University Medical Center
Durham, North Carolina

Kerry Mullenix, PT, LAT, ATC
Physical Therapist
Sports Medicine
Duke University Medical Center
Durham, North Carolina

Gregg Nicandri, MD
Sports Medicine Fellow
Duke Sports Medicine
Durham, North Carolina

Nicholas Potter, DPT, ATC, LAT
Physical Therapist
Duke Sports Medicine
Duke University Medical Center
Durham, North Carolina

Airron Richardson, MD
Clinical Associate
Department of Surgery
Division of Emergency Medicine
Duke University Medical Center
Durham, North Carolina

Craig Rineer, MD
Hand Fellow
Division of Orthopedic Surgery
Duke University Medical Center
Durham, North Carolina

Jamie Robbins, PhD
Associate Professor
Department of Human
Performance and Sport Sciences
Winston-Salem State University
Winston-Salem, North Carolina

Jeffrey Roberts, MD
Clinical Associate
Department of Family Medicine
Duke University Medical Center
Durham, North Carolina

David Ruch, MD
Professor, Department
of Surgery
Division of Orthopedic Surgery
Duke University Medical Center
Durham, North Carolina

Michael Sampson, DO
Associate Professor, Family
Medicine/Sports Medicine
Director, Primary Care Skills/
Family Medicine Clerkship
Philadelphia College of
Osteopathic Medicine
Suwanee, Georgia

Deborah Squire, MD
Assistant Professor
Department of Pediatrics
Duke University Medical Center
Durham, North Carolina

Harry Stafford, MD
Clinical Associate
Department of Family Medicine
Duke University Medical Center
Durham, North Carolina

John Sundy, MD, PhD
Associate Professor
Department of Medicine
Division of Pulmonary Medicine
Duke University Medical Center
Durham, North Carolina

Paul Tawney, MD
Assistant Professor
Department of Surgery
Division of Orthopedic Surgery
Duke University Medical Center
Durham, North Carolina

Dean Taylor, MD
Professor, Department of Surgery
Division of Orthopedic Surgery
Duke University Medical Center
Durham, North Carolina

Alison Toth, MD
Assistant Professor
Department of Surgery
Division of Orthopedic Surgery
Duke University Medical Center
Durham, North Carolina

Priscilla Tu, DO
Sports Medicine Fellow
Duke Sports Medicine
Durham, North Carolina

Symbols and abbreviations

↑	increased
↓	decreased
ABCD	airway, breathing, circulation, disability
AC	acromioclavicular
ACE	angiotensin-converting enzyme
ACL	anterior cruciate ligament
ACOG	American College of Obstetricians and Gynecologists
ACSM	American College of Sports Medicine
ACTH	adrenocorticotrophic hormone
ADH	antidiuretic hormone
ADLs	activities of daily living
ADP	adenosine diphosphate
AED	automated external defibrillator
AHA	American Heart Association
AITFL	anteroinferior tibiofibular ligament
ALS	advanced life support
ALT	alanine transaminase
AMA	American Medical Association
ANA	antinuclear antibody
ANCA	antineutrophil cytoplasmic antibody
AP	anteroposterior
APL	abductor pollicis longus
AR	aortic regurgitation
AS	ankylosing spondylitis; aortic stenosis
ASD	atrial septal defect
ASIS	anterior superior iliac crest
AST	aspartate transaminase
ATFL	anterior talofibular ligament
ATLS	advanced trauma life support
ATP	adenosine triphosphate
AV	atrioventricular
AVN	avascular necrosis
AVPU	alert, verbal, pain, unresponsive
BEH	benign exertional headache
bid	twice a day
BLS	basic life support
BMD	bone mineral density
BMI	body mass index
BMR	basal metabolic rate

BP	blood pressure
BUN	blood urea nitrogen
CAA	coronary artery anomalies
CAD	coronary artery disease
CAQ	certificate of added qualification
CBC	complete blood count
CDC	Centers for Disease Control and Prevention
CFL	calcaneofibular ligament
CHF	congestive heart failure
CHO	carbohydrate
CJD	Creutzfeldt–Jakob disease
CMC	carpometacarpal
CMO	chief medical officer
CN	calcaneonavicular
CNS	central nervous system
CO	cardiac output
COPD	chronic obstructive pulmonary disease
COX-2	cyclo-oxygenase-2
CPPD	calcium pyrophosphate dihydrate disease
CPR	cardiopulmonary resuscitation
CRP	C-reactive protein
CSAI	Competitive State Anxiety Inventory
CSF	cerebrospinal fluid
CT	computed tomography
CTBI	chronic traumatic brain injury
CXR	chest X-ray
D5W	5% dextrose water
DB	dry bulb
DBP	diastolic blood pressure
DCS	diffuse cerebral swelling
DEXA	dual energy X-ray absorptiometry
DF	dorsiflexion
DFA	direct immunofluorescence assay
DIP	distal interphalangeal
DM	diabetes mellitus
ECG	electrocardiogram
ECRB	extensor carpi radialis brevis
ECRL	extensor carpi radialis longus
ECU	extensor carpi ulnaris
EDC	extensor digitorum communis
EEA	energy expenditure for activity
EEG	electroencephalography

EIA	exercise-induced asthma
EIB	exercise-induced bronchospasm
EMG	electromyography
EMS	emergency medical services
ENT	ear, nose, throat
EPB	extensor polaris brevis
EPO	erythropoetin
ER	external rotation
ESR	erythrocyte sedimentation rate
EVH	eucapnic voluntary hyperpnoea
FAI	femoroacetabular impingement
FCR	flexor carpi radialis
FCU	flexor carpi ulnaris
FDA	Food and Drug Administration
FEV_1	forced expiratory volume in 1 second
fMRI	functional magnetic resonance imaging
FPT	functional performance test
FRC	functional residual capacity
FSH	follicle-stimulating hormone
FVC	forced volume capacity
GCS	Glasgow Coma Scale
GERD	gastroesophageal reflux disease
GFR	glomerular filtration rate
GH	growth hormone
GI	gastrointestinal
GIRD	glenohumeral internal rotation deficit
GnRH	gonadotrophin-releasing hormone
GT	globe temperature
Hb	hemoglobin
HEENT	head, eyes, ear, nose, throat
HMB	beta-hydroxy-beta-methylbutyrate
HPV	human papillomavirus
HR	heart rate
HRT	hormone replacement therapy
IA	intrinsic asthma
IBD	inflammatory bowel disease
ICD	implantable cardioverter defibrillator
ICP	intracranial pressure
Ig	immunoglobuliin
IGF-1	insulin-like growth factor 1
IHD	ischemic heart disease
IHS	International Headache Society

IM	intramuscular
IO	intraosseous
IOC	International Olympic Committee
IP	interphalangeal
ITB	iliotibial band
ITBFS	iliotibial band friction syndrome
IV	intravenous
IVP	intravenous pyelogram
J	joule(s)
LAD	left anterior descending artery
LBBB	left bundle branch block
LCL	lateral collateral ligament
LH	luetinizing horming
LMA	laryngeal mask airway
LOC	loss of consciousness
LV	left ventricle
LVH	left ventricular hypertrophy
MCL	medial collateral ligament
MCV	mean corpuscular volume
MDI	metered-dose inhaler
MI	myocardial infarction
MJ	megajoules
MPHR	maximum predicted heart rate
MR	mitral regurgitation
MRI	magnetic resonance imaging
MRSA	methicillin-resistant *Staphylococcus aureus*
MS	mitral stenosis
MSU	mid-stream urine sample
MT	metatarsal
MTBI	mild traumatic brain injury
MTPJ	metatarsophalangeal joint
MVP	mitral valve prolapse
NATA	National Athletic Trainers' Association
NCAA	National Collegiate Athletic Association
NSAIDs	nonsteroidal anti-inflammatory drugs
OA	osteoarthritis
OCD	osteochondritis dissecans
OCP	oral contraceptive pill
OTC	over the counter
PaO_2	partial pressure of arterial oxygen
PCL	posterior cruciate ligament
PCR	polymerase chain reaction

PDA	patent ductus arteriosus
PEA	pulseless electrical activity
PEFR	peak expiratory flow rate
PFJ	patellofemoral joint
PFT	pulmonary function test
PIN	posterior interosseous nerve
PIP	proximal interphalangeal
PLRI	posterolateral rotary instability
PMMD	premenstrual dysphoric disorder
PMR	polymyalgia rheumatica
PMS	premenstrual syndrome
PNF	proprioneurofacilitation
PNS	peripheral nervous system
POMS	profile of mood states
POP	plaster of Paris
PPE	preparticipation exam
PRE	progressive resistive exercise
PRICE	protect, rest, ice, compression, elevation
PS	pulmonary valve stenosis
PSIS	posterior superior iliac crest
PTFL	posterior talofibular ligament
PVC	premature ventricular complex
PVCM	paradoxical vocal cord motion
Q	cardiac output
qid	4 times a day (quarter in die)
RA	rheumatoid arthritis
RBBB	right bundle branch block
RDA	recommended daily allowance
RH	relative humidity
RM	repetition maximum
ROM	range of movement
RR	respiratory rate
RV	residual volume; right ventricular
SA	sinoatrial
SAC	Standardized Assessment of Concussion
SAH	subarachnoid hemorrhage
SAID	specific adaptations to imposed demand
SA/M	surface area to body mass (ratio)
SARA	sexually acquired reactive arthritis
SBP	systolic blood pressure
SCA	sudden cardiac arrest
SCAT	Sports Concussion Assessment Tool

SCD	sudden cardiac death
SEM	sports and exercise medicine
SIJ	sacroiliac joint
SIS	second-impact syndrome
SLAP	superior labrum anterior to posterior
SLE	systemic lupus erythematosus
SLR	straight-leg raise
SPECT	single-photon emission computer tomography
SSRI	selective serotonin reuptake inhibitor
STI	sexually transmitted infection
SVT	supraventricular tachycardia
SV	stroke volume
TBI	traumatic brain injury
TC	talocalcaneal
TCA	tricyclic antidepressant
TENS	transcutaneous electrical nerve stimulation
TFCC	triangular fibrocartilage complex
TLC	total lung capacity
TN	talonavicular
TSH	thyroid-stimulating hormone
TUE	therapeutic use exemption
UCL	ulnar collateral ligament
ULCL	ulnar lateral collateral ligament
URI	upper respiratory tract infection
US	ultrasound
UV	ultraviolet
VCD	vocal cord dysfunction
VF	ventricular fibrillation
VM	vastus medialis
VMO	vastus medialis obliquus
VO_2max	maximal oxygen consumption
VSD	ventral septal defect
VT	ventricular tachycardia
VZV	varicella zoster virus
WADA	World Anti-Doping Agency
WB	wet bulb
WBC	white cell count
WBGT	wet bulb globe temperature
WHO	World Health Organization
WPW	Wolff–Parkinson–White (syndrome)

Acute care and sports injury

Sports first aid

First aid comprises the assessments and interventions that can be performed by a bystander with minimal or no medical equipment.

When an injury occurs

- Assess responsiveness—if the person is unresponsive, call 911 or send someone to activate emergency medical services (EMS).
- Assess the airway, breathing, and circulation (ABCs) and initiate basic life support (BLS) as needed.

If the injured person is alert, is breathing, and has a pulse:

- Immobilize the patient if spinal injury is suspected.
- Control any external bleeding with direct pressure.
- Splint any fractures.
- Treat for shock, hyperthermia, or hypothermia as indicated.
- If no major injuries are suspected, remove the person from the field for cleansing and treatment of other minor wounds and injuries.

Remember:

- Activate EMS if loss of normal function has occurred, or if advanced support beyond first aid is necessary.
- Keep within recognized first-aid guidelines, and respond to emergencies within the limits of your training.
- We all have a duty of care (Good Samaritan) but will have a different standard of care, whether physician, nurse, or trainer.
- Informed consent should be obtained from the injured person, or the person's parents if a minor, before the treatment of any nonemergent injury commences. Authorization to treat in the absence of the parent may be obtained in writing prior to sports participation. Exceptions exist for life-threatening injuries.

Basic life support

Introduction

Following an initial assessment of the possible DANGER to those carrying out the resuscitation and the RESPONSE of the victim, BLS comprises four basic steps:

1. Airway maintenance
2. Breathing
3. Circulation
4. Defibrillation

BLS guidelines listed here are for out-of-hospital, single-rescuer, adult BLS, and imply no equipment is employed (with the exception of the automated external defibrillator [AED])—a simple airway or facemask should be used if available (see Fig. 1.1).

Purpose of BLS

- Adequate ventilation and circulation need to be maintained until means of reversing the underlying cause of the arrest can be obtained.
- BLS is a "holding operation"—on occasion, particularly when the primary pathology is respiratory failure, it may itself reverse the cause and allow full recovery.
- Failure of the circulation for 3–4 minutes (less if the victim is initially hypoxic) will lead to irreversible cerebral damage.
- Current "thoracic pump" theory proposes that chest compression, by increasing intrathoracic pressure, propels blood out of the thorax, and forward flow occurs because veins at the thoracic inlet collapse while the arteries remain patent.
- Even when performed optimally, chest compressions do not achieve more than 30% of the normal cerebral perfusion.
- Assessment of the carotid pulse is time consuming and leads to an incorrect conclusion (present or absent) in up to 50% of cases. For this reason, training in detection of the carotid pulse as a sign of cardiac arrest is no longer recommended for non-health-care persons.
- The risk to the rescuer during cardiopulmonary resuscitation (CPR) is minimal.
- As blood oxygen remains high initially, ventilation is less important than compressions. Thus the priority is to start with compressions.
- Jaw thrust is not recommended for lay rescuers but for more experienced personnel in cases of suspected cervical spine injury.

Guideline changes

The American Heart Association (AHA) updated the BLS guidelines in 2005 to reflect the fact that an interruption in chest compressions is associated with a reduced chance of survival for the victim. The update stresses the need to maximize chest compressions while minimizing interruptions and simplifies the skills to aid lay rescuer resuscitation.

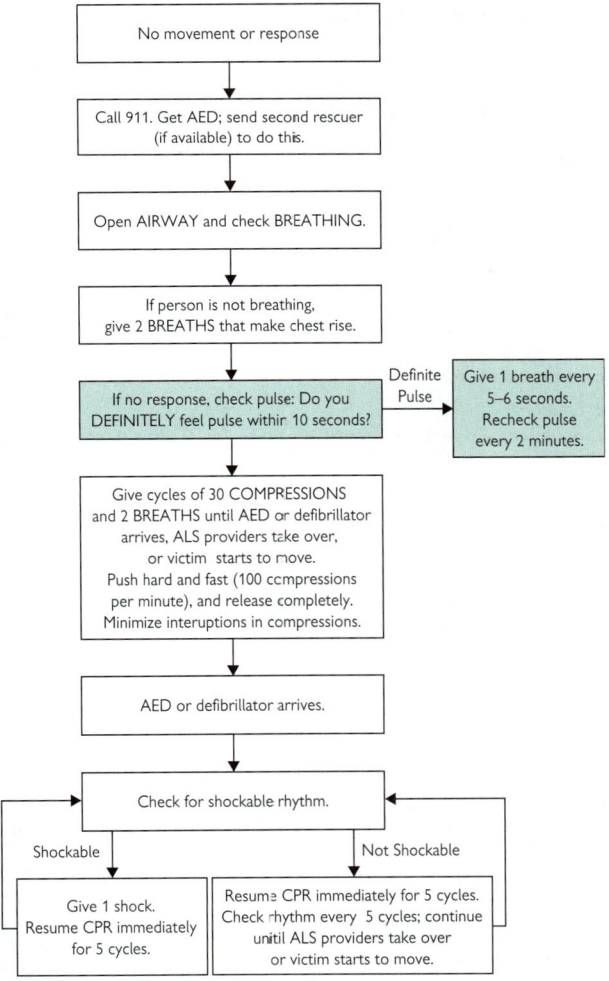

Figure 1.1 Basic life support (BLS) algorithm. Algorithm for BLS for adults by a single rescuer. AED, automated external defibrillator; ALS, advanced life support; CPR, cardiopulmonary resuscitation. Shaded boxes are steps performed by health-care providers, not by lay rescuers. Adapted with permission from the American Heart Association. 2005 American Heart Association guidelines for cardiopulmonary resuscitation and emergency cardiovascular care. *Circulation* 2005; **112**(24 Suppl):IV-19.

Sequence of events for BLS

- Check for response—tap the victim's shoulder and shout, "Are you okay?"
- If the person responds, place the person in the recovery position, send for help if required, and reassess regularly.

IF THERE IS NO RESPONSE:

- Activate EMS and obtain an AED if available. A bystander may be sent, or the lone rescuer should go and call 911 at this time.
- Initiate the four steps in BLS:
  1. Airway maintenance
  2. Breathing
  3. Circulation
  4. Defibrillation

1. Airway maintenance

Open the airway—head tilt, chin lift is recommended for the lay rescuer's evaluation of all victims.

2. Breathing

Look, listen, and feel for normal breathing for at least 5 seconds, but no more than 10 seconds. If in doubt, proceed as if the victim were not breathing.

- Look for chest movement.
- Listen at the person's mouth for breath sounds.
- Feel for air on your cheek.

If the person is breathing, place the person in the recovery position, send for help if required, and reassess regularly.

If the person is not breathing, give two rescue breaths.

3. Circulation

The health-care professional should check for a carotid pulse. The layperson should not check for signs of circulation but should proceed immediately to commence chest compressions.

- Place the heel of one hand on the victim's breastbone at the nipple line, and place the heel of the other hand on top of the first.
- Interlock fingers of both hands, extend arms vertically above the sternum, and depress the sternum 1.5–2 inches, allowing for complete recoil, at a rate of 100 compressions each minute.
- After 30 compressions, open the airway again (head tilt/chin lift), and deliver 2 more breaths while watching for the victim's chest to rise. Each breath in should take 1 second.
- Return hands to the correct position on the sternum and give a further 30 compressions.

4. Defibrillation

When the AED arrives, the pads should be placed on the victim immediately. CPR should be discontinued while the device analyzes the victim's heart rhythm. The device will advise that a shock be delivered to the victim or that CPR be continued if a shockable rhythm is not detected. Follow the AED prompts.

Details regarding defibrillation may be found in Advanced cardiac life support (p. 10) and Automatic external defibrillators (p. 16) in this chapter.

Continue with chest compressions and rescue breaths at a ratio of 30:2. Continue until the following occur:

- More qualified help arrives and takes over.
- The victim shows signs of life.
- Rescuer exhaustion occurs.

When to go for help

When there is more than one rescuer, one of the rescuers should go for help immediately. With a single rescuer, and if the casualty is an adult, then assume the cause is cardiac and go for help before commencing cardiac compressions.

Perform resuscitation for five cycles of CPR (2 minutes) before going for help if

- The cause is likely an asphyxial arrest (e.g., drowning).
- The victim is a child.

Two-person resuscitation

- When another rescuer is available to help, the second rescuer should be sent to activate EMS and obtain an AED while the first rescuer begins CPR.
- When the second rescuer returns, the rescuers take turns delivering chest compressions.
- Rescuers usually work on opposite sides of the victim.
- One rescuer maintains the airway and delivers breaths. The other rescuer performs fast and deep compressions.
- The compression-to-ventilation ratio with two rescuers is 30:2 for adults and 15:2 for children.
- The two rescuers switch roles after every five cycles of CPR to avoid fatigue. The switch should take less than 5 seconds.

Resuscitation of children

The fear of causing harm to a child as a result of resuscitation is unfounded. For ease of teaching and retention, laypeople should be taught that the adult sequence should be used for children who are not responsive and not breathing.

The following minor modifications to the adult sequence (see Fig. 1.2) will make CPR more suitable for use in children (ages 1 year to adolescent):

- Lone rescuers should perform five cycles of CPR before going for help. If the collapse was sudden and witnessed, the rescuer may immediately go for help after verifying that the person is unresponsive (e.g., young athlete who collapses on the playing field).
- Compress the chest by approximately 1/3 to 1/2 of its depth.
- The compression-to-ventilation ratio is 15:2 with two rescuers instead of 30:2 as with adults or with a single rescuer. This is the only time a rescuer would deviate from the 30:2 ratio used everywhere else in BLS.

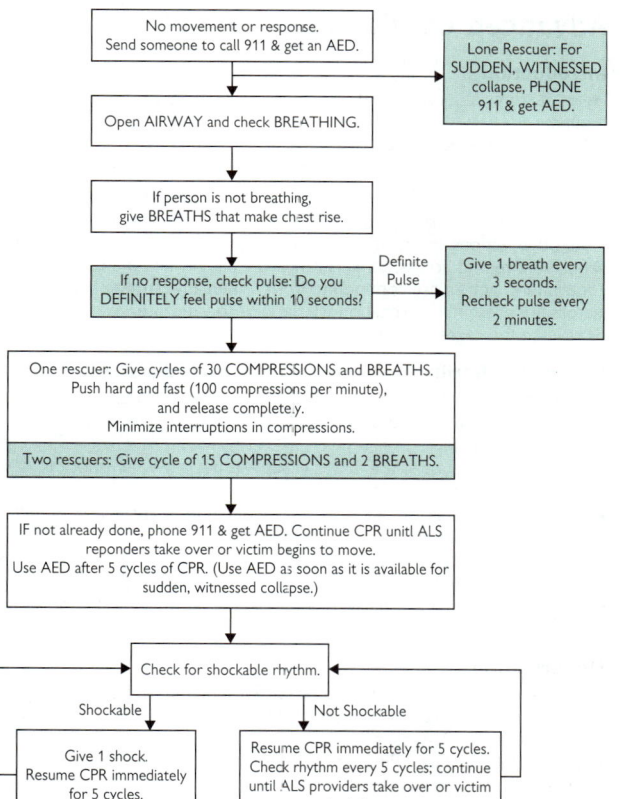

Figure 1.2 Pediatric basic life support (BLS) algorithm. Algorithm for BLS for children >1 year of age. AED, automated external defibrillator; ALS, advanced life support; CPR, cardiopulmonary resuscitation. Shaded boxes are steps performed by health-care providers, not by lay rescuers. Adapted with permission from the American Heart Association. 2005 American Heart Association guidelines for cardiopulmonary resuscitation and emergency cardiovascular care. *Circulation* 2005; **112**(24 Suppl):IV-158.

Advanced cardiac life support

Introduction

Heart rhythms associated with **pulseless arrest** can be divided into two groups:

- Ventricular fibrillation/ventricular tachycardia (VF/VT)
- Other rhythms including asystole and pulseless electrical activity (PEA)

The main difference between the two is the need for defibrillation and the administration of antiarrhythmic medications in those with VF/VT.

All other actions, including chest compressions, airway management and ventilation, venous access, administration of epinephrine, and correction of contributing factors, are common to both. When any of these contributing factors are present, resuscitation will require specific intervention to treat or reverse the cause (see Fig. 1.3).

Ventricular fibrillation/ventricular tachycardia/arrest

- In adults, VF is the most common rhythm at time of arrest.
- Arrest may be preceded by a period of VT or supraventricular tachycardia (SVT).
- The best survival rates are in this group—especially when shock is delivered promptly.
- Survival rates decline by 7%–10% for each minute that the arrhythmia persists—BLS can slow but not halt this decline.
- It is vital that patient rhythm be determined early via monitoring electrodes or defibrillator paddles.
- Start BLS if there is any delay in defibrillation, but this should not delay shock delivery.

Defibrillation

- Give one initial shock; energy selection for biphasic devices is device specific (typically 120–200 joules [J], if unknown use 200 J); energy used for monophasic devices is 360 J.
- Immediately resume CPR after the initial shock, and continue for five cycles of CPR.
- Check rhythm and pulse after five cycles of CPR. If the victim is still in VF/VT, deliver another shock at the same energy (higher energy may be used with biphasic devices) and continue CPR immediately thereafter. If asystole is present treat as asystole (see p. 13). If a pulse is present begin postresuscitation care.
- Once the second shock has been delivered and CPR is resumed, the first dose of epinephrine (1 mg intravenous/intraosseus [IV/IO]) may be administered. This dose of epinephrine should be repeated every 3–5 minutes while in VF/VT arrest. The first dose may be substituted with a dose of vasopressin (40 units IV/IO).
- After five more cycles of CPR, the rhythm and pulse are again reassessed. If the victim is still in VF/VT another shock is given and CPR is immediately resumed. At this time antiarrhythmics are considered.
- If VT/VF recurs after restoration of spontaneous circulation, begin algorithm from the beginning. Start with the initial shock and then begin CPR.

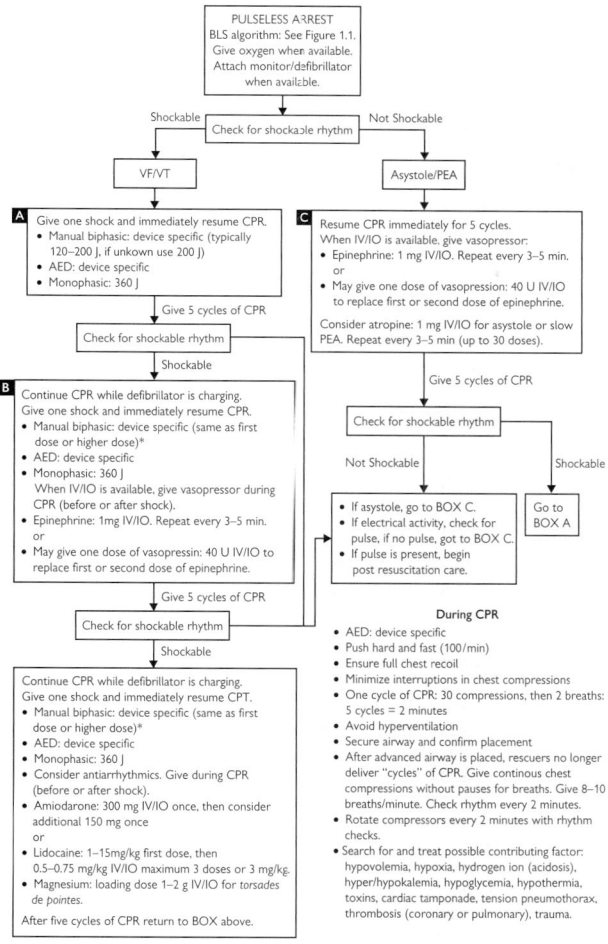

Figure 1.3 Algorithm for advanced life support for adults with pulseless cardiac arrest. AED, automated external defibrillator; BLS, basic life support; CPR, cardiopulmonary resuscitation; IO, intraosseous; IV, intravenous; J, joules; PEA, pulseless electrical activity; VF, ventricular fibrillation; VT, ventricular tachycardia. Adapted with permission from the American Heart Association. 2005 American Heart Association guidelines for cardiopulmonary resuscitation and emergency cardiovascular care. *Circulation* 2005; **112**(24 Suppl):IV-58.

Chest compressions, airway, and ventilation

If ventricular fibrillation persists after the initial shock, the best chance of restoring a perfusing rhythm still lies with defibrillation, but myocardial and cerebral viability must be maintained with chest compressions and ventilation of the lungs (CPR).

- Immediately resume five cycles of CPR at a ratio of 30 compressions to 2 ventilations.
- Consider reversible causes—see p. 14.
- Check electrode/paddle positions, gel pads, etc.

The patient's airway should be secured:

- Tracheal intubation is most reliable if adequate training/experience.
- Alternatives include laryngeal mask airway (LMA).
- The aim is to ventilate the patient's lungs and deliver the highest possible concentration of oxygen, preferably 100%.
- Once the patient's trachea has been intubated, chest compressions, at a rate of 100/minute, should continue uninterrupted (except for pulse checks and defibrillation when indicated), and ventilation should continue at approximately 8–10 breaths/minute (1 breath every 6–8 seconds).
- Performance of chest compressions uninterrupted for ventilation results in a substantially higher mean coronary perfusion pressure.
- LMA is an alternative that should enable uninterrupted compressions and ventilation. If leakage is excessive, revert to 30:2 ratio.

Intravenous access and drugs

- IV access should be established if this has not been achieved already.
- Drugs administered by the peripheral route must be followed by a flush of at least 20 mL of 0.9% saline to assist their delivery into the central circulation.
- Epinephrine is administered, 1 mg by the IV route or 2–2.5 mg via the endotracheal tube (diluted with 5–10 mL normal saline).
- Epinephrine is administered every 3–5 minutes while the victim remains in VF/VT arrest.
- The role of adrenaline is to improve the efficacy of CPR—alpha-adrenergic actions cause vasoconstriction, which increases myocardial and cerebral perfusion pressure.
- There is no evidence that any antiarrhythmic medication increases survival to hospital discharge; however, amiodarone has been shown to increase short-term survival to admission.
- Consider amiodarone (300 mg IV/IO diluted with 20–30 mL of D5W for the first dose, then 150 mg IV/IO once) to treat pulseless VF/VT.
- Lidocaine is an alternative to amiodarone. It has no proven short- or long-term benefit but has fewer side effects than amiodarone (1–1.5 mg/kg first dose, then 0.5–0.75 mg/kg IV/IO, maximum 3 doses or 3 mg/kg).
- Amiodarone or lidocaine is administered after the third shock during a VF/VT arrest and is considered after each additional shock.

- Magnesium can effectively terminate torsades de pointes. 1–2 g of magnesium may be administered as an IV/IO push in 10 mL D5W over 5–20 minutes.
- Magnesium is also indicated in victims with known or suspected low serum magnesium. These victims include patients with a history of alcoholism, poor nutrition, or other hypomagnesemic states.
- There is no evidence that bicarbonate improves likelihood of successful defibrillation or improves survival in VF arrest. Its administration may produce a wide array of adverse effects including worsening intracellular acidosis.
- The use of bicarbonate (1 mEq/kg) may be considered in special resuscitation situations such as preexisting metabolic acidosis, hyperkalemia, or tricyclic antidepressant overdose. Whenever possible, bicarbonate therapy should be guided by blood gas analysis.

When do you stop resuscitation?

- The number of times the loop in the VF/VT arrest algorithm is repeated during any individual resuscitation attempt is a matter of clinical judgment.
- The decision to terminate resuscitative efforts lies with the treating physician.
- Factors to consider include time to CPR and defibrillation, prearrest state, and comorbid diseases, as well as the initial arrest rhythm.
- Witnessed collapse and a short time to resuscitation improve the chances of successful resuscitation.

Asystole and pulseless electrical activity (PEA)

Outcome is very poor unless a reversible cause can be found and treated effectively. If asystole or PEA is confirmed, appropriate drugs are given and a further five cycles of CPR are given to complete the algorithm loop.

Asystole

It is essential that the correct diagnosis be made and, most importantly, that VF is not missed.

Asystole must be confirmed by the following:

- Checking that the leads are attached correctly.
- Viewing the rhythm in more than one lead.
- CPR is initiated and continued for five cycles (2 minutes). The airway is secured, IV access obtained, and the first dose of epinephrine (1 mg IV/IO) given.
- The first or second dose may be substituted with vasopressin (40 units IV/IO).
- CPR is continued and epinephrine is administered every 3–5 minutes. CPR is not interrupted for administration of any medication.
- Rhythm is checked after every five cycles of CPR (2 minutes). If a shockable rhythm (VF/VT) is present, deliver a shock and resume CPR, then continue on the VF/VT algorithm. If an organized rhythm is present check for pulse. If there is no pulse, immediately resume CPR.

- Any reversible or aggravating factors should be identified and treated promptly.
- Consider atropine, 1 mg IV/IO. This may be repeated every 3–5 minutes up to 3 doses.

Pulseless electrical activity

Patients with PEA have mechanical cardiac contractions, but the contractions are too weak to produce a blood pressure that is detectable without invasive blood pressure monitoring. PEA is often caused by reversible conditions, and the patient's best chance of survival will be by prompt identification and treatment of these reversible underlying causes.

- Because of the similarity in causes and management between asystole and PEA, the treatment is the same.
- If PEA is associated with a bradycardia (<60 bpm), atropine 1 mg IV/IO is given. This may be repeated every 3–5 minutes up to 3 doses.

Potential reversible causes or contributory factors

During any cardiac arrest, potential causes or aggravating factors for which specific treatment exists should be considered. For ease of memory, these are divided into two groups on the basis of their initial letter—either *H* or *T*:

The *H*'s:
- Hypovolemia
- Hypoxia
- Hydrogen ion (acidosis)
- Hypo- or hyperkalemia
- Hypoglycemia
- Hypothermia

The *T*'s
- Tamponade (cardiac)
- Tension pneumothorax
- Thrombosis (coronary or pulmonary)
- Trauma
- Toxins (tricyclic antidepressants [TCAs], digoxin, beta-blockers, calcium-channel blockers)

Automated external defibrillators

Electrical defibrillation is well established as the only effective therapy for cardiac arrest due to VF. The scientific evidence to support early defibrillation is overwhelming, the single most important determinant of survival being the delay from collapse to delivery of the first shock. The chances of successful defibrillation decline at a rate of 7%–10% with each minute if no CPR is provided.

BLS alone will help to sustain a shockable rhythm but is not a definitive treatment as it is unlikely to restore a perfusing rhythm. Without CPR, VF rapidly deteriorates to asystole.

The "chain of survival"

The chances of survival following cardiac arrest are considerably improved if appropriate steps are taken to deal with the emergency. These four steps are as follows:

- Early recognition of the emergency and activation of appropriate emergency services
- Early CPR
- Early defibrillation
- Early advanced life support

Manual defibrillation has been widely available for many years, but the requirement for training in arrhythmia recognition limits the application of this technique to medical practitioners, nurses working in critical care areas, and ambulance paramedics.

Recent developments in AEDs have enabled increasing numbers of individuals to perform defibrillation safely and effectively. Increased provision of early defibrillation through the widespread deployment of AEDs is now considered a realistic strategy for reducing mortality from cardiac arrest due to ischemic heart disease.

Equipment

AEDs are reliable computerized devices that are simple to operate and enable both laypersons and health-care providers to deliver safe defibrillation.

AEDs are provided with a sturdy carrying pouch that should contain spare electrodes, strong scissors, and a disposable safety razor.

Training

Any individual with responsibility for the management of cardiac arrest in the hospital or community must be trained in and authorized to perform defibrillation using an AED. The AHA has also integrated the use of AEDs into BLS training.

AHA guidelines recommend adequate training of lay rescuers in AED use, adequate provision of AEDs in settings where sudden cardiac arrest may occur, and sending for and using an AED or defibrillator as soon as possible after a witnessed arrest.

Sequence of actions for AED

AED use is integrated with the use of CPR at the scene of a suspected cardiac arrest. When a rescuer arrives at the scene of a possible cardiac arrest, the victim's ABCs are checked. If the victim has no response, is not breathing, and does not have a pulse (the layperson is not required to check for a pulse), use of an AED is appropriate.

Lone rescuer with an AED

If the lone rescuer has immediate access to an AED, the rescuer should immediately activate EMS and get the AED. CPR is initiated when the rescuer returns. The AED is used if the victim does not respond, is not breathing, and does not have a pulse (the layperson is not required to check for a pulse).

Exceptions are if the victim is likely a victim of an asphyxia arrest (e.g., drowning) or if the victim is a child and the rescuer did not witness the arrest: the rescuer should give five cycles (2 minutes) of CPR before going for help and the AED.

Two rescuers with an AED

When two rescuers arrive at the scene of a likely cardiac arrest, one rescuer checks the victim for response. If the victim does not respond, the second rescuer activates EMS and gets the AED while the first rescuer performs CPR until the AED arrives.

When the AED arrives, CPR is interrupted and defibrillation is attempted.

Exceptions are if the victim is a child and the rescuer did not witness the arrest: finish five cycles of CPR before attaching and using the AED. EMS personnel or other health-care professionals may complete five cycles of CPR before using the AED if the call-to-arrival time is greater than 4–5 minutes.

AED operation

Although there are multiple available models, all AEDs operate following four universal steps:

- Turn the AED **ON**.
- **ATTACH** electrode pads to the victim's bare chest. One pad is placed on the victim's upper-right chest, and the other is placed to the left of the victim's left nipple. If the chest is wet or sweaty it should be wiped dry. Hairy victims may need to be shaven. If the connecting cables are not preconnected, they will need to be plugged in.
- Clear the victim and **ANALYZE** the rhythm. Do not touch the victim during analysis. The AED will tell you if a shock is indicated.
- **SHOCK.** If a shockable rhythm is detected by the device, a shock is advised. Ensure that everyone is clear of the patient before pressing the shock button. Immediately resume five cycles of CPR. CPR should be resumed whether a shock was indicated or not. The AED will automatically prompt the rescuer to repeat the third and fourth steps when 2 minutes of CPR has been performed.

Major emergencies in sport

- Bleeding and shock
- Head injuries
- Cervical spine injuries
- Choking
- Unconscious casualty
- Severe facial injuries
- Hypothermia, heat stroke, and altitude sickness
- Abdominal trauma
- Cardiac and pulmonary emergencies

Major limb injuries

- Fractures and dislocations
- Major ligament injuries

Medical emergencies

- Diabetes
- Seizures
- Acute asthma attack
- Severe allergic reaction
- Poisoning

The unconscious athlete

Unconsciousness results from lack of oxygen or nutrients to the brain.

Causes of unconsciousness
- *Lungs*: respiratory problem, injury or poison
- *Heart*: lack of adequate circulation to brain
- *Metabolism*: diabetes, drugs, alcohol, infection, too hot, too cold
- *Brain*: lack of oxygen, head injury, epilepsy

Management
- Activate EMS for any unresponsive person. Assess ABCs.
- If the person is not breathing, begin BLS.
- If the person is breathing, look for clues as to the cause.
- Treat if possible.
- Monitor the person continuously.

Monitoring the unconscious casualty

The Glasgow Coma Scale (GCS) is the most widely used scale worldwide for assessing level of consciousness but is difficult for the first-aider to understand and use. Simpler versions are available, including the AVPU scale, shown in Box 1.1.

Box 1.1 AVPU scale

A = Alertness	Avpu = **A**lert
V = Verbal	aVpu = responds to **V**erbal cues
P = Pain	avPu = responsive to **P**ain
U = Unresponsive	avpU = **U**nresponsive

Choking

Choking is serious. It may lead to the choking person becoming unconscious, and is potentially fatal if the obstruction is not removed.

Mild airway obstruction

If airway obstruction is mild or partial the person will be conscious, breathing, and be able to cough forcefully.

- Encourage victim to cough.
- Do not interfere with the person's own efforts to expel the foreign body, but stay with the victim to monitor.
- If mild airway obstruction persists, activate EMS by calling 911.

Severe airway obstruction

If airway obstruction is severe there will be little to no air exchange and the person will be unable to cough. The person will be unable to speak and may be turning blue. Many choking victims will make the universal choking sign by clutching their neck with their hands.

- Ask the victim of suspected choking if they are choking. If the person nods and is unable to speak, begin abdominal thrusts (Heimlich maneuver).
- Abdominal thrusts are performed by wrapping your arms around the victim from behind. A clenched fist is made with one hand and grasped with the other. Place the grasped fist just above the navel, and make quick, upward thrusts into the victim's abdomen toward the chest.
- Repeat abdominal thrusts until the object is expelled or the person becomes unresponsive.
- Carry out back blows up to 5 times. These are done with the heel of the hand between the scapulae.
- If the person becomes **unconscious,** proceed to BLS.

The only difference in BLS after choking is that each time the airway is opened to deliver breaths, the mouth should be opened wide to look for the foreign body. If the object is seen it should be removed with the fingers. Never perform a blind finger sweep.

Choking in children and infants

Choking in children (ages 1 year and above) is treated the same as that in adults.

If airway obstruction in an infant is mild, do not interfere with the infant's efforts to cough and expel the foreign body. If the infant is unable to cough or cry, proceed with alternating back slaps and chest thrusts.

- Back slaps are performed by holding the infant face down on your forearm and supporting the infant's head and jaw with your hand. Five slaps with the heel of your hand are delivered between the infant's shoulder blades with enough force to expel the object.
- If the object is not expelled with back slaps, rotate the infant into the supine position on your other forearm and perform five chest thrusts.
- Chest thrusts are delivered in the same fashion as for infant CPR chest thrusts.

- Repeat the sequence of alternating back slaps and chest thrusts until the foreign body is expelled or until the infant becomes unresponsive.
- If the infant becomes unresponsive, place the infant on a firm, flat surface and begin CPR.
- As with adults, each time you open the airway, look for the obstructing foreign body and remove it with your fingers if visible. Do not perform a blind finger sweep.
- After five cycles of CPR, activate EMS.

Management of shock and bleeding

Introduction

Bleeding most commonly arises as a result of trauma:

- *Externally:* direct trauma—wounds, facial and nasal injuries, etc.
- *Internally:* head, chest, or abdominal injury, or from major fractures, particularly to the pelvis and long bones

The major hazard of significant bleeding in sport is the development of shock.

Management of shock

Shock is defined as an inadequate perfusion of the body's vital organs. Inadequate perfusion resulting in shock may occur when blood loss or dehydration decreases circulating blood volume, when the heart is damaged, or any time blood pools in large dilated veins instead of being circulated to vital organs.

The body will use compensatory mechanisms to maintain perfusion and blood pressure initially; thus hypotension is **not** an early sign of shock, especially in children and healthy young adults.

Causes of shock

Hypovolemic

- Blood loss—external or internal hemorrhage
- Other fluid loss such as diarrhea, vomiting, burns, etc.

Cardiogenic—pump failure

- Myocardial infarction or myocarditis
- Thoracic aortic dissection, acute valvular regurgitation
- Cardiac arrhythmias
- Cardiac-depressant drug overdose

Anaphylaxis

- Food allergy, especially peanuts
- Insect stings, especially from bees and wasps

Neurogenic

- May occur in a cervical spine injury

Systemic

- Sepsis
- Liver or adrenal failure
- Drug overdose (e.g., vasodilators)

Management of bleeding

The initial first aid history and assessment may give clues as to the cause, e.g., bleeding wound, chest pain, bee sting, etc.

If the blood pressure is so low that it is unrecordable, treat as a medical emergency and activate EMS by calling 911.

- Assess/open airway—look for obstruction, vomit, or blood and clear if possible.

General management plan for acute sports injuries

Preparation and planning

The successful management of sports injury requires preparation and planning. Factors include the following:

- Equipment and facilities
- First aid kit and doctor's bag
- Liaison with officials, administrators, and coaches
- Membership of the "medical team," which includes a variety of health-care professionals

On-site availability

On-site availability allows

- Initiation of the appropriate management immediately.
- Direct observation of the mechanism of injury—this aids accurate diagnosis.

Ideally such availability includes presence at both practices and games. This can help to build trust with the coaching staff, the training staff, and the athletes. It may also allow further input into the athlete's preparation in the following areas:

- Preseason screening and assessment
- Fitness assessment
- Planning of training schedules
- Monitoring rehabilitation, arranging surgical opinions and operations, etc.

Event management

Medical input may be valuable in planning of events and may include advice on playing surface, equipment, adequate time for warm-up and rest, training facility evaluation, and availability of first aid equipment.

Proper event management will not only limit injury risk (e.g., by not playing on dangerous surfaces) but also ensure prompt and appropriate care at the time of the injury.

Observation

This includes the following:

- Observation of training and warm-up to ensure proper technique
- Observation of the sport so that the doctor is familiar with the rules and likely injuries that will result
- Observation of exact injury mechanism can result in prompt and appropriate treatment.

History

An appropriate history is vital to ensure correct diagnosis and treatment. In the acute setting the athlete may be distressed by the pain or the implications of serious injury.

The exact nature and location of the pain will be a guide as to the structures injured. In Achilles tendon or anterior cruciate ligament rupture, for example, the athlete may describe an audible "pop."

Clinical examination

Early examination, before swelling and the inflammatory response ensue, may aid in the diagnosis, which can be more difficult at a later time. Initial field-side assessment is frequently helpful. However, at times it may be more appropriate to carry out a clinical examination at a more suitable location, e.g., the training room. Protective equipment should be removed with caution to allow full examination, unless this could worsen the injury.

The initial examination should
- Establish a preliminary diagnosis.
- Determine whether the athlete can continue.
- Determine whether further urgent or emergent treatment is required, e.g., in the training room or at the hospital.

Treatment

- *Emergency care*: Injuries to the head, cervical spine, and chest, and those to major joints or bones should be considered an emergency and managed appropriately.
- *Triage*: This includes transport from the field and, if required, to the hospital for X-rays and further evaluation. Open communication with the EMS staff, local hospital, and athlete, coach, and family is crucial.
- *Immediate injury care*: If standard care is appropriate it should follow the PRICE regimen—see Management of acute soft tissue injury (p. 28).

Return to play

Return to training and competition is determined by the following:
- Return will not worsen the injury.
- Return will not increase the risk of further injury.
- The athlete will be able to perform at a pre-injury level.
- The athlete's return will not place other competitors at risk.

This decision should take into account factors such as the importance of the event, time left in the event, future schedule, and playing conditions.

The medical team should observe the athlete closely on return to play, to ensure that recovery is complete and no further damage is taking place. Judgment on return to play should be based solely on the health of the athlete and should take precedence over the wishes of the coach, relatives, club, supporters, and, sometimes, the wishes of the athlete him- or herself.

Management of acute soft tissue injury

The PRICE mnemonic incorporates the various treatment modalities for acute soft tissue injuries:

P = protect
R = rest
I = ice
C = compression
E = elevation

Protect

This refers to a number of types of protection:

- Protect the athlete so he or she does not make the injury worse.
- Protect and support surrounding structures.
- Protect other competitors.
- Protection of the injured part may include crutches, splints, slings, braces, taping, strapping, etc. Protection of an injury is essential if healing and recovery of function are to occur in a timely manner.

Rest

True rest is difficult to enforce and, in practice, usually unnecessary.

Absolute rest

Absolute restriction of activity is only necessary in the acute management of an injury to control inflammation. Severe soft tissue injuries may require a short period of complete rest or immobilization in a cast or a brace to restrict movement and limit further injury. Absolute rest may also be required initially after an operation.

Relative rest

Although absolute rest is important in the acute management of some soft tissue injuries, absolute rest over a prolonged period leads to muscle and ligament atrophy, decreases circulation to the injury, promotes joint adhesions and stiffness, and prolongs healing and repair of injured tissues. Frequently an athlete should maintain some activity in the subacute period. This will usually be part of the rehabilitation program and is often important physically as well as psychologically to the athlete. Relative rest ensures the following:

- Maintenance of muscle strength and joint lubrication as well as a more complete recovery of supporting tendons and ligaments
- Maintenance of general cardiovascular conditioning and aerobic fitness, e.g., swimming, stationary cycling, or jogging

Exercise is a recognized part of the rehabilitation program for soft tissue injury. Damaged ligaments benefit from the "stress" of weight bearing and movement. Excessive rest will prolong the inflammatory phase and lengthen the time to return to play. The length and amount of relative rest will depend on severity of the injury and should be supervised by a trained health-care provider.

Ice

The application of cold (cryotherapy) has been advocated since the classical description of inflammation by Celsus in the first century AD (redness, swelling, heat, and pain), to which Virchow, in 1858, added loss of function.

Theoretical benefits of cryotherapy include the following:

- Limitation of bleeding via vasoconstriction: The theory of reflex vasodilatation remains controversial
- Limitation of swelling
- Limitation of inflammation and further tissue damage: This may be due to the effect of histamine on vascular membranes and on neutrophils and leukocytes
- Reduction in metabolism in local tissues: This reduces enzyme function, inhibits pain, and decreases swelling and oxygen consumption
- Assistance with pain control. However, watch for the athlete who becomes "pain free" with ice and wishes to resume playing; ice inhibits pain in two ways
  - Relief of surrounding muscle spasm
  - Decreases the number and speed of sensory pain impulses

How to apply ice

Ice comes in a variety of forms, including crushed ice (better than ice cubes as the contact is better), chemical ice packs, reusable gel cold packs, and those combined with compression, e.g., Cryo/Cuff.

Coolant sprays work by evaporation, thus reducing skin temperature. They do not achieve sufficient depth of cooling to be effective in reducing muscle temperature.

Debate continues as to the optimum frequency and time of application. An intermittent protocol is more effective than continued application. Repeated applications of 20–30 minutes every 1.5–2 hours for 48–72 hours is usually effective.

Ice works via conduction. Because adipose tissue is an excellent insulator, ice application may have to be extended in those areas with greater body fat.

Contraindications to using ice

- Broken or damaged skin
- Where nerve damage is suspected and sensation altered
- Where altered circulation is suspected
- When ice application increases pain

Compression

The early use of compression will do the following:

- Support the injured area
- Decrease swelling

On an extremity, a wrap should be applied in a distal to proximal direction, and pulses should be checked after applying to ensure the wrap is not too tight.

Ice can be combined with compression. Later, compression can be replaced by a supportive bandage or strapping.

Taping is best done by an experienced sports athletic trainer or physical therapist to achieve maximum benefit.

Elevation

- Contributes to the reduction in blood flow and, as a result, swelling
- Elevate injured extremity above the heart
- Should be combined with support of the elevated part, e.g., pillows
- Should be maintained over the first 24 hours

Care of wounds

A *wound* is defined as a "disruption of the tissues produced by an external mechanical force." Wounds include the following:

- Abrasions
- Contusions
- Lacerations
- Incisions and puncture wounds

Open wounds are very common in contact sports such as football, soccer, lacrosse, ice hockey, etc. They are also common in sports where falls often occur, such as cycling, skateboarding, and horseback riding.

Prognosis is dependent on the type of trauma and the extent of the damage. Watch closely for the following:

- Severe bleeding and clinical shock
- Infection
- Complications secondary to the extent of the damage, e.g., blood vessel, nerve, and tissue damage

Abrasions

An abrasion (Latin *abradere*, "to scrape") is a superficial injury. Damage is only to the epidermis so it should not actively bleed (though in practice abrasions may extend into the dermis). A scratch is linear, whereas a graze suggests a broader impact.

The cause is normally a glancing contact with a rough surface. Tangential impact produces a moving abrasion, which indicates direction by the pattern of damage to the epidermis and may leave trace material such as grit. This type is most common in sports played on artificial surfaces such as AstroTurf.

Direct impact produces an imprint abrasion with the pattern of the causative object.

All abrasions reflect the site of impact (contrast contusions).

Contusions (bruises)

A *contusion* involves bleeding into the soft tissue due to the rupture of a small blood vessel resulting from a direct, blunt force, e.g., a punch. A hematoma is a contusion in which a larger amount of bleeding results in a pool of blood.

Contusions and strains comprise 60%–70% of all sports injuries and are of variable severity from simple skin damage to contusions of internal organs. Most go unreported and untreated. They are typically caused by blunt trauma such as a blow or a fall. Uncomplicated contusions do not breach the skin surface and there is no external bleeding.

It is important to exclude other causes of bleeding, including abnormalities of the clotting system in diseases such as leukemia, thrombocytopenia, liver disease, and vitamin deficiencies (vitamin C).

Pathology

Trauma causes rupture of capillaries and possible venules (arterial damage rare). After impact, bleeding may continue for some time due to circulatory pressure. If the volume of bleeding is sufficient, swelling occurs. If extravisated blood collects in a pool it is known as a *hematoma*. Local inflammatory reaction occurs at a site with necrotic tissue, caused by macrophage infiltration.

The site of bruising does not always indicate the exact site of injury, as blood will track through tissues under the influence of gravity and body movement (e.g., bruising along the lower border of the foot in an ankle sprain and thigh bruising in a fractured hip).

Deeper bruising will result in a slower appearance of surface-skin discoloration. Changes in color do not give an accurate estimate of the time of the initial impact.

Signs and symptoms
- Soreness and pain with active movement
- Visible trauma and swelling
- Unaffected residual function compared to that with injuries such as a muscle rupture
- Bruising requires a formal assessment before return to play

Differential diagnosis
This includes soft tissue injury such as muscle rupture, ligament sprain, etc.

Lacerations
Most lacerations are treated by primary closure with a close approximation of the wound edges, or primary intention. This may involve suturing or items such as steri-strips, staples, or wound glue.

Secondary wound healing occurs when the wound is initially left open. This may occur when there is infection or for a crush injury with extensive tissue damage.

Wound healing may also be affected by the following:
- *Anatomical site*: poor over tibia
- *Vascular supply*: poor in peripheral vascular disease
- *Movement*: e.g., over a joint
- *Wound configuration*: e.g., jagged edges
- *Mechanism of injury*: incised wounds heal quickly.
- *General health and nutrition of the casualty*: older patients, those on steroids, etc.

Assessment of wounds
It is important to obtain an accurate history:
- Time of injury
- Mechanism of injury
- First aid treatment, if any
- Tetanus immunization status, if any
- Allergies or hypersensitivities (especially tapes, dressings, etc.)
- Medication, if any

Physical examination
- Anatomical site
- Size—width and length
- Depth
- Configuration—straight, jagged edge, etc.
- Tissue loss

- Deformity
- Loss of function, including motor and/or sensory loss
- Pain
- Bleeding—actual and estimated

Immediate management
- Elevation with support
- Direct pressure—with sterile dressing if available
- Pressure dressing—not tourniquet

Cleaning
- This is essential to prevent infection and remove foreign-body fragments.
- The protective-barrier effect of skin is broken in wounds, allowing microorganisms to enter deeper tissues.
- Wounds that "look" clean are not necessarily sterile—consider all traumatic wounds contaminated.
- Clean wounds with high-pressure irrigation to remove contaminants. Use sterile water if available; however, there is no evidence of increased infection when using drinking-quality tap water.

Wound closure
A variety of methods are available, and the type chosen depends on the nature of the wound and the amount of time since injury, among other factors. Some wounds may be best treated by delayed closure.
- Sutures
- Steri-strips
- Staples
- Adhesive

Dressings
Many types are now commercially available. The choice of dressing depends on factors such as the following:
- Nature and location of wound
- Presence and risk of infection
- Amount of exudates

Tetanus
All patients should have current tetanus status established and be immunized as per current Centers for Disease Control and Prevention (CDC) guidelines.

Return to sport
This will depend on a number of factors:
- Nature of wound—size, method of closure, edges, etc.
- Site of wound, especially if over a joint
- Nature of sport

Nonsteroidal anti-inflammatory drugs (NSAIDs)

As the level of competition increases and greater competitive performance is required, there is a point at which the strain on the skeletal framework exceeds that which the body can withstand, resulting in damage to connective tissues and joints.

The inflammatory response

This response enables the body's defensive and regenerative resources to be channeled into tissues that have suffered damage or are contaminated with abnormal material (e.g., invading microorganisms). The term *inflammation* is derived from the Latin *inflammare*—to set on fire. It is used to describe the pathological process that occurs at the site of tissue damage. Classical description was first made by Celsus in first century AD.

There are four signs of inflammation—redness, swelling, heat, and pain. Virchow (1858) added loss of function (see Box 1.2).

Prior to the 20th century *phagocytosis* was considered the primary movement of inflammatory reaction with specialized cells being able to move "amoeba-like" to the site of the noxious agent, to ingest and destroy foreign material such as bacteria. The importance of a vascular system was later recognized—without this there would be no redness or heat associated with the inflammatory response.

Inflammation is a dynamic process that may, at times, cause more harm to the organism than the initiating noxious stimulus itself. Hayfever, for example, can be incapacitating but occurs as a consequence of our defense system's response to harmless airborne pollen.

Not all inflammatory reactions are useful; there are no benefits from the inflammatory reactions that occur in diseases such as rheumatic fever or rheumatoid arthritis.

Vascular changes

The immediate reaction of skin is redness due to increased blood flow through the inflamed area. Its duration depends on the severity of the stimulus. Skin temperature rises and approaches that of the deep body temperature.

The whole capillary bed at the damaged site becomes suffused with blood at an increased pressure as capillaries dilate and closed ones open up. Venules open up with increased venous flow.

Thus two of the cardinal signs of inflammation, *heat* and *redness*, are caused by this increase in blood flow to the affected area.

Swelling

Swelling results from changes in the permeability of the blood vessel wall to protein. Normally the tissue fluid is composed of water with some low-molecular-weight solutes. The very low protein content, compared to that of the blood, is because of the impermeability of the blood vessel wall, which inhibits protein movement from the blood vessel to the surrounding tissues.

Box 1.2 The inflammatory response

1. An influx of blood giving rise to the characteristic *heat* and *redness*
2. A movement of plasma protein and associated water into the tissue, causing *swelling*
3. An influx of phagocytic cells that have the potential to cause tissue destruction
4. *Pain*, perhaps due to pressure on the nerve ending by the swelling or to the effect of chemical mediators of pain being released
5. Finally, and perhaps most important to sports, *loss of function*—Virchow's fifth sign

Normally the vascular pressure generated from the heart forces water out of the blood at the arteriolar end, while the colloid osmotic pressure exerted by the protein in the blood draws water back at the venous end. Without the presence of the plasma protein, blood volume would rapidly diminish because of net movement of water from the blood to the tissues.

Pain

- May also be due to release of pain-inducing chemicals at the site of the reaction
- Is due in part to the increased pressure on sensory nerves that is caused by accumulation of the edematous fluid

Mediators

Lewis first proposed the *mediator* concept in 1927; he called this the H-substance. The first class discovered were prostaglandins, which are formed by the action of cyclo-oxygenase on arachidonic acid.

- Prostaglandins are abundant in the body, stored in granules in mast cells. They are found in high levels in lungs, the gastrointestinal (GI) system, and skin.
- They produce vasodilatation—redness and temperature and increased blood vessel permeability to protein, and swelling.
- At high concentration they can also produce pain.

Leukocytes in inflammation

More persistent inflammatory reactions involve the influx of leukocytes, the most important in inflammation being the polymorph/neutrophil. Normal extravascular tissue contains few polymorphs, but in inflammation these cells pass from the blood into damaged tissue.

Polymorphs are the first inflammatory cells to accumulate at the site of injury. They are *phagocytic* and ingest and digest invading microorganisms and tissue debris.

Acute inflammation will gradually resolve in time with no damage or, if more severe, synthesis of connective tissue to form a scar.

Use of anti-inflammatory drugs to treat inflammatory conditions

Hippocrates mentions chewing of willow bark. MacLagan (1876) used an extract of willow bark, called *salacin,* to treat rheumatic fever. In 1899, a synthetic analogue of salacin, produced by Bayer, called *acetylsalacilic acid,* was given the trade name *aspirine*. Now 20 or so aspirin-like drugs are available—aspirin and ibuprofen are two of the least expensive medications that can be bought over the counter.

There is no clear evidence of any single agent being more effective than others.

Mechanism of action

In 1971, John Vane and colleagues published three papers in *Nature* that outlined the ability of anti-inflammatory drugs to suppress the synthesis of prostaglandins. The activity of these drugs is as follows:

- Reduce the symptoms of heat and redness, as prostaglandin normally promotes an increased blood flow
- Reduce pain, as there will be no hyperalgesia without prostaglandin
- Reduce edema and swelling, as the permeability-increasing effect of chemical agents on blood vessel walls would not be subject to the normal exaggerating action of prostglandin

The use of NSAIDs in inflammatory conditions is well established. They are a simple and relatively safe means of reducing the inflammatory response to injury and assisting return to competitive fitness more rapidly.

There are advantages to NSAID use in the early treatment of inflammatory responses to injury. Effectiveness of treatment over longer periods is less apparent, however. In self-limiting injuries, the differences between treatment and placebo groups diminish with time.

Whereas early NSAIDs were all based on aspirin, now there are more than 20 individual drugs available. Ibuprofen is most widely used and available for purchase over the counter.

Newer drugs were developed to lessen the gastric side effects, in particular GI bleeding, which is an especially important factor in the elderly. The most recently developed drugs that selectively inhibit cyclo-oxygenase-2 (COX-2) appear to have an excellent initial side-effect profile. Recent reports suggest an increased risk of cardiovascular events, however.

Strains and sprains

A *strain* is a partial or complete tear of a muscle or tendon. The most commonly strained muscles are those that cross two joints during an eccentric, rather than concentric, contraction. Lower limb muscles such as rectus femoris, biceps femoris, semitendinosus, adductors, hamstrings, and medial head of the gastrocnemius are frequently injured. Muscle strain more commonly occurs at the myotendinous junction, the weakest link in the muscle.

Ligament injury is also common in sports medicine. The knee, ankle, elbow, shoulder, and fingers are the most common joints affected.

- *Grade 1 injury:* A small number of fibers is damaged, resulting in some pain and swelling, with minimal loss of strength, function, or stability.
- *Grade 2 injury:* More fibers are damaged, with moderate pain, swelling, and loss of function in the form of muscle weakness or subtle joint instability.
- *Grade 3 injury:* There is complete tear of the tissue, which may result in complete instability of a joint or a gap in the muscle fibers.

Diagnosis is by clinical examination. An ultrasound or magnetic resonance scan may be helpful in some situations.

Ligaments

Anatomy and physiology

Ligaments are of variable shapes and sizes with fibers running parallel between two bony points of insertion. Some appear as less distinct sheets of connective tissue.

Most ligaments are extra-articular (though cruciates are intra-articular). They have variable blood supply—e.g., it is poor for cruciates, but good for medial collateral of the knee.

Most research is conducted on the cruciate ligaments because of their vital role in knee stability.

Ligament tensile strength is lost with immobility; plaster cast immobilization for 8 weeks requires a 9-month rehabilitation to recover tensile strength. Conversely, there may be increased ligament strength with a formal training program.

Histology

- Parallel collagen fibers run in a wave pattern to allow a spring-like stretch and lengthening. This allows an adjustment of tension and reduces the risk of injury.
- At the ligament insertion into the bone, there is a transition from fibrous tissue to fibrocartilage, which becomes mineralized as it attaches to bone.

Composition

- Ligaments are mainly type I collagen (some type II), elastin, and proteoglycans; 65% by weight is water.
- The stiffness of the ligament increases with loading, which allows limited movement but resists excessive load.

Function of ligaments

- Maintenance of joint alignment and the gliding motion of joint surfaces—ligament disruption will result in malalignment and subsequent early joint degeneration
- Proprioception around the joint
- Supporting the skeleton, e.g., spinal ligaments
- Maintenance of pressure on articular cartilage

Classification of ligament injuries

- *Grade I:* mild sprain with ligament stretched but not torn, no instability and a firm end point on stressing
- *Grade II:* partial tear with mild instability and softer end point on stressing
- *Grade III:* complete tear associated with significant instability

Mechanism of injury

Injury may occur as a result of direct trauma, or indirectly when there is a sudden mechanical stress to the joint. One of the most common ligament injuries is to the medial collateral ligament of the knee when there is a forced valgus injury. This may occur even when the point of contact is distal, because of the long levers of the lower leg.

If, for example, the athlete is struck on the lateral side of the lower leg when the foot is fixed, the knee joint is forced medially. This tends to stress the medial side of the joint and may also damage the meniscus and cruciate ligament(s).

Ligament healing

Classically, ligament healing is divided into three phases.

Inflammatory or substrate phase

This begins immediately after the acute injury with the classical inflammatory response of bleeding, swelling, cellular infiltrate of inflammatory cells, and white blood cells with later fibroblast aggregation.

Cellular proliferation phase

This phase occurs from 4 days until 2–3 weeks after injury. Fibroblasts proliferate and collagen is produced. Macrophages and mast calls are abundant. A new capillary network is established.

Remodeling phase

This phase is ongoing and probably continuous. Fibroblast infiltration and collagen production peak and diminish. Collagen scar forms, which gradually remodels from the healing type III to type I collagen fibers.

Factors affecting ligament healing

The degree of injury

The injury itself is the initial stimulus for repair. Traumatically torn tissue usually disrupts the length of the ligament and incomplete tears repair more easily.

Wound stress

This is a topic of much debate and research. Initial protection of the site (for about 2 weeks) allows some strength to be regained. Later, however, mobilization and a degree of stress are essential if maximal repair is to be achieved.

Adequate blood supply and nutrition

Adequate blood supply is important for the following:
- Transport of inflammatory cells that initiate wound healing
- Ensuring optimum wound healing
- Decreasing the risk of infection
- Improving wound healing if infection ensues

It has also been suggested that vitamin C, protein, and cystine may facilitate tissue healing.

Prevention of ligament injury

Factors that may help to prevent or limit damage and consequently time lost from sport include the following:
- *Understanding the risk*: high-risk sports are those played at high velocity and in which direct trauma is more likely to occur. Playing these sports results in a higher risk of ligament injury.

- *Rules of the sport*: modification of the rules in contact sports may reduce the risk of injury.
- *Sporting environment*: certain climatic conditions, such as heavy rain or ice, will alter the surface on which sport is played and thus the injury risk.
- *Use of protective equipment and devices*: these include both protection to prevent injury, such as protective padding, and the use of protective braces and supports to minimize repeated injury to an already damaged, incompletely healed ligament.
- *"Prehabilitation"*: while the immediate goal of training programs is to optimize performance, it will also have the additional benefit of reducing the incidence of injury. This can be achieved by the following:
  - High standard of coaching and training
  - Warm-up and stretching programs
  - Endurance and strength training
  - Proprioceptive, flexibility, and agility training
- *Medical screening of the athletes*: assessment of the following:
  - Previous injury and degree of rehabilitation achieved
  - Excessive ligamentous laxity, which may be picked up on screening examination
  - Incompetence of other supporting ligaments
  - Poor muscle strength
  - Other factors such as alcohol or drug use, which may increase injury risk

As with all febrile illness, athletes should not return to active play in the sport until fever subsides.

Bone

The human body comprises a variety of different materials, which can be divided into two groups based on function:
- Active structures, which produce force—muscles
- Passive structures, which do not produce force—bones, cartilage, ligaments, and tendons

Functions of bone

The adult human skeleton consists of 206 individual bones. These bones
- Provide support.
- Act with muscles as levers to transfer force.
- Protect the internal organs.
- Have a metabolic function—calcium storage and metabolism.

Types of bone

1. Cortical

Cortical is Latin meaning "bark"; it is also known as compact bone.
- Predominant in limbs—appendicular skeleton
- Surrounds trabecular bone as a protective covering
- Main role is to provide skeletal strength
- Has 3 layers—outer periostium, middle intracortical layer, and inner endostium, next to the marrow cavity
- Contains neurovascular "haversian canals" with capillaries and nerve fibers

2. Trabecular

In Latin *trabs* means "timber." This is also known as cancellous or spongy bone.
- Forms bones of axial skeleton, e.g., skull, rib cage, and spine
- Minimal part of skeletal strength
- Has a Major metabolic role
- Made up of strands or trabeculae of bone whose pattern is determined by the forces applied to the bone

Classes of bones

- *Long bones* have a hollow shaft and two extremities, e.g., humerus and tibia. They are found in limbs and act as levers to transmit force generated by the muscles.
- *Short bones* are cubical in shape, have a cortical cover, and have a spongy core. They include carpal and tarsal bones.
- *Flat bones* are layers of cortical bones with a spongy center. They include the sternum, skull bones, ribs, and scapula. Flat bones provide a large area for tendon attachment and protective function.
- *Irregular bones* have an adapted shape for a particular function. They include the pubis, maxilla, and vertebrae.

Bone metabolism

Bone composition
- Bone cells—osteoclasts and osteoblasts
- Bone matrix
  - 40% organic—type 1 collagen, proteoglycans, and growth factors
  - 60% inorganic—calcium hydroxyapatite

Calcium metabolism
- Regulated by parathyroid hormone (PTH) and vitamin D
- Recommended daily intake = 1000 mg
- Excreted by kidneys

Bone turnover
- Balance of osteoblast and osteoclast activity
- Affected by hormones such as estrogen, glucocorticoids, and thyroxine
- Bone "stress" is important.

Normal bone metabolism
- Peak bone mass in early adulthood
- Plateau until 35–40 years
- Rapid annual decline (1%–2%/year) in women after menopause
- Male bone loss begins later (45 years) and at a slower rate

Osteoporosis is the decrease in bone mass (per unit volume). Primary osteoporosis is normally postmenopausal and is determined by reduced estrogen. Other risk factors include the following:
- Caucasian race
- Heredity
- Early menopause or hysterectomy
- Smoking and alcohol or drug abuse
- Low calcium intake

Standard diagnosis includes measurement of bone density (DEXA scan) and calcium metabolism. Treatments include dietary measures, calcium and vitamin D, hormone replacement therapy (HRT), and bisphosphonates. Screen for osteoporosis in those with a fracture or two or more risk factors.

Secondary osteoporosis can result from a variety of causes:
- Poor diet
- Endocrine causes
- Drug induced, e.g., steroids
- Chronic disease, e.g., rheumatoid arthritis and chronic renal disease
- Malignancy

Bone biomechanics

Wolff's law (1892) states: "The shape of bone is determined only by the static stressing." While in general terms this is largely true, the effect of stress on bone is not as simple. Stress can have a variety of effects, as seen in a healing fracture or in bone atrophy. Wolff did not take into account the effect of heredity, where stress will not influence an inherited bone deformity.

When loaded, bone becomes increasingly "stiff," thus less likely to fracture under load (spine). Fracture will occur, however, when the load exceeds the ultimate strength of the bone.

Stress fractures are clinical manifestations of bone fatigue. This occurs from increased load repetitions that, individually, are within the normal acceptable load. Animal studies, for example, show a 5-fold increase in stress fractures from walking to jogging. The bones of the lower limb are more highly loaded and react with less strain at a given level of stress.

Fracture, which is the pathological result of load, may result from the following:

- Excessive force
- Weakened bone
- Small bone diameter
- Excess frequency of load
- Reduced recovery time between repeated loading

Bone remodeling is a slow process. A gradual progression in training intensity allows bone response that prevents stress fractures.

Bone shape is optimal for a normal load pattern so that bone deformity or an excessive load can contribute to the risk of skeletal injury.

Bones in children and adolescents deform at a lower load than in adults. The bone is weaker than the attached ligaments or tendons and is thus more likely to suffer avulsion fractures.

Bone and physical activity

- *Effect of gravity:* Bone mass has a positive correlation to body mass. Astronauts suffer an increased excretion of calcium and decreased bone mineralization that is not reversed by exercise in non-weight-bearing conditions.
- *Effect of inactivity:* Bed rest induces a weekly loss of bone mass with a mineral loss of up to 30%. The effects of prolonged bed rest may not be reversible.
- *Effects of muscular activity:* Muscular activity has a positive loading effect on the skeleton. Less activity and deteriorating muscle mass in the elderly increase fracture risk.
- *Effects of physical activity:* Multiple studies show a positive correlation between bone mass and physical activity benefits at any age.
- *The female athletic triad:* Female athletes who do not balance the demands of their sports with the needs of their bodies may develop this triad, which has negative effects on bone metabolism: (1) osteoporosis, (2) amenorrhea, and (3) disordered eating.

Sports injury in children

- Acute sports injuries occur 1.8–2.5 times more often in boys than in girls.
- The highest incidence of sports injuries is in children between the ages of 5 and 15 years (twice that of the general population).
- Peak rate of injury is age 12 years in girls and 14 years in boys.
- In contact sports, injuries occur more commonly in postpubertal than prepubertal children.
- Peak fracture incidence coincides with time of peak height velocity.
- Winter sports appear to be more injurious than summer sports for children.

Mechanisms of injury

How children differ from adults

- An immature skeleton requires special consideration.
- Identical mechanisms of injury produce different pathologies in children from those in adults.
- The existence of growth plates and apophyses (insertion of muscle–tendon units into immature bone) largely accounts for the different injury profile observed in children.
- Ligaments and tendons are stronger than bone in children.
- In children growth plate injuries and avulsion fractures are more common than ligament and tendon tears.

Osteochondroses

Pathology

- Group of conditions affecting the growing skeleton and articular cartilage
- May be intra-articular (e.g., osteochondritis dissecans), physeal (e.g., Scheuermann's disease), or extra-articular (e.g., traction apophysitis)

Cause and prognosis

- They vary in etiology and frequency of occurrence.
- They are more common in boys than in girls.
- Causative factors are not fully understood.
- Stress, ischemia, and genetics are all implicated to varying degrees.
- They differ in treatment and prognosis—some resolve spontaneously, others require surgical intervention.

Traction apophysitis

Cause

A combination of growth and excessive loading of the vulnerable tendon-growth plate interface occurs.

Treatment
- Local anti-inflammatory measures
- Unloading the inflamed tendon–bone interface by avoiding or reducing provocative activities (usually running and jumping)
- Improving flexibility of the involved muscle–tendon unit
- Graduated strengthening program
- Gradual reintroduction of activity

The specifics of these conditions will be discussed later in the book under the region they affect.

Further reading

Conn JM, Amnset JL, Gilchrist J (2003). Sports and recreation related injury episodes in the US population, 1997–99. *Inj Prev* **9**:117–123.

Head and face

Traumatic brain injury (TBI)

TBI is an injury to the brain or central nervous system and incorporates injuries to other structures of the head (skull bones, soft tissues, and vascular structures of the head and neck).

The incidence for all TBIs varies among countries and is approximately 300/100,000 per year, with 80% of those injuries being mild. In the United States there are approximately 1.4 million cases per year. Of those, about 235,000 are hospitalized with 50,000 deaths. Males are more than twice as likely to suffer a TBI as females. Sporting injuries comprise approximately 10% of all cases of TBI.

General management

The major priorities at the early stage are the basic principles of first aid. The simple mnemonic *ABCD* may be useful (see Table 2.1).

Only after these basic aspects of care are achieved and the patient is stabilized should you consider moving the patient from the field to an appropriate facility. Before moving the patient, carefully assess for cervical spine or other injuries.

Indications for urgent referral to the hospital

Any player who has or develops the following:
- Fractured skull
- Penetrating skull trauma
- Deterioration in conscious state following injury
- Focal neurological signs
- Confusion or impairment of consciousness lasting >30 minutes
- Loss of consciousness >5 minutes
- Persistent vomiting or increasing headache post-injury
- Any convulsive movements
- More than one episode of concussive injury in a session
- When there is assessment difficulty (e.g., an intoxicated patient)
- Children with head injuries
- High-risk patients (e.g., hemophilia, anticoagulant use)
- Inadequate post-injury supervision
- High-risk injury mechanism (e.g., high-velocity impact)

Table 2.1 Initial on-field assessment of concussion

A	Airway	Ensure clear, unobstructed airway. Remove mouthguard or dental device.
B	Breathing	Ensure the patient is breathing adequately.
C	Circulation	Ensure adequate circulation.
D	Disability	Evaluate for any neurological disability.

Glasgow Coma Scale (GCS)

The most widely used TBI severity scale throughout the world is the Glasgow Coma Scale (GCS) (see Table 2.2). It is useful in categorizing the acute injury as well as mild, moderate, and severe injuries, and is performed serially to monitor progress over time. Deterioration in the GCS score may herald intracranial complications requiring neurosurgical or neurointensive care intervention.

Table 2.2 Glasgow Coma Scale

Category	Response	Score
Eye opening response (E)	Spontaneous	4
	To speech	3
	To pain	2
	No response	1
Verbal response (V)	Oriented	5
	Confused, disorientated	4
	Inappropriate words	3
	Incomprehensible sounds	2
	No response	1
Motor response (M)	Obeys commands	6
	Localizes	5
	Withdraws (flexion)	4
	Abnormal flexion (posturing)	3
	Extension (posturing)	2
	No response	1

Management of traumatic brain injury

Acute management of sporting TBI

- An eyewitness account or, in the case of professional sports, videotape analysis may be available.
- Vital signs must be recorded following an injury. Abnormalities may reflect brainstem dysfunction.
- An acute rise in intracranial pressure with central herniation usually manifests rising blood pressure and falling pulse rate (the Cushing response).
- Hypotension is rarely due to brain injury, except as a terminal event, and alternate sources for the drop in blood pressure should be aggressively sought and treated. (Cerebral hypotension and hypoxia are the main determinants of outcome following brain injury and are treatable.)

A thorough neurological examination should be performed, including measurement of the GCS. It serves as a reference to which other repeated neurological examinations may be compared. Record your findings. Skull palpation should be a quick and simple component of every physical examination in head trauma. It is important to check for any evidence of cerebrospinal fluid (CSF) leakage through the nose or ears.

When time permits, a more thorough physical examination should be performed to exclude coexistent injuries and to detect signs of skull injury (e.g., Battle sign). Restlessness can frequently accompany brain injury or cerebral hypoxia and may be confused with a belligerent patient who is presumably intoxicated. If the patient has a decreased level of alertness but is restless, attention should be given to the possibility of increased cerebral hypoxia, a distended bladder, painful wounds, or tight casts. When these have been ruled out with certainty, drug therapy may be considered in consultation with a neurotrauma expert.

Diagnosis in head trauma

Indications for emergent head computed tomography (CT) in the initial evaluation of the head-injured patient include the following.

Indications for emergent neuroimaging

- History of loss of consciousness
- Depressed level of consciousness
- Focal neurological deficit
- Deteriorating neurological status
- Skull fracture
- Progressive or severe headache
- Persistent nausea/vomiting
- Post-traumatic seizure
- Mechanism of injury suggesting high risk of intracranial hemorrhage
- Examination obscured by alcohol, drugs, metabolic derangement, or postictal state

- Patient inaccessibility for serial neurological examinations
- Coagulopathy and other high-risk medical conditions

Obtain CT images as soon as the patient is hemodynamically stable and immediate life-threatening injuries have been addressed. Any deterioration in the neurological examination warrants prompt evaluation by CT, even if a previous study was normal.

Compared with CT, magnetic resonance imaging (MRI) is time consuming, expensive, and less sensitive to acute brain hemorrhage. Moreover, access to critically ill patients is restricted during lengthy periods of image acquisition, and the strong magnetic fields generated by the scanner necessitate the use of nonferromagnetic resuscitative equipment. Presently, MRI is best suited for electively defining associated parenchyma injuries following the acute event.

Plain skull radiographs are inexpensive and easily obtained and often demonstrate fractures in patients with epidural hemorrhage. However, the predictive value of such films is poor. Other, more traditional diagnostic tools have largely been supplanted by brain CT in the initial assessment of the head-injured patient.

Management of post-traumatic seizures

Impact seizures or concussive convulsions are well-recognized sequelae of head trauma. These are not epileptic and require no specific management beyond the treatment of the underlying concussive injury.

Post-traumatic epilepsy may also occur and is more common with increasing severity of brain injury. A convulsing patient is at increased risk of hypoxia with resultant exacerbation of the underlying brain injury. Maintenance of cerebral oxygenation and perfusion pressure (blood pressure) is critical in the management of such patients. Convulsions may cause a dramatic increase in intracranial pressure, so they should be prevented during the recovery phase of acute head injury.

Phenytoin (or fosphenytoin) is usually the drug of choice because a loading dose can be administered intravenously to rapidly achieve therapeutic concentrations and phenytoin does not impair consciousness. Benzodiazepines (e.g., lorazepam, clonazepam, diazepam) can be used for the acute treatment of post-traumatic seizures but they produce at least transient impairment of consciousness. Phenytoin, benzodiazepines, or any other anticonvulsant drug has been shown to prevent the development of post-traumatic epilepsy.

Post-traumatic epilepsy should then be managed in the same manner as symptomatic partial-onset epilepsy. Carbamazepine, phenytoin, and valproate are the drugs of choice for the initial management of secondarily generalized convulsions. Carbamazepine and phenytoin are drugs of choice for complex partial seizures, but valproate is also effective. New agents, such as gabapentin, lamotrigine, and topiramate, are also effective in the management of partial-onset seizures and generalized convulsions.

Treatments do change and it is important to keep up to date with current practice management standards.

Non-brain head injury

Various soft-tissue, bony, ocular, and other injuries may occur to the head. Scalp wounds, although dramatic in appearance, usually heal well with good wound management. Blood loss from scalp wounds may be extensive, particularly in children, but rarely causes shock.

Use the usual precautions against blood-borne infections such as hepatitis B and C and HIV infection. All open fractures or depressed skull fractures should have specialty consultation once at the hospital.

The wound should be irrigated with copious amounts of saline before closing and any debris, including hair, must be removed from the wound. Bony fragments should not be removed until surgery. The galea should be closed first using interrupted sutures and then the superficial layer of the scalp can be sutured or closed with staples.

Traumatic intracerebral hematomas and contusion

Subtypes

Traumatic intracerebral hematomas can be divided into acute or delayed types. Delayed traumatic intracerebral hemorrhages may take up to several weeks for signs to present.

Presentation

Clinical signs and symptoms depend on the size and location of the intracerebral hematoma as well as the rapidity of its development. In most cases, there is a brief period of confusion or loss of consciousness. Only one-third of these patients remain lucid throughout their course. Impaired alertness is found frequently on initial examination.

The prime aim is to reduce post-traumatic edema and ischemia. Treatment includes adequate circulation and ventilation, aggressive monitoring and control of intracranial hypertension to ensure adequate cerebral perfusion pressures, close intensive care monitoring, correction of any coagulopathies or electrolyte abnormalities, and seizure prophylaxis. Interventions to control elevated intracranial pressure include mechanical hyperventilation, osmotic diuresis, and emergency ventriculostomies.

Head-injured patients should be monitored for a coagulopathy for at least 24–48 hours after injury.

Prognosis

The overall cognitive impairment and the speed and quality of recovery are strongly related to the associated diffuse axonal injury. When occurring in isolation and when the volume is <30 cc, an intracerebral hematoma is compatible with a favorable recovery.

Brainstem compression and loss of consciousness significantly worsen prognosis regardless of treatment. Overall, mortality rates are in the range of 25%–30%.

Subdural hematoma

Subdural hematomas can be the result of either nonpenetrating or penetrating trauma to the head. There is bleeding into the subdural space due to stretching, and subsequent rupture of bridging cerebral veins. These injuries are typically seen following falls on hard surfaces or assaults with non-deformable objects rather than with low-velocity injuries.

In many cases there is a brief period of confusion or loss of consciousness. There is frequently impaired cognitive function and/or attention on initial examination.

Soft tissue injuries are seen at the site of impact. Other signs of significant head trauma that can suggest subdural hematomas include periorbital and postauricular ecchymosis, hemotympanum, CSF otorrhea or rhinorrhea, and facial fractures.

Focal neurological deficits depend on the location and size of the lesion. Hematoma enlargement or an increase in edema surrounding the hematoma produces additional mass effect. This leads to further depression of the patient's level of consciousness, increases the motor or speech deficit, and eventually compresses the ipsilateral third nerve and midbrain.

The impact that produces acute subdural hematoma frequently causes severe injury to the cerebral parenchyma. This coexisting severe brain injury explains, in large part, the better outcome for epidural hematomas than for acute subdural hematomas. Indeed, in most cases of acute subdural hematoma, it is likely that the extra-axial collection is less important in determining outcome than the parenchyma injury sustained at the time of impact.

Epidural hematoma

A direct blow to the head is required for epidural hematoma formation. As the skull is deformed by the impact and the adherent dura is forcefully detached, hemorrhage may occur into the pre-formed epidural space.

This injury is most commonly seen in children because of their more pliable skull. While the source of bleeding is most likely arterial from the middle meningeal artery, it can be venous, or both.

Presentation

There is remarkable clinical variability with epidural hemorrhage. In rare cases, epidural hematomas can be asymptomatic. However, most present with nonspecific signs and symptoms referable to an intracranial mass lesion. Presentation depends on the size and site of the hematoma, rate of expansion, and presence of associated cerebral pathology. Epidural hematomas involving the temporal lobe may cause a more precipitous decline than those at other sites because of their proximity to the brainstem.

Alterations in consciousness can be quite variable in extent and duration. The so-called lucid interval occurs in less than one-third of patients and thus is not a sensitive diagnostic clinical sign.

Treatment

An unrecognized or untreated large traumatic epidural hematoma leads to progressive neurological dysfunction due to the expanding mass lesion. This ultimately results in transtentorial or uncal herniation, brainstem compression or ischemia, and death.

Rapid diagnosis and prompt surgical evacuation offer the best chance of a favorable outcome. If treatment begins prior to obtundation, pupillary dysfunction, and vegetative motor posturing, the probability of full functional recovery is high.

Prognosis

The expanding epidural lesion only partially accounts for the neurological morbidity observed with epidural hematomas. Concomitant cerebral pathology is encountered in up to 50% of cases and is associated with lower admission GCS, more substantial and prolonged intracranial pressure (ICP) elevation, and higher mortality.

In general, it is the sequelae of these lesions that dictate the degree of residual functional impairment in patients who survive epidural hematomas.

Traumatic subarachnoid hemorrhage

Traumatic subarachnoid hemorrhage (SAH) is usually classified according to the site of arterial rupture and bleeding. It is usually due to vertebral artery injury—either a tear or dissection—although it may also be due to tearing of meningeal vessels.

Subarachnoid bleeding typically presents with frank meningeal symptoms such as headache, neck stiffness, and photophobia.

The most common initial symptoms are neck pain and occipital headache that may precede the onset of neurological symptoms from seconds to weeks. Clinical symptoms and signs often develop with a "stuttering" onset over days or weeks following the original injury or "sentinel bleed."

Treatment

Medical management of SAH is the same as for intracerebral hematomas with intracerebral monitoring and control of ICP. Vasoactive substances released by the hematoma may promote further ischemia, and the calcium-channel blocker nimodipine can be used to prevent vasospasm.

Operative treatment is directed toward control of ICP or treatment of hydrocephalus. The prognosis is variable and many cases have fatal outcomes.

Diffuse cerebral swelling

DCS or second-impact syndrome?

DCS is a rare but well-recognized complication of mild TBI in sports that occurs predominantly in children and teenagers. It is unlikely that a single impact of any severity may result in this rare complication. However, participation in sports often draws attention to concussive injuries in this setting.

Pathophysiology

The injured brain swells within the cranium. This increase in brain volume eventually increases ICP. In the first few hours and days following severe head injury, ICP is often raised from increased cerebral blood flow. Later brain swelling is due to an increase in brain tissue water content.

Anecdotal evidence suggests massive traumatic cerebral edema, documented on CT scanning, occurs within 20 minutes of cerebral injury. A significant increase in ICP can lead to brain herniation.

Post-injury DCS can occur within minutes or be delayed for days or even weeks. Because of this theoretical risk, no athlete with a concussive injury should be allowed to return to play or training until ALL clinical symptoms have fully resolved and cognitive function has returned to normal.

Prognosis

In cases of cerebral herniation complicated by ischemia, patients may suffer permanent neurological sequelae if coma duration is 6 hours or longer. Most patients with a maximum ICP increase of <30 mmHg experience good recovery.

Head injury advice card

All patients, athletes or nonathletes, should be given a head injury card upon discharge from medical care. An example is shown in Box 2.1.

Box 2.1 Head injury advice

This patient has received an injury to the head. A careful medical examination has been carried out and no sign of any serious complications has been found.

It is expected that recovery will be rapid, but in such cases it is not possible to be quite certain.

If you notice any change in behavior, vomiting, dizziness, headache, double vision, or excessive drowsiness, please call:

....

or the nearest hospital emergency department immediately.

Other important points:
- No alcohol
- No analgesics or pain killers
- No driving

Patient's name ....

Date and time of injury ....

Date of medical review ....

Treating physician ....

CLINIC PHONE NUMBER ....

Sports concussion

Definition

Concussion is derived from the Latin, *concussus*, which means to shake violently. Concussion is defined as a complex pathophysiological process affecting the brain, induced by traumatic biomechanical forces. It is due to a direct blow to the head, face, neck, or elsewhere on the body with an impulsive force transmitted to the head.

Changes in alertness, concentration, or memory and development of physical symptoms following an impact to the brain are characteristic of concussion. It results in rapid onset of short-lived impairment of neurological function that resolves spontaneously with a graded set of symptoms that may or may not involve loss of consciousness.

Resolution of clinical and cognitive symptoms typically follows a sequential course.

Typically concussion is associated with grossly normal structural neuroimaging studies.

Epidemiology (conservative estimates)

- 2%–4.5% of all athletic injuries
- The Centers for Disease Control and Prevention (CDC) reports 300,000 sports-related concussions annually in the United States.
- >100,000 occur in football alone each year.
- 20% of all high school football players sustain at least one each year.
- There are an estimated 900 sports-related TBI deaths per year.
- Other sports are: boxing, ice hockey, wrestling, gymnastics, lacrosse, soccer, basketball.
- Fewer than 10% result in loss of consciousness.
- Risk of concussion is 4–6 times higher in players with a history of previous concussion.
- Risk factors for concussion include male gender, younger athletes, history of multiple concussions, dangerous style of play for the athlete, high-risk sport, or having a comorbid mental health disorder.
- *Many cases go unreported.*

Typical concussion symptoms

- Headache
- Dizziness or vertigo
- Nausea
- Visual changes
- Lightheadedness
- Easy fatigability or lethargy
- Irritability
- Sleep disturbance
- Sensitivity to light or sound
- Weakness

Cognitive features

- Amnesia
- Disorientation
- Confusion
- Easily distracted
- Poor concentration
- Memory difficulties

Signs of concussion

- Impaired attention
- Vomiting
- Vacant stare
- Delayed responses, poor focus
- Decreased alertness
- Disorientation
- Slurred, slowed, or incoherent speech
- Gross incoordination
- Emotional lability
- Inappropriate playing behavior
- Poor coordination

Concussion pathophysiology

Concussions occur mostly when momentum of the head is changed abruptly by either

- Blunt trauma or
- Accelerative, decelerative, or rotational forces.

It may also result from trauma to the torso or axial skeleton. The force of injury is transmitted indirectly to the brain.

Categories of brain injury

Focal (coup)

- Blunt trauma to the cranial vault (forceful blow to a stationary head)
- Maximal brain injury is beneath the point of cranial impact
- Results in brain contusions, lacerations, and hemorrhage (epidural, subdural, subarachnoid, intracerebral spaces)

Diffuse (contra-coup)

- Shearing forces due to acceleration or deceleration with angular rotation (moving head striking a stationary object)
- Maximal brain injury is opposite the site of cranial impact
- Known as "diffuse agonal injury"

Theories of pathophysiology

Currently, concussion pathobiology is incompletely understood. Recent studies point to neurochemical and neurometabolic dysfunction.

Injured cells are exposed to changes in the extracellular and intracellular environments. Brain cells that are not irreversibly destroyed remain alive in a vulnerable state during the minutes to few days after concussion injury.

A vulnerable state is theoretically linked to second-impact syndrome. Loss of consciousness does not necessarily imply increased severity.

Acute concussion management

The following management guidelines generally follow the recent third International Conference on Concussion in Sport held in Zurich, November 2008.

Initial evaluation
- Assess airway, breathing, circulation (ABC).
- Assess general level of consciousness and mental status.
- Conduct secondary survey for skull, neck, or back injuries. For airway protection, removal of helmets or other head protectors should only be performed by individuals trained in this trauma management.
- Assess Glasgow Coma Scale (see p. 55).

Sideline evaluation
- Determine mechanism of injury.
- Check for prior concussion injury history (previous symptoms, number of concussions, postconcussive convulsions), past medical history, medications, drug or alcohol use.
- Brief neuropsychological test batteries such as the Maddocks questions, Sports Concussion Assessment Tool 2 (SCAT2), or the Standardized Assessment of Concussion (SAC) have been validated in this setting.

Neurological screening
- Speech should be assessed for fluency and lack of slurring.
- Check eye motion and pupils and perform visual examination.
- Pronator drift is performed by asking the patient to hold both arms in front of the patient palms up, with eyes closed.
  - Positive test is pronating the forearm, dropping the arm, or drift away from midline.
- Examine coordination, fine movements, gait, and balance.

Mental status testing/cognitive function (see SCAT2 card, p. 70)

Orientation (modified Maddocks questions)
- At what venue are we at today?
- Which half is it now?
- Who scored last in this game?
- What team did you play last week or game?
- Did your team win the last game?

Memory recall
- Select any 5 words for memory recall, but choose a different set of words each time you perform a follow-up examination with the same candidate.
- Recite months of the year in reverse order.
- For digits backwards, if correct, go to the next string length. If incorrect, read trial 2. Stop after incorrect on both trials.

Exertional maneuvers

- Provocative tests to elicit possible postconcussion symptoms (BESS, see SCAT2 card, p. 70).
- Use the following if considering return to play for an athlete who is oriented and asymptomatic (5 repetitions)
  - Jumping jacks
  - Push-ups
  - Sit-ups
  - Up-downs
  - Single-leg balance with eyes closed, arms at 90° abduction
  - Running (40 yard dash) or stationary bike

Monitor

- Carefully watch for any deterioration of signs or symptoms.
- Repeat testing in 15 minutes.
- Provide instructions for home, follow-up
- If any symptoms of concussion occur during exertional maneuvers, the athlete should not be allowed to return to the game.

The SCAT2 (Sport Concussion Assessment Tool 2)

The SCAT2 card is a standardized method for evaluating concussion for people over 10 years of age. The SCAT2 card includes a symptom evaluation along with a physical sign score, GCS, Maddocks score, and SAC score. It also includes a balance and coordination examination. All of these assessments are compiled for a total SCAT2 score.

The entire SCAT2 may be obtained from the Zurich Consensus document. There is also a pocket SCAT2 tool (see Fig. 2.1).

Pocket SCAT2

Concussion should be suspected in the presence of any one or more of the following: symptoms (such as headache), or physical signs (such as unsteadiness), or impaired brain function (e.g. confusion) or abnormal behaviour.

1. Symptoms

Presence of any of the following signs & symptoms may suggest a concussion.

- Loss of consciousness
- Seizure or convulsion
- Amnesia
- Headache
- "Pressure in head"
- Neck Pain
- Nausea or vomiting
- Dizziness
- Blurred vision
- Balance problems
- Sensitivity to light
- Sensitivity to noise
- Feeling slowed down
- Feeling like "in a fog"
- "Don't feel right"
- Difficulty concentrating
- Difficulty remembering
- Fatigue or low energy
- Confusion
- Drowsiness
- More emotional
- Irritability
- Sadness
- Nervous or anxious

2. Memory function

Failure to answer all questions correctly may suggest a concussion.

"At what venue are we at today?"
"Which half is it now?"
"Who scored last in this game?"
"What team did you play last week/game?"
"Did your team win the last game?"

3. Balance testing

Instructions for tandem stance

"Now stand heel-to-toe with your non-dominant foot in back. Your weight should be evenly distributed across both feet. You should try to maintain stability for 20 seconds with your hands on your hips and your eyes closed. I will be counting the number of times you move out of this position. If you stumble out of this position, open your eyes and return to the start position and continue balancing. I will start timing when you are set and have closed your eyes."

Observe the athlete for 20 seconds. If they make more than 5 errors (such as lift their hands off their hips; open their eyes; lift their forefoot or heel; step, stumble, or fall; or remain out of the start position for more that 5 seconds) then this may suggest a concussion.

Any athlete with a suspected concussion should be IMMEDIATELY REMOVED FROM PLAY, urgently assessed medically, should not be left alone and should not drive a motor vehicle.

Figure 2.1 Pocket SCAT2. From McCrory P, Meeuwisse W, Johnston K, et al. (2009). Consensus statement on concussion in sport, 3rd International Conference on Concussion in Sport held in Zurich, November 2008. *Clin J Sport Med* **19**:185–200.

Footnotes for flow chart (Fig. 2.2)

The flowchart is a conceptual management approach to provide advice on return to work and sport.

This management algorithm provides general guidance only. The letters in parentheses correspond to the flowchart (Fig. 2.2).

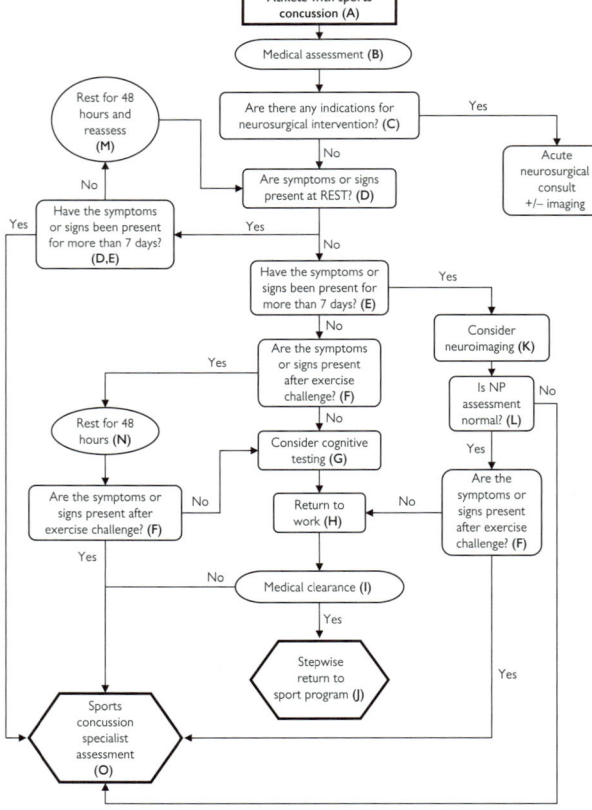

Figure 2.2 Sports concussion algorithm. NP, neuropsychological.

(A) "Athletes with sports concussion" refers to those with no evidence of previous concussion and no history of behavioral, neurological, or psychological problems or learning disorder. In any return to sport the athlete must be free of any drugs, alcohol, or medication that may mask symptoms or interfere with cognitive performance.

(B) Initial medical assessment involves history, neurological examination, physical examination including examination of the face, skull, and cervical spine, and SCAT card assessment.

(C) Indications for neurosurgical intervention are detailed in the section Glasgow Coma Scale (GCS) (p. 55).

(D) Symptoms and signs of concussion

(E) The Zurich guidelines allow 7–10 days for symptoms and signs of most concussions to resolve.

(F) An exercise challenge requires the athlete to exercise until the heart rate is >60% of maximum predicted heart rate (MPHR). MPHR = 220 – age in years. As a simple rule of thumb, this corresponds to a heart rate of >120 beats per minute.

(G) Formal neuropsychological testing is not required for most concussions. However, the athlete must be able to score normally on the SCAT2 card mental status assessment. If the score is abnormal, more formal neuropsychological assessment may be warranted.

(H) Return to work or school depends on complete resolution of symptoms, signs, and cognitive function both at rest and after exercise. Athletes should be medically reassessed after return to work or school to ensure functional recovery before proceeding to the stepwise return-to-play guideline. When considering return to school, it is prudent for the teachers and parents to be aware of potential problems that may arise at this stage.

(I) Medical clearance involves an assessment of symptom recurrence after return to school and documentation that the athlete has completed all steps appropriately in the management plan and, in particular, is asymptomatic at rest and following exercise challenge.

(J) Stepwise return to a sports program under the return-to-play recommendations. All six steps must be completed, as described in the next section, Return to play (p. 74). We emphasize the important role of physician clearance at this stage.

(K) Athletes with symptoms or signs lasting ≥7 days may require brain CT or MRI.

(L) Neuropsychological (NP) assessment is recommended in all athletes with complex concussion.

(M) At 48 hours the athlete should be reassessed. Obviously, if there are any persistent symptoms or signs, the rest period will be >48 hours. Once 7–10 days is reached and the patient is still symptomatic, consideration may be warranted for assessment by a concussion specialist.

(N) At this stage in the flowchart the athlete is asymptomatic at rest, but symptomatic after exercise. The athlete must return to complete rest for another 48 hours before repeating the exercise challenge.

(O) A "sports concussion specialist" is a neurologist, neurosurgeon, or sports medicine physician with specific expertise in managing sport-related concussion and who has access to specialized formal neuropsychological assessment and generally works in a multidisciplinary management setting.

Return to play

One of the most challenging aspects of managing sport-related concussion is recognizing the injury, especially in athletes with no obvious signs. When a player shows any signs or symptoms of concussion:

- There is no return to play in the current game or practice.
- The player shouldn't be left alone, and needs regular monitoring.
- Medical evaluation must occur following injury.
- Return to play must follow a medically supervised stepwise process.
- The player must NEVER return to play while symptomatic!
- "When in doubt, sit them out."

Post-concussive observation

- Recommended for at least 24 hours after a concussion
- Observer should be given explicit instructions on patient monitoring
- Awaken patient from sleep every 2 hours
- Patient should avoid strenuous activity for at least 24 hours

Warning signs to seek medical attention

- Inability to awaken patient
- Severe or worsening headaches
- Confusion or somnolence
- Restlessness, unsteadiness, or seizures
- Difficulties with vision
- Vomiting, fever, or stiff neck
- Urinary or bowel incontinence
- Weakness or numbness involving any body part

Return-to-play protocol

1. No activity, complete rest (exertional and cognitive)
2. Light aerobic exercise (walking, stationary bike), no weight lifting
3. Sport-specific exercise with progressive addition of resistance training (may add resistance training progressing from light to heavier weights at steps 3 or 4)
4. Non-contact training drills
5. Full-contact training after medical clearance
6. Game play

- With a stepwise progression, the athlete may proceed to the next level only if completely asymptomatic at the current step.
- Each step should take a minimum of 1 day.
- If symptomatic, the athlete should drop back to the previous asymptomatic level for 24 hours.
- Athletes should avoid medications that may mask, affect, or modify symptoms.
- Physical and cognitive rest is required, as activities that require attention and concentration may exacerbate symptoms and delay recovery.

Neuroimaging

Positive findings on neuroimaging studies mandate termination of play for the season. Evaluation is for brain swelling, contusion, or other intracranial pathology.

Emergent CT scan

This is required if there is prolonged loss of consciousness (LOC) or signs or symptoms of concern for epidural or subdural hematoma.

Nonemergent CT scan/MRI

If post-concussion symptoms persist 1–2 weeks after injury or are worsening, imaging is nonemergent. Such symptoms include headache, confusion, lethargy, amnesia, focal neurological deficits, seizures, etc.

Use clinical judgment.

Radiographs

These include C-spine series and evaluation of facial bones for fractures.

CT

CT is widely available and quick to perform. It is better for detecting acute bleeding, fracture, or intracerebral edema.

MRI

MRI is more sensitive than CT for detecting traumatic brain injuries (contusion or axonal shear injury).

Electroencephalography (EEG)

If there is concern for an underlying seizure disorder EEG should be performed.

SPECT scan (single photon emission CT)

Assesses regional blood flow and metabolic activity with SPECT. A larger number of abnormalities can be detected with this imaging modality.

It is not yet validated for use in clinical practice.

Functional MRI (fMRI)

This is a viable tool for assessment of neural processes following concussion without using radiation exposure. It measures brain activation through cerebral blood flow and oxygenation and can be used to measure "in-scanner" neurocognitive tasks.

fMRI provides validity data about sensitivity and specificity of neuropsychological testing to detect subtle changes in brain function.

Neurocognitive testing

This is an objective measure to detect and follow subtle cognitive deficits post-concussion and track recovery for safe return to play. Such testing should not be the sole basis of a return-to-play protocol.

It is administered as a battery of tests with several scales that evaluate cognitive functioning, with attention to recall, concentration.

Neurocognitive testing may be valuable in documenting cognitive deficits in patients with ongoing complaints. Clinical usefulness depends on obtaining baseline measurements for comparison with post-injury values.

Disadvantages
- Possible practice effect, long duration, examiner training necessary

Computerized neurocognitive testing

This testing has been developed in response to the time, cost demands, and limitations in neuropsychological expertise of traditional testing.

Advantages
- Test more athletes at baseline in shorter duration with less expense
- Highly sensitive tests for concussion when including attention, concentration, and memory functioning
- Serial examinations for comparison purposes with normative values

Disadvantages
- Practice or learning effect
- Observation that players may return to baseline while still symptomatic
- Players purposely do poorly on the baseline test
- Distractions during testing

Concussion grading scales

No single system is endorsed; over 20 scales have existed, including the Cantu, Colorado Medical Society, and American Academy of Neurology scales. Return to play should be based on individualized assessment.

It is possible for the severity of concussion to be determined only in retrospect, thus after symptoms have resolved.

Concussion complications

Immediate

Concussive convulsions
- Nonepileptic phenomena due to loss of cortical inhibition and release of brainstem activity
- CT/MRI typically normal
- Good long-term prognosis

Epidural hematoma
- Laceration of middle meningeal artery

Subdural hematoma
- Tearing of bridging veins

Delayed

Post-concussive syndrome
- Constellation of physical and/or cognitive symptoms that last from months to days
- Nearly 15% of patients with mild head injury continue to complain of post-concussive symptoms 1 year after their injury.
- Often triggered or aggravated by exercise or sport-specific activity

Symptoms
- Low-grade headache, dizziness, fatigue, emotional lability, and neurocognitive impairment; coordination disturbances; sleep problems; changes in appetite

Imaging
- Neuroimaging if symptoms last greater than 1–2 weeks
- Exclude possibility of underlying radiographically evident brain injury

Treatment
- Rest and close follow-up
- If persistent headache and negative imaging: nonsteroidal anti-inflammatory drugs (NSAIDs), β-blockers, tricyclic antidepressants (TCAs), calcium-channel blockers
- Symptoms must have resolved before return to play.

Cumulative neurocognitive impairment
- Chronic traumatic brain injury (CTBI)
- In the boxing world = dementia pugilistica
- Characterized by parkinsonism, ataxia, dysarthria, behavioral changes and Alzheimer's disease

Risk factors
- Repeated concussions, long duration of exposure to mild traumatic brain injury (MTBI)
- Apolipoprotein E4 (ApoE4) allele genetic marker

Second-impact syndrome (SIS)
- Rare catastrophic brain injury associated with premature return to play from concussion
- Occurs while still symptomatic and healing from previous concussion
- Rapid, massive brain swelling due to cerebral vasculature autoregulatory dysfunction
- Deterioration can be rapid (2–5 minutes after second impact to brainstem failure) and fatal
- Studies show that the magnitude of trauma and severity of concussion do not seem to correlate with incidence of SIS
- Risk factors are young age and history of head injury
- Unknown incidence
- SIS underscores the importance of not returning to play before the brain has had a chance to heal
- Higher risks of long-term memory and attention impairments

Concussion prevention

Mouthguards

There is no published evidence that mouthguards will prevent concussion, but they should be mandatory to prevent orofacial injuries.

Mouthguard types include the following:

- "*Stock*" mouthguards may be purchased from sporting goods stores.
- "*Mouth-formed*" or "*boil and bite*" guards are heated and then immediately worn by the athlete, allowing some adaptation to the dentition to occur. They do not provide much protection and they tend to fit poorly. They often interfere with breathing and speech. They are nonetheless cheaper and more widely available than other types.
- "*Custom-made*" guards come in several types but all require a dentition impression cast, with the guard made from this cast. They are fitted by a dentist or dental technician.

Helmets and head protectors

Helmets theoretically reduce the risk of brain injury. There is published evidence for the effectiveness of sport-specific helmets in reducing head injuries in sports with high-speed collisions, missile injuries (e.g., baseball), and falls onto hard surfaces (e.g., gridiron, ice hockey).

No sport-specific helmets have been shown to be of proven benefit in reducing head injury in sports such as soccer, Australian football, and rugby. Most commercially available soft helmets fail to meet impact-testing criteria that would be typical of sports-related concussion. Randomized controlled trials in various football codes have failed to show a protective effect against concussion.

Other means of preventing sports concussion

Rule changes, such as banning spear tackles in American football, reduce the incidence of catastrophic head and neck injury. Neck muscle conditioning may also reduce impact forces transmitted to the brain.

On-field recognition of concussive injury is a priority as well as application of appropriate validated guidelines in returning athletes to sport. Education of athletes and their health-care providers on how to detect concussion, its clinical features, assessment techniques, and principles of safe return to play is crucial.

Concussion and the preparticipation exam

Each athlete should have a thorough concussion history obtained. This should also include any facial or cervical injuries. Specific questions include the severity and symptom duration along with previous number of concussions. If available, preseason neuropsychological baseline testing should also be done for high-risk athletes and/or sports.

The SCAT2 form may also be used to obtain a preseason baseline if computer testing is not available.

Pediatric concussions

Children (<18 years old) should be treated more conservatively than adults for concussion. The Zurich guidelines should be used for children over 10 years old.

Many studies have shown that children take longer to recover from concussions than adults and they score lower on neurocognitive assessment when recovering from a concussion, even when asymptomatic. They are also more likely to have SIS.

It is not appropriate for children to return to play the same day with a concussion.

Post-traumatic headache

Post-traumatic headache generally has a good prognosis for recovery, although some patients may remain affected for considerable periods of time.

Paradoxically, headaches may occur more often and be of longer duration in patients with concussive injury than in patients with more severe TBI.

Classification of post-traumatic headache (International Headache Society [IHS] criteria)

1. *Post-traumatic (or trauma-triggered) migraine*: in sports such as soccer, where repetitive heading of the ball gives rise to the term "footballer's migraine." Even mild head trauma may induce migraine.
2. *Extracranial "vascular" headache*: these are periodic headaches at the site of head or scalp trauma
3. *Dysautonomic cephalgia*: an unusual consequence of trauma to the anterior part of the neck, triggering autonomic symptoms from local injury to the sympathetic trunk and adjacent ganglia. This entity may be successfully treated with propranolol.
4. *Headache overlap syndrome*: this is persistent low-grade occipital headache

Diagnostic workup

The rate of significant neuropathological injury is between 1% and 3% in patients with headache, and the typical headaches found, even in life-threatening conditions, were nonspecific in nature.

Post-traumatic headaches are generally treated in the same fashion as primary headache syndromes. Analgesic-rebound headache can complicate a post-traumatic headache disorder. For post-traumatic migraine, aspirin and NSAIDs can be used with mild episodes and ergot preparations and sumatriptan can be used to treat severe attacks.

Chronic post-traumatic migraine or recurrent episodes requiring prophylactic agents may be treated with amitriptyline or propranolol if no contraindications exist. Alternative agents include nadolol, timolol, amitriptyline, nortriptyline, doxepin, verapamil, NSAIDs, valproic acid, methergine, methysergide, fluoxetine, or phenelzine.

Prognosis

Acute post-traumatic headache has a good prognosis; in most cases, symptoms resolve within 1–3 months. Education and support can help patients deal with transient cognitive difficulties associated with headaches.

The chronic post-traumatic syndrome with prolonged disability is difficult to treat and generally requires specialist intervention.

Headaches and sport

Classification of exercise-related headache

The IHS in conjunction with the World Health Organization (WHO) has determined this classification.

Clinical approach to headache

1. Exclude possible intracranial causes on history and physical examination. If intracranial pathology is suspected an urgent workup is required, which may include neuroimaging studies and laboratory work.
2. Exclude headaches associated with viral or other infective illness.
3. Exclude a drug-induced headache (see below) or headache related to alcohol and/or substance abuse.
4. Consider an exercise (or sex-related) headache syndrome.
5. Differentiate between vascular, tension, cervicogenic, and other causes of headache.

Many commonly used drugs can provoke headaches. Some of these drugs, such as NSAIDs, are in widespread use by athletes. If not recognized, this may be the reason for treatment failure.

Drugs that may cause headache include the following:

- Alcohol
- Anabolic steroids
- Analgesics
- Antibiotics
- Antihypertensives
- Caffeine
- Corticosteroids
- Dipyridamole
- Nicotine
- Nitrazepam
- NSAIDs
- Oral contraceptives
- Sympathomimetics
- Theophylline
- Vasodilator agents

Clinical evaluation of headaches

History

- Age of onset of the headaches
- Frequency and duration
- Time of onset of headache
- Mode of onset
- Site of pain and radiation
- Headache quality
- Associated symptoms
- Precipitating factors
- Aggravating and relieving factors
- Previous treatments
- General health

- Past medical history
- Family history
- Social and occupational history
- Drug and medication use

Physical examination
A complete neurological and general physical examination is required with particular attention to the cervical spine as a potential source of headache. General appearance (including skin lesions such as rashes), vital signs (pulse, blood pressure, and temperature), mental status and speech, gait, balance and coordination, cranial nerve and spinal tract examination, visual fields, acuity and fundiscopic examination, and skull palpation should all be assessed.

Key symptoms to flag

Certain symptoms may indicate the presence of more serious pathology, such as a mass lesion or infective process, and require urgent neurological assessment. These include the following:

- Sudden onset of severe headache
- Headache increasing over a few days
- New or different headache
- Persistently unilateral headaches
- Chronic headache with localized pain
- Stiff neck or other signs of meningismus
- Focal neurological symptoms or signs
- Atypical headache or change in the usual pattern of headache
- Headaches that wake the patient during the night or early morning
- Local extracranial symptoms (e.g., sinus, ear, or eye disease)
- Systemic symptoms (e.g., weight loss, fever, and malaise)

Specific common headache syndromes

Migraine
Migraine is an episodic headache that is usually accompanied by nausea and photophobia and that may be preceded by focal neurological symptoms. It has a prevalence of 12%–18% in community populations.

In elite athletes, there are specific management considerations related to the use of "banned" drugs. Many conventional headache medications (such as β-blockers, caffeine, codeine-containing preparations, dextropropoxyphene, narcotics and opioids, etc.) are restricted agents and their use, if detected, may result in severe penalties for the athlete.

Tension-type headache
Tension-type headache results in a constant tight or pressing sensation that may initially be episodic and related to stress, but can recur almost daily in its chronic form without regard to any obvious psychological factors.

Cervicogenic headache
This type of headache involves abnormalities of the neck, including synovial joints, the intervertebral disks, ligaments, muscles, nerve roots, and the vertebral artery. Cervicogenic headache shares many of the clinical fea-

tures of chronic tension-type headache. It is usually occipital in onset and may radiate to the anterior aspect of the skull and face.

The headache is usually constant in nature, lasts for days to weeks, and has a definite association with movement or manipulation of cervical structures.

Benign exertional headache (BEH)

The formal criteria for BEH are as follows:

a. The headache is specifically brought on by physical exercise.
b. The headache is bilateral, throbbing in nature at onset, and may develop migraine-like features in those patients susceptible to migraine.
c. It lasts from 5 minutes to 24 hours.
d. It is prevented by avoiding excessive exertion.
e. It is not associated with any systemic or intracranial disorder.

Exertional headache may be due to dilatation of pain-sensitive venous sinuses at the base of the brain as a result of increased cerebral arterial pressure. A similar type of vascular headache is described in relation to sexual activity and has been termed *benign sex headache* or *orgasmic cephalgia*.

Treatment strategies include NSAIDs such as indomethacin at a dose of 25 mg three times per day. Other pharmacological strategies that have anecdotal support include the prophylactic use of ergotamine tartrate, methysergide, or propranolol pre-exercise.

These headaches tend to recur over weeks to months and then slowly resolve, although some cases may be lifelong. In the recovery period, a graduated symptom-limited weight-lifting program is appropriate.

Effort headache

Effort headaches differ from the exertional headaches in that they are not necessarily associated with a power or straining type exercise and occur in a variety of sports. The clinical features include the following:

a. Onset of mild to severe headache with aerobic type exercise
b. More frequent in hot weather
c. Vascular-type headache (i.e., throbbing)
d. Short duration of headache (4–6 hours)
e. Provoking exercise may be maximal or submaximal
f. Patient may have prodromal "migrainous" symptoms
g. Headache tends to recur in individuals with exercise
h. Athlete may have a past history of migraine
i. Normal neurological exam and diagnosis

Epilepsy and sports

See Table 2.3.

Specific syndromes

Concussive convulsions

A *concussive convulsion* is defined as a convulsive episode that begins within 2 seconds of impact associated with concussive brain injury. Following impact, there is typically a phase of brief tonic stiffening followed by myoclonic jerking.

The convulsive movements may be transient but can last up to 3 minutes in some cases. These episodes are not associated with structural or permanent brain injury and are a nonepileptic phenomenon.

Post-traumatic epilepsy

Seizures are common after severe head injury and account for 2% of the total cases of epilepsy. Post-traumatic epilepsy is categorized into immediate (within 24 hours of injury), early (within 1 week), and late (after 1 week) subtypes (see Table 2.3).

Risk factors are prolonged unconsciousness, skull fracture, intracerebral hematomas, hemorrhagic cerebral contusion, and focal neurological signs. Children have almost three times the risk of early post-traumatic epilepsy compared to that of adults for the same severity of brain injury.

Idiopathic epilepsy

One of the peaks of incidence of epilepsy is in the late teens and early 20s, the time when many men and women are actively involved in athletic pursuits. Exercise does not increase seizure frequency, affect antiepileptic drug levels or induce epileptiform EEG changes.

There is no evidence that epileptics are more prone to seizures after head injury or are more prone to injury than other athletes.

Other less common causes of convulsions in sport

- *Syncope:* Patients who faint often have convulsive movements of the extremities that are thought to be due to a brainstem reflex phenomenon.
- *Cardiac rhythm disturbances:* An anoxic convulsion may occur with a transient arrhythmia.
- *Movement disorders:* Episodic involuntary movement disorders may be precipitated by movement or exercise.
- *Metabolic disturbances:* Convulsive activity, dystonia, and syncope may occur secondary to hypoglycemia, hyponatremia, hypocalcemia, and hypomagnesemia, all conditions recognized in sports—particularly in endurance running and ultra-marathons.
- *Illicit drug use and/or alcohol use*
- *Pseudoseizures*

Table 2.3 Sports-related seizures

	Timing of event	Type of seizure	Likely etiology
Immediate	Seconds to hours post-injury	Generalized/ myoclonic	Nonepileptic
Early	Hours to 7 days post-injury	Focal	Epileptic
Late	>7 days post-injury	Generalized	Epileptic

Fractures

Skull fracture

Athletes with a cranial fracture usually have a headache and may or may not have symptoms of an underlying brain injury. Local soft-tissue swelling may also indicate an underlying fracture. Palpation of the skull should be a mandatory part of the clinical assessment of all head injuries. Percussion of the skull may result in a characteristic "cracked pot" sound.

Rhinorrhea and otorrhea are classic signs of skull fracture with torn dural membranes. If a glucose stick test of nasal or ear fluid leak is positive, the fluid is CSF.

In all cases of skull fracture, especially if a CSF leak is present, an urgent neurosurgical consultation is required. When a skull fracture is suspected, the patient should always be hospitalized for observation and neurosurgical evaluation. The physician should cover the injured area of an open cranial fracture with a sterile dressing.

Nasal fractures

Displaced nasal fractures have a clinically obvious deformity; however, non-displaced fractures can be diagnosed radiographically, using lateral images.

The patient should be referred to a maxillofacial surgeon or otolaryngologist. Septal hematomas must be evacuated immediately because of the risk of septum necrosis.

Closed nasal bone repositioning is the most common treatment. This should be done either immediately after the injury or 3–7 days later, when the swelling is reduced. The patient should wear a protective splint or facemask for 4 weeks when participating in training or competition.

Mandibular fractures

Mandibular fractures are the second most common group (13%–45%) of sport-related facial injuries and are usually caused by a blow to the lower jaw, such as may occur in combat and team sports, or in a fall in which the lower jaw or the chin hits a hard surface.

Symptoms include swelling and hematoma, problems with occlusion, mucous membrane tears, differences in the level of the tooth row, mobility in the area of the fracture, and hypoesthesia with nerve damage in the mental nerve area. The standard radiographic image is a panoramic X-ray, also known as a panorex.

Most lower-jaw fractures should be treated by a specialist. The prognosis is good if proper occlusion is achieved after the operation.

Zygomatic fracture

Typical cheekbone fractures involve the zygomaticomaxillary complex: the infraorbital rim, the orbital floor, and the lateral orbital rim. Cheekbone fractures are the third most common sport injury to the face.

The clinical presentation is a flattening of the prominence of the cheekbone. If the cheekbone is pressed inward, it may be difficult for the patient to open the mouth wide. Double vision and nerve injury corresponding to the infraorbital nerve are symptoms of a fracture in the orbital floor. A CT scan with axial and coronal views with appropriately thin cuts provides the best imaging.

Eye injuries

Contusion of the eyeball

Contusion of the eyeball may be caused by direct blows to the eye (boxing), a ball in the eye (squash), crashing into a hard object, and falling accidents. Tearing, light sensitivity, and blepharospasm (cramps of the eyelid) are signs and symptoms of contusion of the eyeball.

Carefully evaluate for swelling and bleeding in the eyelid, subconjunctival bleeding, corneal edema, corneal damage, bleeding in the anterior chamber (hyphema), separation of the iris (iridodialysis), traumatic paresis of the pupil (mydriasis, oval pupil), accommodation paresis, lens damage or dislocation, bleeding in the vitreous, retinal damage (bleeding or edema), or damage to the optic nerve.

Visual acuity MUST be assessed in every eye injury and the threshold for referral to an ophthalmologist should be low.

Perforation of the globe (eyeball)

Ski poles in the eye, bow and arrow shooting accidents, and accidents with other sharp objects frequently cause globe rupture. Ruptures of the eye may also be caused by powerful blunt contusion trauma. In that case, the globe ruptures at the weak points (along the limbus and the optic nerve).

A teardrop-shaped pupil is pathognomic for a globe perforation. If perforation is suspected, the patient should be sent to the nearest emergency department to receive an emergent ophthalmology consultation.

Boxing and head injury

Boxing-related neurological injury

In amateur boxing, the rate of acute head injury (in contested bouts) varies between 0.14 and 0.4 injuries per 1000 exposures, whereas in professional boxing the rate is up to 40 per 1000 exposures. The risk of such events is relatively low when compared to other sports. No studies have been reported to suggest that female boxers are at increased risk.

Few prospective studies enable a true estimate of the incidence or prevalence of chronic boxing-related neurological injury in either amateur or professional boxing.

The "punch drunk" syndrome

In 1928, Harrison Martland anecdotally described a syndrome in prizefighters that was known in lay boxing circles as the "punch drunk" or "slug nutty" state, although he did not actually examine any boxer with this condition. It was later labeled *dementia pugilistica*, *traumatic encephalopathy*, or *chronic traumatic encephalopathy of boxers*.

In the early stages, the clinical syndrome is mixed because of lesions affecting the pyramidal, cerebellar, and extrapyramidal systems. In the latter stages, cognitive impairment becomes the major neurological feature. Throughout the course of the condition, various neuropsychiatric and behavioral symptoms may occur.

Compared to professionals, amateur boxers show milder neurophysiological and neuroimaging evidence of chronic traumatic encephalopathy. There are many differing symptoms with variable degrees of severity. Neuroradiological imaging techniques have not shown any systematic evidence of brain injury in boxers.

Neurophysiological studies show variable results. EEG abnormalities may occur in one-third to one-half of punch drunk professional boxers, and consist of diffuse slowing or flat, low-voltage records.

There is indirect evidence of compromise of the blood–brain barrier as revealed by increases in creatine kinase isoenzyme BB from astrocytes during the first 9 minutes after a boxing match and as suggested by increased CSF protein. Similar changes are noted with creatine kinase and neuron-specific enolase, with elevations following a single bout of amateur boxing.

Surprisingly few detailed reports of neuropathological changes in ex-boxers are available.

Risk factors for chronic boxing-related neurological injury

The putative risk factors fall into two broad areas—exposure and genotype. Chronic boxing-related neurological injury is described in boxers who began fighting at a young age, had several hundred professional fights, and had a long (>10 year) career. In addition, the *ApoE4* phenotype has been associated with an increased risk of chronic boxing-related neurological injury in boxers.

Prevention

There are no scientifically validated means by which chronic boxing-related neurological injury may be prevented. Neuroradiological studies are not useful as a sole screening tool.

1. Monitoring of bout frequency—high exposure (>20 bouts) correlates with risk of chronic boxing-related neurological injury. A boxing "passport" is recommended.
2. Regular, preferably annual, neuropsychological and neurobehavioral assessment is recommended.
3. Regular, preferably annual, neurological examinations are recommended that focus on the cerebellar, pyramidal, and extrapyramidal systems and gait rather than simply being a generic neurological examination.
4. An initial MR scan should be conducted at first registration to exclude boxers with pre-existing CNS abnormalities and to serve as a baseline for future comparison.
5. Ideally, testing for a boxer's *ApoE* genotype should be performed at the outset of his or her career, along with genetic counseling to discuss the implications of a positive finding.

A boxer's career should be terminated with the development of neurological signs.

A "high-risk" notification system is to be encouraged in the following cases:

- Boxers who have had >20 fights (including amateur fights)
- Boxers who have had >6 losses or knockdowns
- Active boxers >35 years
- Boxers who have an *ApoE4* genotype
- Active boxing career >10 years
- Boxers experiencing neurological symptoms post-bout

Screening alone will not lead to injury reduction. Injury prevention, appropriate medical advice, and corrective programs, where indicated, must be implemented. Unless boxers, medical staff, trainers, and boxing officials act on the deficits discovered during the screening process, pre-participation screening will act solely as a predictor of injury, rather than as a preventive measure.

Paradoxical vocal cord motion (PVCM) or vocal cord dysfunction (VCD)

This condition results in inappropriate movement of the vocal cords that in turn leads to functional airway obstruction as well as inspiratory and expiratory stridor. It is often confused with asthma because it can sound like wheezing.

Normally, vocal cords abduct with inspiration, sniffing, or panting. Phonation, swallowing, and Valsalva maneuvers induce adduction. Conversely, the vocal cords in PVCM adduct during inspiration and/or expiration. In addition, the posterior laryngeal wall can move forward to further compress the airway.

PVCM has been associated with psychosocial disorders, stress, exercise, neurological injury, gastroesophageal reflux, and irritant inhalational exposure.

The exercise-related form occurs predominantly in young female athletes. They may present with dsyspnea and stridor that is triggered with exercise. Patients suffering from the PVCM may also complain of a choking sensation, dysphonia, and cough. The symptoms last on the order of several hours to days. Albuterol has little to no effect on symptoms.

Chest X-rays exclude other causes, but are of little value. The best diagnostic modality is laryngoscopy with direct visualization of the cords during the respiratory cycle.

Other diagnoses that should be excluded are laryngeal angioedema, laryngospasm (much shorter duration—seconds to minutes), structural lesions (e.g., vocal cord polyps), and vocal cord paralysis or fixation.

Acute management includes supportive care, reassurance, and panting to abduct the posterior cricoarytenoid muscle. Continuous positive airway pressure and heliox therapy may also be of benefit. Long-term prevention may include speech therapy and psychological counseling.

Dental injuries

Tooth fracture classification

Ellis I: Involves only the enamel of tooth, can be smoothed with an emery board or referred to a dentist

Ellis II: Involves the yellow dentin and the tooth is sensitive to air and temperature. Zinc oxide/eugenol paste should be used to protect the tooth until a dentist is seen.

Ellis III: Involves the pulp and a dot of blood can be seen within the tooth. The tooth should be dressed with zinc oxide/eugenol paste and a dentist should follow up within 24 hours.

Tooth concussion

The tooth is tender to percussion but does not move. Treatment is with NSAIDs and a soft diet, and a dental referral is needed.

Subluxation

The tooth is tender and mobile, but not dislodged. Treatment is the same as for tooth concussion.

Luxation

Intrusive: Forced below the gum line. Do not pull it out, because this can further damage underlying bone. A dental referral is needed.

Extrusive: Partially avulsed. Reduce the tooth gently and stabilize with zinc oxide/eugenol paste until a dentist can see the patient.

Avulsion

The tooth has been knocked completely out. Do not replace a primary tooth in a child because it can prevent permanent teeth from erupting properly.

Try to get the tooth in liquid, such as Hank's solution, sterile saline, or milk. A dry tooth quickly becomes a dead tooth.

Tooth reimplantation has a far less favorable outcome when it is out for more than 60 minutes. Stabilizing paste should be used and close dental follow-up arranged.

External ear injuries

Blunt trauma

Pinna hematomas are quite common in sports that expose the ear to continuous friction or strong impact (e.g., wrestling and rugby). They should be aspirated and covered with a compressive dressing to prevent recurrence. This may have to be repeated several times over days to weeks. See Chapter 23, Auricular hematoma aspiration/incision (p. 756), for description.

Antibiotics and an ear, nose, thoat (ENT)/plastic surgery referral are recommended. These hematomas can progress to a hardened deformity known as "cauliflower ear."

Lacerations

The goal is to preserve cartilaginous structures. After anesthetizing and irrigating copiously, wound margin debridement should be minimal. If cartilage realignment is necessary, it is done with absorbable sutures, after which the skin is closed with 5–0 or 6–0 nonabsorbable suture.

The blood supply to the cartilage is poor, which increases the risk of infection. Antibiotics should strongly be considered.

Avulsions

The avulsed portion should be wrapped in gauze moistened with saline. It can be placed in a resealable plastic bag and then the bag placed on ice. The athlete needs to go to an emergency department and ENT/plastic surgery should be contacted emergently.

Shoulder

Anatomy

Important areas of shoulder anatomy (see Figs. 3.1, 3.2, and 3.3) are the following:

- Musculotendinous units of the rotator cuff and biceps
- Bony landmarks of the humerus, scapula, and clavicle
- Four joints of the shoulder

Rotator cuff

The rotator cuff is composed of the tendons of four muscles:

- The subscapularis is located anteriorly on the scapula (see Fig. 3.4).
- The supraspinatus, infraspinatus, and the teres minor are located posteriorly on the scapula (see Fig. 3.5).

All are closely associated with the glenohumeral capsule, as is the biceps tendon. The primary function of the rotator cuff is to position the humeral head in the glenoid, allowing larger muscles to provide necessary power.

Humerus

Important bony landmarks include the following:

- *Greater tuberosity* of the humerus
  - This is the insertion site of the supraspinatus, infraspinatus, and teres minor.
  - This prominence is often associated with impingement.
- The *bicipital groove* is a palpable indentation immediately medial and anterior to the greater tuberosity of the humerus.

  It houses the tendon of the long head of the biceps. It is easily identified if the humerus is alternately internally and externally rotated while palpating this area.
- On the anterior and inferior border of this groove is the *lesser tuberosity*, the insertion site of the subscapularis.

Articulations

There are three true joints of the shoulder:

- Glenohumeral joint
- Acromioclavicular (AC) joint
- Sternoclavicular joint

All three may have a fibrocartilagenous disc present within the articulation. As with all true joints, they are susceptible to arthritides and trauma.

The scapulothoracic articulation is not a true joint, but may be associated with pain syndromes, bursitis, and neuropathies.

Glenohumeral joint

The glenohumeral joint sacrifices the bony and ligamentous stability of other joints for increased range of motion.

There are both dynamic and static stabilizers of the joint. The dynamic stabilizers are the musculotendinous complex of the rotator cuff. The static stabilizers are the glenohumeral ligaments (superior, middle, and inferior) and the joint capsule.

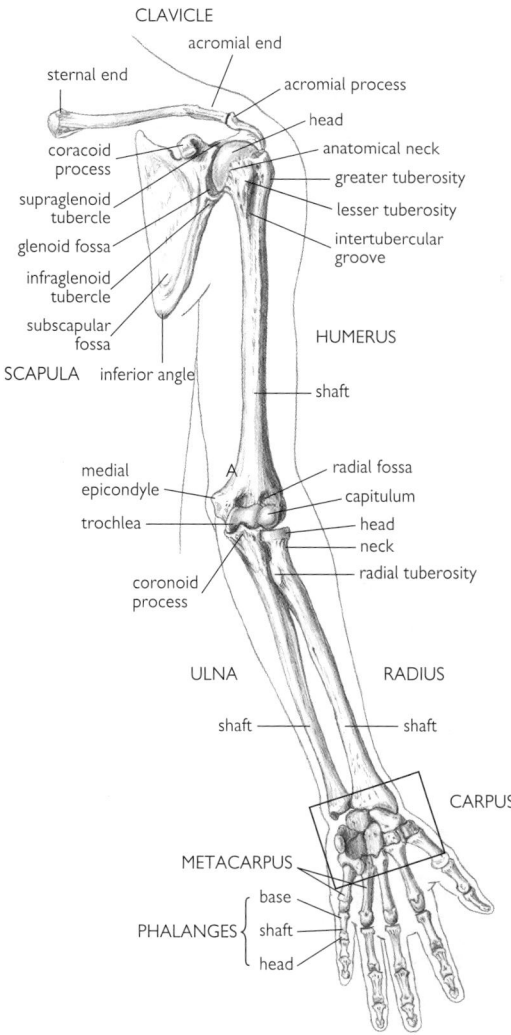

Figure 3.1 Bones of shoulder girdle and upper limb, anterior view. Reproduced with permission from MacKinnon P, Morris J (2005). *Oxford Textbook of Functional Anatomy*, Vol. 1. Oxford, UK: Oxford University Press. ©2005.

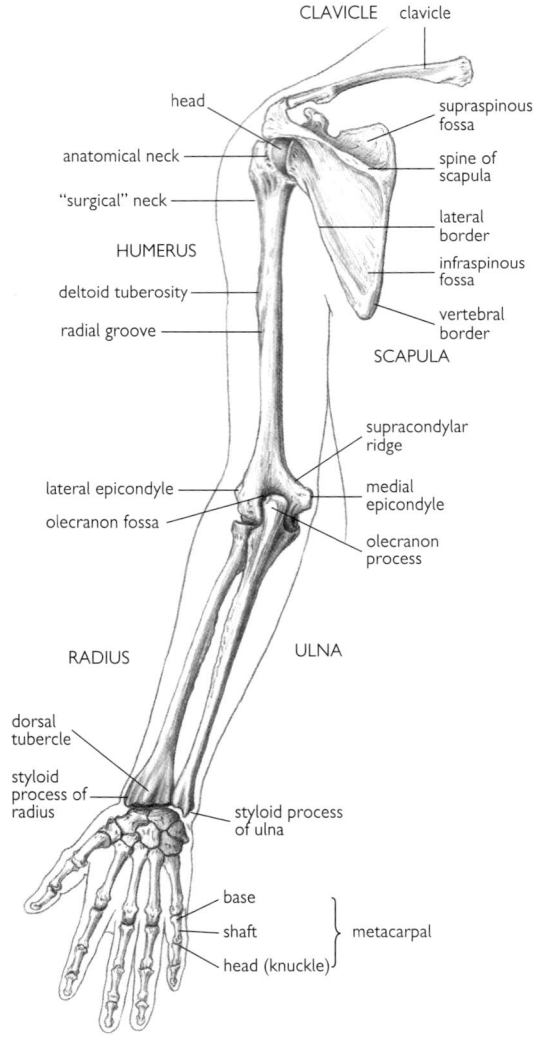

Figure 3.2 Bones of shoulder girdle and upper limb, posterior view. Reproduced with permission from MacKinnon P, Morris J (2005). *Oxford Textbook of Functional Anatomy*, Vol. 1. Oxford, UK: Oxford University Press. ©2005.

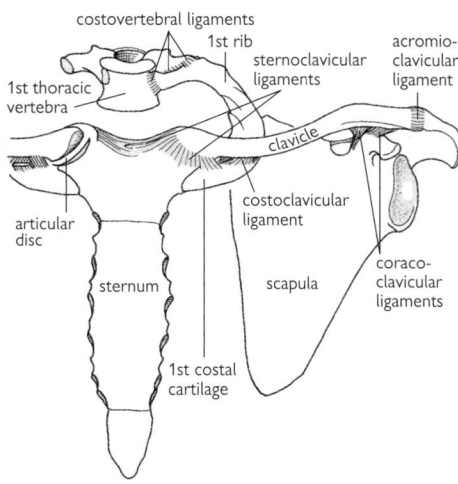

Figure 3.3 Bones and ligaments of the shoulder girdle. Reproduced with permission from MacKinnon P and Morris J (2005). *Oxford Textbook of Functional Anatomy*, Vol. 1. Oxford, UK: Oxford University Press. ©2005.

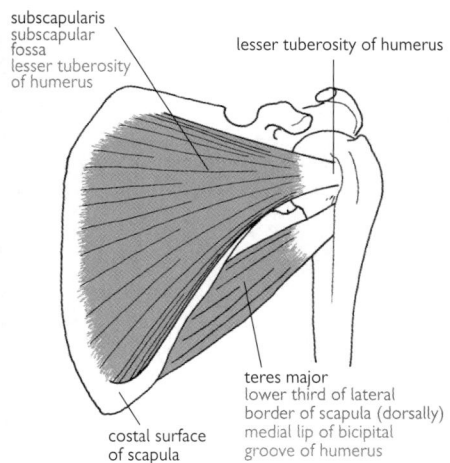

Figure 3.4 Subscapularis and teres major. Reproduced with permission from MacKinnon P, Morris J (2005). *Oxford Textbook of Functional Anatomy*, Vol. 1. Oxford, UK: Oxford University Press. © 2005.

Clavicle

The clavicle acts as a strut and is the only true osseous connection between the shoulder and the thorax.

Bursae

There are four important bursae in the shoulder.

Subacromial bursa

- It is located immediately inferior to the AC joint and superior to the glenohumeral joint.
- It can become inflamed (bursitis) in impingement syndrome.
- Injection into this bursa to eradicate symptoms is the basis of the impingement test.

Subdeltoid bursa

- It is located inferior to the deltoid tendon on the lateral shaft of the humerus

Subscapular bursa

- It is located between the joint capsule and the tendon of the subscapularis muscle

Subcoracoid bursa

- It is located between the joint capsule and the coracoid process of the scapula

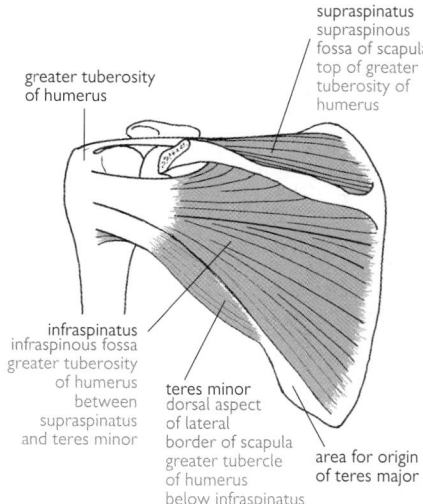

greater tuberosity
of humerus

supraspinatus
supraspinous
fossa of scapula
top of greater
tuberosity of
humerus

infraspinatus
infraspinous fossa
greater tuberosity
of humerus
between
supraspinatus
and teres minor

teres minor
dorsal aspect
of lateral
border of scapula
greater tubercle
of humerus
below infraspinatus

area for origin
of teres major

Figure 3.5 Supraspinatus, infraspinatus, teres minor; acromion removed.
Reproduced with permission from MacKinnon P, Morris J (2005). *Oxford Textbook of Functional Anatomy,* Vol. 1. Oxford, UK: Oxford University Press. ©2005.

History

The key to developing an effective differential diagnosis for the patient with shoulder pain is a thorough history. Key questions in the evaluation are as follows:

- What is the chief complaint or symptom? Chief complaints may range from pain to instability to weakness.
- How long have the symptoms been present?
- How did it develop? Was there a history of trauma or injury?
- Has it changed since the onset?
- Have you had similar symptoms in the past?

If pain is the chief complaint, ask the patient the following:

- Where is the point of maximal tenderness (location)?
- How would you characterize your symptoms (sharp, dull, aching)?
- How would you rate the severity of your symptoms on a scale from 1 to 10? This helps to establish a baseline, which can be used to assess the success of treatment.
- What activities or positions exacerbate discomfort?
- Do you experience pain at night?

The aim of the initial questions is to localize the anatomical area of interest and to help establish a differential diagnosis. Knowledge of the mechanism of injury can assist in making a diagnosis. For example, a pain with a history of shoulder dislocation or recurrent subluxations suggests instability. The history can also indicate whether the problem is acute or chronic.

Night pain or pain with overhead activities may signify impingement or rotator cuff pathology, whereas pain with lifting, pushing open a car door, or carrying luggage may be due to instability.

Ask the patient about the type and extent of activity involving the shoulder:

- What do you do for work and hobbies?
- What type of sports do you play?

Knowing the activity demands of the patient is important. Overuse shoulder injuries are often seen in workers whose jobs require them to perform repetitive overhead tasks. They are especially susceptible to impingement syndrome, subacromial bursitis, and AC problems.

Certain athletes, especially those involved in throwing, racquet sports, swimming, or volleyball, place increased demands on their shoulder and as a result have an increased incidence of shoulder injuries.

Screen for referred pain

- Cervical spine
- Cardiopulmonary
- Abdominal
- Do you experience neck pain?
- Does your pain radiate down one or both of your arms?
- Do you experience weakness in your arm?
- Have you had changes in sensation in your hand or upper extremity?

Cervical myelopathy or radiculopathy may present with upper extremity manifestations. It is important to ask patients about their cervical spine.

It is also important to ask about the following:

- Is there associated abdominal pain, or chest pain?
- Is there a history of weight loss, fatigue, or fevers?

Shoulder pain can be referred from the gastrointestinal (air under the diaphragm) or cardiovascular (myocardial infarction) systems. Recognizing this possibility can lead to timely treatment for these patients. Constitutional signs of malignancy or a septic arthritis are rare, but may be helpful in guiding the workup.

Finally, ask about previous injuries and treatment:

- What prior treatments have you had for your symptoms?
- Have there been any previous injuries to either of your shoulders?

These are important questions to ask. Prior injuries may alter the physical examination of the affected or contralateral shoulder. Knowledge of previous treatments can assist the physician in deciding on the next best step in management.

Examination

Inspection

Exposure (including scapulae)

It is important to visualize both shoulders and scapulae, looking for deformity or asymmetry. Women may tie their gown around the neck with the arms out.

Muscle atrophy

Biceps atrophy may be due to musculoskeletal nerve injury.

Scapular winging may be due to long thoracic nerve injury with a serratus anterior nerve palsy or a spinal accessory nerve (CN XI) injury with a trapezius palsy. Symptomatic throwing athletes may also exhibit asymmetric scapulothoracic motion that manifests as scapular winging.

Asymmetry

Prominence in the distal anterior arm may indicate a proximal biceps tendon rupture, often referred to as "Popeye" deformity. Prominence of the scapular spine suggests muscle atrophy secondary to denervation or disuse.

Asymmetry can be caused by a brachial plexus injury, spinoglenoid notch cyst, brachial neuritis (Parsonage–Turner syndrome), or, in an older patient, possibly a chronic, retracted rotator cuff tear.

Palpation (see Table 3.1)

Localize the point of maximum tenderness only after the remainder of the examination is complete. Palpation may produce discomfort and cause the patient to guard, making the remainder of the examination difficult.

Active and passive movements

Movements described in the shoulder (see Table 3.2):

- Abduction (normal 180°)
- Forward elevation (normal 180°)
- Extension (normal 45°)
- Internal rotation (normal 70°)
- External rotation (normal 75°)
- Scapular protraction, retraction, and elevation

Assess fluidity of the scapulohumeral and scapulothoracic movement. This is best done by observing the patient's shoulder movements while standing behind the patient.

A painful arc of motion may suggest rotator cuff pathology, a labral tear, glenohumeral arthritis, or the inflammatory phase of adhesive capsulitis.

Impingement pain is encountered between 90 and 120° of abduction. Restricted or painful internal rotation at 90° of abduction may also signify shoulder impingement. Internal rotation is best assessed by measuring the vertebral level that can be reached by the patient behind their back. It requires at least 55° of internal rotation to perform this test (i.e., T7 is at the inferior angle of the scapula).

Table 3.1 Areas of palpation in the shoulder

Bony palpation	Palpation of the soft tissues
• Suprasternal notch	• Rotator cuff muscles
• Sternoclavicular joint	• Subacromial and subdeltoid bursa
• Clavicle	• Axilla
• Coracoid process	• Major muscles of the shoulder
• AC joint	
• Acromion	
• Greater tuberosity of the humerus	
• Bicipital groove	
• Spine of the scapula	
• Medial border of the scapula	

Table 3.2 Shoulder (glenohumeral) joint: movements, principal muscles, and their innervation

Movement	Principal muscles	Peripheral nerve	Spinal root origin
Flexion	Pectoralis major (clavicular part)	Pectoral nerve (medial and lateral)	C 5, 6
	Deltoid (clavicular part)	Axillary nerve	C 5, 6
Extension	Latissimus dorsi	Nerve to latissimus dorsi (thoracodorsal nerve)	C 6, 7, 8
Abduction	Supraspinatus (initial 20°)	Suprascapular nerve	C 5, 6
	Deltoid	Axillary nerve	C 5, 6
Adduction	Pectoralis major	Pectoral nerves (medial and lateral)	C 5, 6
	Latissimus dorsi	Nerve to latissimus dorsi	C 6, 7, 8
Medial (internal) rotation	Pectoralis major	Pectoral nerves (medial and lateral)	C 5, 6
	Latissimuss dorsi	Nerve to latissimuss dorsi	C 6, 7, 8
	Subscapularis	Subscapular nerves (upper and lower)	C 5, 6
	Teres major	Lower subscapular nerve	C 5, 6
Lateral (external) rotation	Infraspinatus	Suprascapular nerve	C 5, 6
	Teres minor	Axillary nerve	C 5, 6
	Deltoid (posterior fibers)	Axillary nerve	C 5, 6
Circumduction	Combinations of the above		

Special tests

Glenohumeral joint stability

Anterior apprehension test

With the scapula stabilized (or in the supine position), the arm is passively moved to 90° of abduction and gently externally rotated until there is apprehension and the patient resists further external rotation. Apprehension (the feeling that the joint is going to dislocate) constitutes a positive test. Pain alone does not necessarily signify instability.

Caution should be exercised not to completely dislocate the joint with this maneuver.

Relocation test

The patient is supine and in the apprehension position as described above. With a positive test, a posterior directed force placed on the anterior humerus will relieve the apprehension. Further external rotation may then be possible. If the posterior force is removed, apprehension returns.

Load and shift test

While stabilizing the scapula, the humeral head is loaded medially against the glenoid while in the plane of scapula. A posterior and anterior stress is applied to the humeral head as if to shift it anteriorly and posteriorly.

Grading is based on translation in relation to the anterior and posterior glenoid rim. A 3+ is completely dislocated.

Posterior apprehension

The shoulder is passively moved to 90° of abduction and gently internally rotated until the patient is apprehensive and resists further internal rotation. A posteriorly directed force placed on the humeral shaft may intensify the feeling of instability.

Jerk test for posterior instability

The shoulder is passively elevated to 90° of forward flexion and internal rotation. The arm is axially loaded and brought into horizontal abduction. A positive test is indicated by a "clunk" as the humeral head, which was dislocated/subluxated at the starting position, is reduced as the arm is brought posteriorly in the horizontal plane.

Sulcus sign

The arm is passively at the side in the standing or sitting position. The humerus is distracted inferiorly. The sulcus sign is an indentation seen immediately inferior to the AC joint and signifies an inferior instability.

The sulcus sign should be quantified in terms of distance, in millimeters, between the edge of the acromion and humeral head.

Impingement syndrome

Neer's sign (impingement sign)

In this test the examiner attempts to force the greater trochanter under the AC joint to compress the bursa, rotator cuff, and biceps tendon. The arm is placed into maximum forward flexion and internal rotation while stabilizing the scapula. The sign is positive if pain is experienced.

Hawkin's sign

With the elbow flexed at 90° and the shoulder forward flexed at 90°, the humerus is progressively internally rotated in order to grind the proximal humerus against the edge of the acromion. The test is positive if pain is experienced.

Duke impingement test

The patient is asked to hold the arm abducted at 30° in the plane of the scapula with the elbows extended and palm directed toward the floor. The patient tries to resist a downward-directed force on the extended arm by the examiner. Pain in the shoulder indicates a positive test.

Impingement test

The impingement test involves injecting of 10 cc of a 1% lidocaine solution into the subacromial space. Improvement of the pain with repeat testing for impingement signs is a positive test and suggests impingement syndrome.

Rotator cuff

Drop arm test

With the arm straight, the shoulder is abducted past 90° in the plane of the scapula, then the patient is asked to slowly lower it to the side. With a supraspinatus tear the patient is unable to lower the arm slowly and the arm drops to the side.

Empty can test

With the arm straight and the shoulder abducted to 90° in the plane of the scapula, the humerus is internally rotated to 45° (as if emptying a beverage can). With a supraspinatus tear the patient is unable to maintain the position against resistance. The shoulder must be compared to the opposite side.

In a recent study, the position of supination (full can position) provided improved isolation of the supraspinatus. It is therefore recommended that both pronation and supination be used.

Lift off test

With the dorsum of the hand placed over the sacrum, the patient is asked to push away from the back against resistance. With subscapularis weakness or tear, the patient is weaker on the affected side than on the contralateral side.

Belly press test

The patient flexes the elbow 90° and internally rotates their arm until their hand is on the abdomen. The patient is asked to apply force toward the abdomen with their hand. In the setting of subscapularis weakness or a tear, the patient will drop the elbow posteriorly and extend the arm in an effort to generate the force.

External rotator test

With elbows at the side and at 90° of flexion, the patient is asked to externally rotate the arm against resistance. With infraspinatus weakness, a discrepancy is seen between the affected side and the contralateral side.

AC joint

Cross body adduction test

With the elbow extended, the arm is brought across the chest, stressing the AC joint. Pain is felt in the AC joint if the test is positive.

Extension test

The posterior AC joint can be tested by asking the patient to actively extend the arm while it is adducted at the side. This movement will elicit pain if the AC joint is the source of the symptoms.

Biceps

Yergason's test

With the elbow at 90° and the wrist held in pronation, the patient will experience pain if he or she attempts to supinate the wrist against resistance.

Speed's test

With the elbow flexed at 30°, the shoulder at 60° of flexion, and the wrist supinated, the patient will experience pain if he or she attempts to flex the arm against resistance.

Labral tears

Crank test

With the patient in the sitting or standing position, the arm is elevated to 160° in the scapular plane. An axial load is applied to the humerus while simultaneously internally and externally rotating the humerus. Pain or reproduction of the patient's symptoms (usually pain or catching) is considered a positive test.

O'Brien test

With the patient in the sitting position, the shoulder is forward flexed to 90° with the elbow in full extension. The forearm is then pronated with the thumb pointing down. A downward force is placed on the arm by the examiner. The force is repeated with the forearm in the supinated position with the thumb pointing upward.

Pain or clicking inside the shoulder joint is considered a positive test for a labral lesion. Pain over the AC joint indicates pathology in the AC joint.

Thoracic outlet syndrome

Adson's test

While feeling the radial pulse, the arm is passively abducted, extended, and externally rotated (abduction and external rotation of the arm compresses the brachial plexus against the scalene muscles). The head is extended and turned to the side of the lesion while the patient holds their breath. Loss of pulse is a positive test.

Wright's test
This test is similar to Adson's maneuver but the arm is hyperabducted over the head while externally rotated and extended (this simulates compression of the neurovascular bundle beneath the pectoralis tendon). Loss of or a diminished radial pulse is a positive test.

Other peripheral nerves that can be injured include the musculocutaneous, suprascapular, and the long thoracic nerves.

Nerves

The brachial plexus is a complex array of nerve roots, trunks, divisions, cords, and branches. Any of these areas may be injured with a traction injury to the brachial plexus.

Because of the high incidence of anterior dislocations, the most likely peripheral nerve to be injured is the axillary nerve.

Shoulder disorders

Epidemiology

Shoulder pain is the second most common musculoskeletal complaint seen by primary care practitioners.

Common diagnoses
- Rotator cuff lesions
- Pericapsular soft tissue pain
- AC joint pain

Factors related to early recovery
- Mild trauma
- Acute onset
- Overuse problems
- Early presentation

Problems related to prolonged recovery
- Diabetes mellitus
- Cervical spondylolysis
- Radicular symptoms
- Advancing age
- Involvement of the dominant extremity

Etiology

Causes of increased susceptibility to injury include the following:
- The shoulder is an inherently less stable joint to allow for the increased range of motion.
- Overuse injuries of the shoulder are common, especially in those involved in repetitive overhead activities.

Differential diagnosis

Acute problems with rapid onset over days to a few weeks include the following:
- Trauma
- Acute overuse
- Cervical nerve root compression

The age of the patient and the history may narrow the differential diagnosis.

Patients younger than 45 often have a biomechanical cause to their problem such as instability or tendonopathy. Those older than 45 are more likely to have degenerative conditions such as osteoarthritis or rotator cuff tears.

Adhesive capsulitis can present with progressive pain and concomitant loss of motion. Patients with diabetes mellitus are at increased risk for this condition.

Acute traumatic causes

Anterior glenohumeral instability

This is graded on a scale from 0 to III on the basis of percentage of humeral head translation in relation to the glenoid on load and shift testing of the shoulder.

- *Grade 0*: normal motion
- *Grade I*: translation of the head to the glenoid rim
- *Grade II*: translation of the head over the rim with spontaneous reduction
- *Grade III*: complete dislocation of the humeral head, which does not spontaneously reduce

Anterior dislocation

The mechanism of injury is most commonly forced external rotation while the upper extremity is abducted. It is also possible to occur from an anterior directed during a fall onto the posterior shoulder forcing the humeral head anteriorly. The impaction of the anterior glenoid on the posterior humerus during dislocation may cause a compression fracture or divot on the posterior humeral head known as a *Hill-Sach's lesion*.

When the humeral head dislocates anteriorly, the anteroinferior labrum is avulsed off the underlying glenoid, termed a Bankart lesion, which can lead to recurrent anterior instability.

A fracture of the anterior glenoid rim may also occur during a dislocation and is termed a bony Bankart lesion. The resultant pear-shaped glenoid is a cause of recurrent shoulder instability and may require open reduction and internal fixation of the fractured fragment or autograft vs. allograft bone to replace any bony deficiency that may result.

History and examination

Patients usually present with pain in the anterior and lateral shoulder. They will often complain of significant pain with any movement of the affected upper extremity.

With an acute anterior dislocation, a sulcus may be visible between the edge of the acromion and the dislocated humeral head on examination.

Patients will splint the arm in an adducted and internally rotated position.

If the shoulder has relocated the patients may have signs of instability on examination.

Diagnosis

Diagnosis of dislocation is usually obvious on inspection.

A radiographic trauma series of the shoulder must include anteroposterior (AP), axillary lateral, and scapular Y views.

A thorough neurovascular examination should be documented in all cases.

Treatment

Immediate reduction is done, preferably after evaluation by X-ray.

Surgical intervention after the first dislocation is unusual but may be appropriate to consider in certain patient populations:

- Young patients (<25 years old), who are at high risk for recurrent dislocations
- High-performance contact athletes at risk for repeated dislocations (football, hockey, rugby, or other collision sport)
- Worsening symptoms of instability despite conservative treatment

Consider a rotator cuff tear in a patient with dislocation for the first time who is older than 45 years of age.

Posterior glenohumeral dislocation

Posterior dislocations account for only 4% of dislocations. Posterior dislocations generally require great force and are often seen after motor vehicle accidents, repetitive weight lifting, or in football linemen. The mechanism is usually a force applied to an arm that is forward flexed to 90° and internally rotated, which forces the humerus posteriorly.

It may also occur after an anterior blow to the shoulder. It can occur with seizure activity or electrocution injuries where a violent subscapularis contraction overpowers the external rotators of the shoulder. As the humeral head dislocates posteriorly, an avulsion of the posterior glenoid labrum (a posterior Bankart lesion) and/or an anterior impaction fracture of the humeral head (a reverse Hill–Sachs lesion) may occur.

History and examination
- Patients with posterior dislocations will present with the arm in internal rotation and held close to the thorax.
- They are generally unable to abduct or externally rotate the shoulder.
- The coracoid may be prominent and the humeral head difficult to palpate.

Diagnosis
Routine shoulder AP shoulder film may miss this injury. An axillary lateral view is critical for identifying a posterior dislocation.

Treatment
Treatment is with closed reduction. Cases of recurrent instability may require surgery for repair of the posterior labrum or to address bony defects in the posterior glenoid or anterior humeral head.

Inferior glenohumeral dislocation

Inferior glenohumeral dislocations are unusual because of the protection given by the acromion. This may represent a generalized laxity and be associated with multidirectional instability. The mechanism is usually a forced abduction injury. The acromion can act as a fulcrum and force the humeral head inferiorly.

History and examination
- With chronic instability there is pain while the arm is down by the side or overhead.

- These patients may also complain of easy fatigability while carrying loads.
- On inspection, the acromion may be prominent.
- There may be a positive sulcus sign.
- Forced abduction may cause pain or apprehension.

Treatment
- Treatment is by immediate reduction with pre- and post-reduction films.
- Rehabilitation
- Surgical stabilization may be possible even if multidirectional instability is present.

Nonoperative management of shoulder dislocation

For elite athletes, in season, treatment should be rehabilitation. They may return to full competition once the strength and range of motion on the injured side is comparable to that in their other shoulder. A brace is recommended for contact or collision sport athletes. At the end of the season or if the athlete is out of season at the time of injury, early operative intervention should be considered because of the high recurrence rate in young athletes (<25 years old).

In the nonathlete or patients who are than 25–30 years older, the primary treatment is rehabilitation, with an anticipated lower rate of recurrence.

During all rehabilitation programs following shoulder dislocation, it is important to ensure the appropriate balance and restoration of scapulothoracic stabilization, glenohumeral stabilization and humeral control, and the various neuromuscular mechanisms involved in their modulation.

Rehabilitation

Initial

Provide a sling for comfort. Note that a sling has no effect on recurrent instability. In general, the athlete's rehabilitation should begin with a focus on regaining range of motion and advance to strengthening. The focus should then be on functional and sport-specific rehabilitation.

Early stage: weeks 0–3

Goals
- Begin joint approximation/proprioceptive exercises
- Achieve full passive range of motion
- Enhance static and dynamic control of the shoulder complex
- Improve shoulder-complex positional awareness

Aims
- Minimize atrophy of the shoulder muscles
- Regain shoulder motion
- Maintain elbow mobility and strength
- Maintain wrist mobility and strength

Treatment
- Passive shoulder mobilizations within the limits of pain
- Strengthening of scapular stabilizers

General exercises

Mobility
- Progress active assisted exercises up to full elevation through flexion

Shoulder complex control
- *Postural correction*: The athlete focuses on finding and maintaining a neutral position of the shoulder complex.
- *Strengthening*: With all strengthening exercises, the athlete is encouraged to maintain a neutral shoulder position.
  - Isometric strengthening of all muscle groups

After 2 weeks, the athlete should perform these exercises in various degrees of shoulder flexion and/or abduction, ensuring at all times that neutral scapular position is maintained.

Middle stage: weeks 4–10

Aims
- Progress strengthening
- Increase joint approximation and joint positional sense

Exercises

The focus is on joint approximation and positional sense and balance. Throughout all exercises, the athlete is encouraged to maintain a neutral shoulder position, e.g., avoiding protraction and winging.

Strengthening
- Once the athlete has gained a good baseline of shoulder control and strength in a neutral position, strengthening through range is essential, and the athlete should focus on improving rotator cuff strength.

End stage: return to sports (11–12 weeks)

Aims
- Increase strength of gross shoulder movements
- Begin sports-specific rehabilitation

Strength and conditioning
Initially the athlete should carry out each activity using dumbbells; form and fatigue can be compared with the uninjured side.

A typical circuit might include the following:
- Bench press
- Shoulder press
- Chin-ups
- Upright rows
- Bicep curls
- Tricep extensions

Athletes returning to contact sports may have a higher risk of reoccurrence; thus other higher demanding conditioning drills may be of benefit in the later stages of rehabilitation.

Return to play
Before safe return to play, the athlete must have achieved the following:
- Full pain-free range of motion
- Regained or improved static and dynamic control of the shoulder complex through all resisted movements and weight-bearing movements
- Strength equal to that of uninjured side
- Full participation in strength and conditioning

The very nature of contact and collision sports increases the risk of injury. Prior to a full return to training, athletes must be strong enough and confident enough to perform in every potential scenario that may involve direct or indirect shoulder contact. In each of these drills, the athlete should be technically and tactically proficient. The lead rehabilitation therapist may thus require input and advice from coaching staff.

AC joint sprains and dislocations

Acute AC sprains are a common traumatic injury usually resulting from a fall onto the lateral shoulder.

Type 1 is a mild sprain to the acromioclavicular ligaments. There is no separation of the AC joint compared to the unaffected side.

Type 2 involves rupture of the AC ligament, but the coracoclavicular ligaments are at least partially intact. There is <1 cm displacement of the clavicle from the acromion.

Type 3 involves complete rupture of both acromioclavicular and coracoclavicular ligaments.

Type 4 is a posterior displacement of the clavicle into the trapezius

Type 5 is a more severe form of type 3 secondary to the deltotrapezial fascia being stripped off the clavicle. This results in a 100%–300% increase in the clavicle–acromial distance.

Type 6 is an inferior dislocation and may be located in the subacromial or subcoracoid region. It is often the result of severe trauma and can be associated with paresthesias.

History and examination

Patients will usually present with pain in the lateral shoulder, often localized to the AC joint. Motion is usually intact, but limited by pain.

Palpation over the AC joint may indicate tenderness.

Asymmetry may be noted between the two shoulders if a high-grade sprain is present.

The cross-body adduction test may be positive.

Diagnosis

The diagnosis is usually made on physical examination. However, accurate grading of sprains may require plain radiographs with comparison views of the opposite shoulder. A Zanca view is good for specifically evaluating the AC joint.

Use of weighted films to overcome splinting from pain has not been shown to be necessary.

Treatment

Treatment is primarily symptomatic for types 1–3. The shoulder should be immobilized for comfort for a brief period of time, a few days to 1 week, depending on severity.

Braces and long-term slings are not recommended as they will contribute to shoulder stiffness.

Range-of-motion exercises should be started as soon as can be tolerated by the patient.

For the low-grade sprains, surgical stabilization is usually not necessary and only indicated for chronic pain, instability, or aesthetic reasons. In cases of aesthetics, the patient may only be trading a bump for a scar.

Surgery is often indicated for the higher-grade lesions (types 4–6). These lesions are usually higher energy and may compromise skin or muscle integrity or be associated with neurovascular compromise, as in the case of type 6 dislocations.

Sternoclavicular joint sprains and dislocations

Sternoclavicular joint sprains and subluxations or dislocations are much less common than acromioclavicular injuries. Anterior dislocations are seen much more frequently than posterior ones. The injury involves disruption of both the sternoclavicular and costoclavicular ligaments. They are graded as first-, second-, or third-degree injuries depending on the degree of associated capsular disruption.

The most common mechanism is a fall onto the lateral or posterolateral shoulder often with a concurrent force applied to the opposite shoulder. This may be seen in a takedown in wrestling or a pile-up in football or rugby.

Less commonly, a posteriorly directed force directly over the sternoclavicular joint may occur, which can result in a posterior dislocation.

History and examination

While elevating the shoulder there may be an observable or palpably obvious subluxation accompanied by a "pop" or "click."

Diagnosis

The dislocation is more easily seen on the *serendipity view* during plain-film examination.

If suspicion is high, but not obvious on plain film, an MRI or CT may be helpful in making the diagnosis.

Treatment

Treatment for an anterior dislocation is nonoperative. Symptomatic treatment is with rest, ice, and NSAIDs. There is a high rate of recurrence with reductions of anterior dislocations.

Posterior dislocations are rare, but serious if present, because of the possibility of compression of the trachea, esophagus, or neurovascular structures in the neck. These cases must be closed reduced emergently in the operating room with a cardiothoracic surgeon available for assistance.

Glenoid labrum tears

Glenoid labrum tears are most often seen after a glenohumeral dislocation. These patients typically have fallen onto an outstretched arm or have an overuse injury such as that in throwing athletes. During an anterior dislocation, the humeral head may tear the anteroinferior labrum off the underlying glenoid, termed a *Bankart lesion*.

If a lesion is present in the superior labrum extending anteriorly to posteriorly beneath the biceps tendon, it is referred to as a *SLAP lesion* (superior labrum anterior to posterior). SLAP lesions are associated with anterior instability.

Superior labral lesions are graded as follows:
- *Type 1*: fraying of the superior labrum
- *Type 2*: fraying plus separation from glenoid
- *Type 3*: bucket-handle tear of the superior labrum
- *Type 4*: bucket-handle tear extending into the biceps tendon

Internal impingement

Often, throwing athletes experience a glenohumeral internal rotation deficit (GIRD) from a contracture of their posterior capsule and posterior rotator cuff. This can lead to abnormal glenohumeral mechanics secondary to anterior and superior humeral translation.

Posterior-superior labral tears and partial articular-sided tears of the rotator cuff may result.

History and examination

The pain is usually present in the posterior shoulder. Popping, clicking, and snapping are also common complaints.

Patients may notice that they cannot throw as hard or as long as they could previously.

On examination, patients with labral tears can have a positive O'Brien's or Speed's test. They may be tender to palpation around the anterior and posterior glenohumeral capsule.

There may be scapulothoracic dyskinesis seen on examination as well with mild winging and asymmetry during motion. The scapula on the affected side may be lower and protracted. Patients may also have anterior tenderness over a contracted pectoralis minor tendon insertion on the coracoid process.

Signs of anterior instability may also be present.

Diagnosis

Routine X-rays are usually normal. A magnetic resonance arthrogram is the best test to evaluate for a labral tear.

Treatment

Any patient with an internal rotation deficit and scapular dyskinesis would benefit from a trial of physical therapy to work on posterior capsular stretching and scapular stabilizer strengthening.

If this fails to resolve symptoms, referral for further evaluation is appropriate. A magnetic resonance arthrogram is the test of choice to confirm the diagnosis of a labral tear and can also be used to evaluate the integrity of the rotator cuff. The need for surgical treatment depends on the patient's symptoms and the level of activity.

For high-level throwing athletes, superior labral tears are often repaired arthroscopically, and partial-thickness rotator cuff tears are frequently treated with debridement.

Biceps tendon rupture

Complete disruption of the tendinous fibers of the biceps occurs most often within the bicipital groove. Occasionally, it presents at the distal tendinous pole. Proximal ruptures occur most often during overhead activity and are the result of gradual attenuation of the tendon.

History and examination

The patient has immediate pain either in the shoulder and proximal biceps or in the distal biceps. Occasionally there is swelling and ecchymosis. Patients may feel a pop or snap during the initial injury.

On examination they usually have an obvious bulging defect in the biceps, caused by the retraction of the muscle belly, called a "Popeye deformity."

Patients may have mild weakness to resisted flexion of the elbow and supination of the forearm if there is a proximal rupture. This may be quite pronounced if there is a distal rupture.

Diagnosis

Plain films are usually normal. An MRI is necessary only if the diagnosis is uncertain.

Treatment

Treatment of biceps ruptures is generally nonoperative with good results, especially in the elderly. The patient is often left with a "Popeye deformity" in the anterior distal arm, which is usually not painful. Occasionally, some patients may note cramping of their biceps.

A biceps tenodesis can be performed for the rare patient who experiences pain after a proximal rupture.

Surgery is indicated if there is a distal tendon rupture at the elbow.

Fractures of the shoulder

Clavicle fractures

History and examination

Mid-shaft clavicle fractures are common injuries and usually are the result of a fall or a direct blow to the clavicle. There is immediate pain.

Shortness of breath or respiratory distress may herald a tension pneumothorax if the mechanism of injury is high energy.

With severe displacement, the brachial plexus may be injured.

Evaluate the patient for swelling and deformity of the clavicle, any subcutaneous crepitation, pneumothorax, or neurovascular deficits of the upper extremity.

X-rays should include clavicular views and a chest film as part of the workup if the patient was involved in a high-energy trauma.

Treatment

Fractures of the middle third of the clavicle will most often heal with nonoperative management, even when displaced. Management of uncomplicated clavicular fractures includes a sling until the patient is comfortable, followed by range-of-motion exercises.

Referral is necessary with comminuted or displaced fractures, as newer studies suggest that these types of fractures may be best served by surgical fixation.

Treatment of very proximal and very distal fractures is controversial and referral may be appropriate.

Scapular fractures

Fractures of the scapula are rare. Because of the high energy required to fracture the scapula, patients with this fracture should always be assessed for associated injuries (i.e., rib fractures, pulmonary contusions).

The treatment of most scapular fractures involves immobilization in a sling for 2–3 weeks accompanied by early range-of-motion exercises as tolerated.

Significantly displaced scapular fractures or those that involve the glenoid, neck, acromion, or coracoid require orthopedic referral for possible surgical intervention.

Fractures of the proximal humerus

One-part proximal humeral fractures in elderly, low-demand patients can often be treated by immobilization in a sling for 1–3 weeks. The patient should start range-of-motion exercises as soon as tolerated.

In about 20% of fractures there is displacement of the humeral head, the lesser or greater tuberosity, or the humeral shaft. These should be referred for possible surgical intervention.

Fractures of the anatomic neck or epiphyseal plate, greater-tuberosity avulsion fractures, or fractures of the humeral head also need to be referred for possible surgical treatment.

Management of proximal humerus fractures depends on the degree of comminution and displacement, the vascularity of the humeral head, the age of the patient, and the patient's functional demands.

Surgical options can include closed reduction and percutaneous pinning, open reduction and internal fixation, or hemiarthroplasty vs. total shoulder arthroplasty.

Chronic overuse disorders

Symptomatic multidirectional laxity

History and examination

Patients with multidirectional laxity may have signs of anterior, posterior, and/or inferior instability. These patients may have generalized joint laxity (assess the knees and elbows for hyperextensibility, the ability to abduct the thumb to the forearm when the wrist is flexed, or extension of the metacarpophalangeal joints past 90°).

Often patients may present with pain but no history of trauma. This is often seen with repetitive throwing or other overhead activities such as swimming. These repetitive activities can cause injuries to the labrum or capsule and place extra stress on the rotator cuff muscles. Recurrent microtrauma may lead to impingement syndrome or osteoarthritis.

Those with anterior instability typically have a positive apprehension sign, relocation test, and possibly an anterior load-and-shift test.

In posterior instability there may be a positive posterior apprehension sign, and perhaps a positive posterior load-and-shift test. Having the patient do a push-up against the wall may reproduce symptoms associated with posterior instability.

Inferior instability may show up on examination as a positive sulcus sign. Carrying weights or suitcases may reproduce symptoms.

Diagnosis

Routine X-rays may show signs of chronic subluxation such as erosion of the glenoid rim.

An MRI may be useful in diagnosing small labral tears and demonstrate a rotator cuff tear.

Treatment

Eighty percent of patients with nontraumatic instability respond well to physical therapy but do poorly with surgical intervention.

If the initial dislocation occurred before the age of 30, only about one-third of patients need operative treatment.

Impingement syndrome and rotator cuff tendonopathy

Impingement syndrome is an overuse injury with compression of the rotator cuff between the greater tuberosity of the humerus and the acromion.

The rotator cuff, biceps tendon, and the subacromial bursa may all be affected. The supraspinatus and biceps tendons are at particular risk because of their position under the coracoacromial arch. It occurs with overuse of the shoulder or in chronic instability.

The combination of laxity and impingement is often seen in swimmers and overhead throwers. If the humeral head is allowed to move superiorly due to laxity, the instability may accentuate impingement symptoms.

Impingement syndrome may also result from direct trauma (such as a fall onto an elbow or an outstretched hand), muscular imbalances, posterior capsular tightness, or anatomical overgrowth (spurring) of the acromion process.

Athletes at particular risk are baseball pitchers, swimmers, tennis players, weight lifters, and golfers, especially if patients are overtraining or have poor technique or mechanics.

Impingement syndrome is rarely seen in patients <40 years of age, unless there is a trauma injury or they are involved in overhead sports.

Increased mechanical irritation of the bursa and rotator cuff over time leads to increased fibrosis and partial-thickness rotator cuff and/or biceps tendon tears. Eventually this may lead to a full-thickness tear of the rotator cuff and biceps tendon.

History and examination

The onset of pain is usually gradual and may be present for weeks or months. It is usually located in the lateral deltoid just distal to the tip of the acromion. Patients may also present with pain in the biceps radiating down to the elbow.

Pain is usually worsened with overhead activities or when lying on the involved side; symptoms may be worse at night. The patient may complain of popping, snapping, or grinding.

On examination there may be pain between 90° and 120° of abduction (painful arc). There may be tenderness with internal and external rotation while the shoulder is at 90° of abduction.

Hawkin's and Neer's tests may be positive. The impingement test is usually positive.

There may be signs of rotator cuff and biceps tendon irritation as well as frank weakness due to pain. This must be re-evaluated after treatment to rule out a complete or partial tear of these tendons.

Diagnosis

Radiographic evaluation is usually normal unless there is acromial overgrowth or degenerative joint disease.

Radiological evidence of calcification suggests calcific tendonitis (see Calcific tendonitis, p. 130).

MRI can detect a partial- or full-thickness rotator cuff tear.

Treatment

Treatment is with rest, range-of-motion exercises, and strengthening exercises of the scapula and thorax.

Injection of corticosteroids into the subacromial space can alleviate symptoms in many patients.

If conservative measures fail after 6 weeks or if partial or complete tears are present, surgical intervention may be warranted.

To prevent impingement syndrome improper techniques that are used in overhead sport activities should be avoided and offending activities minimized.

Rotator cuff tears

Rotator cuff tears occur when there is a complete separation of the tendinous fibers from their insertion onto the greater tuberosity of the humerus.

Most cases are seen in patients over 40 years of age and many have chronic impingement symptoms. Contributing factors may be patient age, vascular changes within the cuff, trauma, attrition, or impingement.

If acute trauma is involved, it usually involves a fall onto an abducted arm or a direct blow to the lateral shoulder.

The most likely tendon to be affected is the supraspinatus. The tear may then extend to the infraspinatus, and in severe cases, it may involve the teres minor and biceps tendon. The subscapularis is rarely involved.

History and examination

The patient usually presents with weakness and poorly localized pain that may radiate down the humerus. Pain is exacerbated by overhead activities. About 50% of patients associate their pain with a specific trauma.

Inspection may demonstrate wasting of the supraspinatus and infraspinatus if the problem has been long standing. The rotator cuff may be tender to palpation or there may be crepitus in the subacromial bursa.

Direct testing of the muscles of the rotator cuff will find weakness when compared with the unaffected side (open can test, lift-off/belly press, or resisted external rotation).

The strength of the external rotators may be affected in extensive tears because of involvement of the infraspinatus.

Patients usually have less tenderness with passive than with active range of motion. Most patients will have one or more of the lag signs present and possibly a positive drop arm test.

Tests for impingement are often positive.

Diagnosis

Plain films may show only acromial overgrowth. MRI is now used to evaluate complete and partial tears and even visualize other shoulder conditions such as articular cartilage damage or tears of the glenoid labrum.

Unless a complete rotator cuff tear is suspected, an MRI or CT need not be obtained unless the patient has failed 6–8 weeks of conservative therapy. An MRI adds little information unless intervention is being planned. Ultrasound is less expensive, but the specificity and sensitivity of this test are highly technician dependent.

Treatment

Initial treatment is usually with rest and avoidance of all overhead activities, along with physical therapy.

If symptoms persist for more than 6–8 weeks or the patient has high demands of the shoulder, an MRI should be ordered earlier and the patient referred for an orthopedic assessment. These patients may be candidates for repair of a full-thickness tear or debridement of a partial tear (<50% of rotator cuff tendon footprint on the humerus).

Acute traumatic tears of the rotator cuff should be referred as soon as possible for surgical consideration.

Little Leaguer's shoulder

This is a stress injury to the proximal humeral physis secondary to shear forces associated with throwing and pitching. It may be the first stage of a continuum leading to a physeal stress fracture.

History and examination
- Usually presents in adolescence with shoulder pain on throwing
- No history of specific injury
- Usually full range of motion
- Swelling uncommon

Diagnosis
An AP X-ray in external rotation demonstrates widening of the proximal humeral physis (epiphysiolysis). It may need to be compared with the contralateral physis to appreciate this finding.

Treatment
- Rest from throwing (usually >2 months required)
- Graduated return to throwing when asymptomatic
- Adhere to age guidelines regarding pitching limits and education of proper throwing technique to prevent recurrence

Prognosis
- Usually good
- Small risk of premature growth plate closure and subsequent humeral length discrepancy

Biceps tendinopathy

Biceps tendonitis is characterized by pain and inflammation of the long head of the biceps tendon within the bicipital groove. These patients are usually young or middle aged.

This condition is often due to repetitive elbow flexion or supination and occurs particularly in activities that require reaching and overhead lifting, such as tennis, swimming, golf, or throwing sports. It is often associated with impingement syndrome and/or rotator cuff tears.

History and examination
- The patient will present with anterior shoulder pain.
- The pain is usually worse during and directly after activity and improves with rest.
- There is usually no pain at night.
- Symptoms may be present for a variable length of time.
- On examination the patient may experience pain with resisted flexion of the elbow and supination of the wrist (Speed's and Yergason's tests).
- There may be tenderness to palpation within the bicipital groove and along the long head of the biceps tendon.
- There may also be limitation of the extremes of abduction, internal rotation, and external rotation.
- There may be biceps weakness secondary to pain.

Diagnosis
X-rays are usually normal. An MRI is usually not warranted unless a repairable biceps or rotator cuff tear is suspected.

Treatment
- Rest, ice, local heat, and protection
- Gentle stretching and exercise

- The patient may benefit from a formal physical therapy program if a quick return to activities is important
- Oral NSAIDs may be of benefit

Calcific tendonitis

With degeneration of the collagen fibers of the rotator cuff tendons, calcium salts may infiltrate the substance of the tendon and cause inflammation. This may be associated with acute or chronic symptoms and may secondarily involve the bursa.

The most common site is the supraspinatus tendon, but it may also involve the biceps tendon, infraspinatus, or subscapularis.

History and examination

There may be severe pain affecting sleep. If calcification is chronic, the patient may have symptoms more like those of impingement syndrome.

On examination, the patient may hold the arm splinted against the body and have intense, global shoulder pain that limits the patient's ability to move the extremity and precludes an accurate examination.

Any palpation over the affected area produces significant tenderness, which may affect range of motion.

Diagnosis

X-ray examination of the shoulder may show calcifications within the tendons of the rotator cuff.

AP views in external rotation and internal rotation will show the rotator cuff best.

Bicipital groove views may show biceps tendon calcifications.

Treatment

Injection of a lidocaine and corticosteroid preparation may be effective and provide dramatic relief. Oral anti-inflammatories rarely provide significant improvement acutely.

Once pain has subsided, physical therapy may be beneficial for rotator cuff and periscapular muscle strengthening.

Surgical intervention may be required in recalcitrant cases.

AC degenerative joint disease

Degenerative joint disease of the AC joint is common and often can develop at a much earlier age than that of the glenohumeral or sternoclavicular joint.

History and examination

The patient usually complains of intermittent pain, often gradual in onset, but may present after trauma. There may be intermittent swelling, popping, clicking, or grinding.

On examination the patient is usually tender over the superior and anterior aspect of the AC joint There may be a prominence of the AC joint on inspection.

The cross-body adduction test is usually positive.

Diagnosis

Radiographs can demonstrate degenerative changes within the AC joint.

An injection of lidocaine into the joint that relieves the pain supports the diagnosis.

Treatment

- Treatment is usually symptomatic.
- Injection with a corticosteroid may be of benefit.
- Surgical intervention consists of resection of the distal clavicle, which can be done arthroscopically or open.

Adhesive capsulitis (frozen shoulder)

This condition is of unknown etiology and results in progressive restriction of passive and active range of motion of the shoulder with associated pain. It is self-limited and often resolves within 18–30 months. There are three stages: inflammatory, freezing, and thawing.

It is characterized by a thickening and contracture of the shoulder joint capsule, glenohumeral ligaments, and the coracohumeral ligament.

Adhesive capsulitis most frequently is idiopathic. However, it is associated with diabetes mellitus, conditions that require prolonged immobilization as in post-traumatic conditions, autoimmune or endocrine diseases, stroke, and myocardial infarction. It also occurs in patients with HIV who are being treated with protease inhibitors.

Eighty percent of patients with this condition are female, and most patients are over 40 years old.

The nondominant arm is often affected.

History and examination

The pain is usually gradual in onset but can be acute and can be referred to the insertion of the deltoid. Patients may report difficulty sleeping on the affected side.

On examination, there is limitation to active and passive range of motion, especially in abduction, internal rotation, and external rotation, which distinguishes it from other shoulder pathologies.

The limited range of motion is secondary to capsular thickening and adhesions.

There is often no specific point tenderness but rather diffuse pain is present, especially with the end-ranges of motion.

Treatment

Corticosteroid injections into the glenohumeral joint and possibly subacromial space may be effective in treating the pain experienced during the early inflammatory phase.

Once the acute pain has been controlled, painless physical therapy should be recommended to regain motion and strength. The condition may take up to 2–3 years to completely resolve.

Arthroscopic capsulotomy with manipulation under anesthesia may be required in recalcitrant cases.

Osteolysis of the distal clavicle

This is often caused by chronic overuse, but it may also be initiated by an acute traumatic injury. Weight lifters appear to be prone to this condition.

Osteolysis of the distal clavicle usually presents with chronic pain in the lateral superior shoulder lasting longer than 4 months.

History and examination

Pain is usually a dull ache over the AC joint. There may be weakness and pain with flexion and adduction.

Diagnosis

Diagnosis is usually by plain X-ray, which may show osteopenia with tapering of the distal clavicle, and associated osteophytes, subchondral erosions, and cysts.

Treatment

Lidocaine and corticosteroid injections can be both diagnostic and therapeutic.

Arthroscopic distal clavicle resection is often performed if the symptoms are not relieved by an injection. This increases the space between the clavicle and acromion and prevents impaction of the two bone ends.

Atraumatic causes

Thoracic outlet syndrome

There are four areas of potential compression:

1. Compression of the subclavian vein between the anterior scalene, clavicle, and first rib
2. Compression of the brachial plexus and subclavian artery between the anterior scalene, middle scalene, and first rib
3. Compression of the neurovascular bundle between the clavicle and the first rib
4. Compression of the neurovascular bundle as it passes under the tendinous portion of the pectoralis minor

Cervical ribs are the most common bony anomaly seen with thoracic outlet syndrome. However, 10% of these cases are asymptomatic. Trauma, as a precipitating factor, is not uncommon.

History and examination

Patients may complain of neurological, vascular, or combined symptoms. Neurological symptoms consist of pain, often sharp but sometimes aching, that radiates from the neck or shoulder into the forearm or hand, often following an ulnar nerve distribution. Paresthesias and hyperaesthesias may also be present.

Symptoms may be exacerbated by overhead activity. Vascular symptoms that originate from the subclavian artery may cause pain over the supraclavicular space. There may be associated pale, cold, or numb fingers. Activities that involve elevation or abduction of the arm may worsen such symptoms.

Compression of the subclavian vein may cause pain over the supraclavicular space or the feeling of pressure in the extremity.

On examination, the extremity may appear dusky, swollen, mottled, or blue, or it may appear entirely normal.

The patient may have a positive Wright's maneuver, Roos maneuver, and/or Adson's test.

Diagnosis

X-ray evaluation of the cervical spine and chest is required. If there is vascular compromise, Doppler studies will usually define the area of concern. Angiograms are usually necessary if there are abnormalities seen on Doppler imaging.

Electrodiagnostic studies may be needed if neurological compromise is suspected.

Treatment

Treatment consists of shoulder-strengthening exercises concentrating on posterior scapular stabilization if the patient's symptoms are not disabling or consistent with vascular compromise.

If there is vascular compromise or conservative treatment fails, refer the patient for possible surgical intervention, which can consist of resection of the first rib.

Septic arthritis

Septic arthritis of the shoulder is rare. It is most frequently seen in infants and children 2 years of age or younger, but may be seen at any age.

This condition represents a surgical emergency. If left untreated it can lead to septic shock, chondrolysis, or arthritis.

There is an increased incidence in patients with diabetes mellitus, cancer, hypogammaglobulinemia, or chronic liver disease and in those receiving corticosteroid or immunosuppressive drugs.

The more common organisms to infect the joint are *S. aureus* (most common in adults), *N. gonorrhoeae*, *Strep. pneumoniae*, *Strep. pyogenese*, *H. influenza* (most common in neonates), and gram-negative bacilli.

History and examination

The patient usually presents with pain, swelling, and loss of range of motion of the joint with no apparent portal of entry.

Occasionally patients may present following an aspiration or injection procedure of the joint.

Diagnosis and treatment

Diagnosis is by aspiration of joint fluid.

If frank pus is present, immediate surgical incision and drainage should be performed and the patient should be started on intravenous antibiotics after cultures are obtained. If the clinical suspicion is high and the joint fluid appears normal or the lab results are equivocal, the patient should be started on intravenous antibiotics until the culture results return.

Osteonecrosis (ischemic necrosis, avascular necrosis)

Ischemia of the humeral head is typically referred to as avascular necrosis (AVN) of the humeral head. It is associated with hemoglobinopathies, pancreatitis, alcoholism, and connective tissue disease. It has also been documented in gout, osteoarthritis, burns, Goucher's disease, prolonged immobilization, pregnancy, hyperparathyroidism, and cytotoxic treatments.

The patient will usually present with chronic shoulder pain and limited range of motion.

X-ray changes are often not seen until several months after the onset of symptoms. An MRI scan is the test of choice for detecting early ischemic changes in the bone.

Treatment is often limited to supportive care, but in cases of severe pain, total joint arthroplasty may be necessary. Some studies suggest that core decompression can be helpful for focal lesions.

Cervical radiculopathy

Always consider the cervical spine in any evaluation of shoulder pain. Cervical radiculopathy causes deep burning pain that radiates from the shoulder to the fingertips and may be associated with paresthesias.

It is often relieved by forward shoulder elevation or repositioning of the neck.

Range of motion of the cervical spine should be tested. Spurling's maneuver and an atlanto-occipital axial compression test should be performed.

Motor function should be evaluated in the upper extremity, arm, and hand. Fine movements of the hand should be evaluated.

Deep tendon reflexes should be tested in the upper extremity and a sensory examination conducted.

An appropriate cervical workup should precede a shoulder workup if any abnormalities are found.

Tumors of the shoulder

The most common malignant bony tumors of the humerus are Ewing's sarcoma and osteosarcoma. These tend to occur in adolescence.

Chondrosarcomas, though rare, tend to occur during the third to seventh decade. Most cases in adults, however, represent metastatic lesions or multiple myeloma.

Other lesions seen include osteochondromas, chondroblastomas, giant cell tumors, aneurysmal bone cysts, and Pancoast tumors.

Tumors may present with pain that is worse at night and in some cases may be significantly improved with NSAIDs.

Plain radiographs may identify the lesions, but MRI is usually needed for clarification.

Referred pain from the chest and abdomen

The phrenic nerve arises from the fourth cervical nerve but also receives branches from the third and fifth nerves. It begins at the posterior scalene muscle, descends the chest in the lateral part of the pericardium, and ends at the diaphragm. Branches of this nerve provide sensory innervation to the mediastinal and diaphragmatic pleura, diaphragmatic peritoneum, and probably the liver, gallbladder, and inferior vena cava.

Irritation of the diaphragm or the innervated areas of the pleura or peritoneum will stimulate the phrenic nerve. Since these nerves also innervate the skin of the neck, supraclavicular area, and shoulder, pain may be referred to these areas.

Pneumonia, pulmonary infarction, empyema, neoplasm, hepatobiliary disease, subphrenic abscess, splenic injury, or a pseudocyst of the pancreas can all produce shoulder pain.

Elbow and forearm

History

- Ascertain the location, quality, and severity of the patient's symptoms.
- Establish symptom onset and mechanism of injury, as well as any exacerbating or relieving factors.
- Are there any neck, forearm, or hand symptoms?

Examination

Inspection (see Fig. 4.1)
- Look at soft tissue contour for evidence of wasting or asymmetry of muscle bulk, muscle fasciculation, scars, or deformities. Over-development of the dominant arm is common.
- Look for swelling, bruising, and soft tissue masses.
- Examine limb alignment and estimate the carrying angle with the arm extended.
- Inspect posteriorly for evidence of dislocation, olecranon bursitis, effusion, and triceps tendon tear (excessively bony prominence, with a gap just above).
- Inspect laterally for synovitis or effusion, which may be evident in the triangular space between the lateral epicondyle, the head of the radius, and the tip of the olecranon.
- Normally, neither synovium nor bursa is palpable.

Palpation
- Examine the bony landmarks with the arm flexed at 70°.
- Palpate posteriorly along the triceps and olecranon.
- Palpate the medial epicondyle and ulnar collateral ligament (UCL).
- Examine the flexor-pronator muscle group.
- Check the biceps tendon and brachial pulse.
- Palpate the radial head.
- Palpate the lateral epicondyle and lateral collateral ligament (LCL).
- Examine the common extensor origin.
- Palpate the ulnar nerve posterior to the medial epicondyle for thickening and/or irritability.

Range of motion
- Assess passive and active range of motion and movement against resistance (for specific muscle groups) and compare sides.
- Normal elbow range of motion is from –5 to 145° of flexion and should be symmetric to the contralateral side.
- Normal forearm pronation and supination is 70 and 85°, respectively.

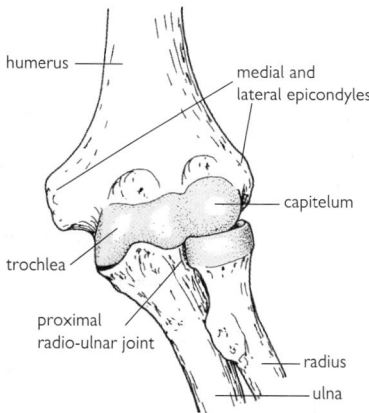

Figure 4.1 Articular surfaces of elbow joint (anterior aspect). Reproduced with permission from MacKinnon P, Morris J (2005). *Oxford Textbook of Functional Anatomy*, Vol 1. Oxford: Oxford University Press, ©2005.

Special tests

UCL injury

Valgus stress test

The patient's hand is placed between the examiner's elbow and body while the medial joint line and UCL are palpated. A valgus stress is applied to the elbow in 30° of flexion. Tenderness and opening of the medial joint line indicate UCL injury.

Moving valgus stress test

The patient brings the shoulder into abduction and external rotation. The examiner flexes and extends the patient's elbow while applying a valgus force. In the patient with a UCL injury, this should reproducibly cause pain in the arc between 80 and 120°.

Posterolateral rotatory instability (ULCL injury)

Lateral pivot shift test

The pivot shift test is performed with the patient supine and the examiner standing above the patient's head. The extremity being tested is brought into 90° of forward flexion, and the shoulder is externally rotated. The patient's forearm is held in maximal supination, and a valgus force is applied with the examiner's other hand as the elbow is flexed from a starting point of full extension. Subluxation is maximized as the elbow reaches 40°.

When positive for posterolateral rotary instability (PLRI), this maneuver results in apprehension and guarding and occasionally a sudden clunk due to the reduction of the radiocapitellar joint.

Medial epicondylosis (golfer's elbow)

History

This is a tendinosis of the common origin of the flexor-pronator muscle group. It commonly occurs with repetitive flexion and pronation and less commonly with valgus stresses. It is often seen in throwing sports, racket sports, and in golfers ("golfer's elbow").

Patients complain of inner elbow pain that is worse with certain activities (throwing, serving, hitting a forehand). They may complain of a weak grip, and some patients may present with paraesthesias in the ring and little fingers suggestive of an ulnar neuropathy.

Examination

There is tenderness at the medial epicondyle. There may be a reduced range of motion at the elbow because of pain on stretching of the flexor-pronator group with full extension.

Patients have increased pain with resisted wrist flexion or pronation, as well as with passive wrist extension.

Imaging

Imaging studies are not routinely performed. X-rays are often normal.

Ultrasound shows decreased echogenicity, inhomogeneity and thickening of the tendon, and, more rarely, a local fluid collection.

MRI may demonstrate an increased signal intensity of the extensor tendons close to their origin on the medial epicondyle.

Treatment

Nonoperative

Relative rest, ice (10–20 minutes every 2 hours in the acute stages), compression, and NSAIDs (topical NSAIDs such as voltaren gel are preferable) are first-line treatment. If these conservative measures fail, an injection of lidocaine and corticosteroid may be considered. A combination of 2 mL of bupivicaine and 1 mL of 40 mg/mL depomedrol is used.

Only one injection is given over the course of therapy. Repeated injections may result in tendon compromise and other complications. Care must be taken not to inject into the ulnar nerve.

Following the injection, a comprehensive rehabilitation program is initiated and the patient is reminded that continuing rehabilitation exercises and proper mechanics are important for prevention of recurrence.

If the injury is related to athletics, patients should be encouraged to seek professional instruction to identify biomechanical errors in form.

Operative

Most patients respond to conservative treatment. If symptoms persist after at least 10 weeks of appropriate conservative treatment, then surgery is considered.

Standard approaches include releasing of the flexor/pronator origin, excising the granulation tissue, decorticating the medial epicondylar bone, and reconstructing the medial musculotendinous unit. Decompression of the ulnar nerve is also commonly performed as part of the procedure.

Medial epicondylar apophysitis

History

The valgus force imparted to the elbow when throwing causes compression of lateral elbow structures and stretching of medial elbow structures. This results in traction of the wrist flexors on the apophysis of the medial epicondyle.

This repetitive traction may result in overgrowth of the apophysis, inflammation, and pain.

This is an overuse injury that often presents in a skeletally immature throwing athlete. Patients typically complain of the gradual onset of medial elbow pain that is exacerbated by pitching, bowling, or throwing long distances.

Examination

A flexion contracture of more than 15° is often present. Pain is elicited upon palpation of the medial epicondyle (common flexor origin).

Pain is reproduced by passive dorsiflexion of the wrist with the elbow in the extended position and with resisted wrist flexion.

Imaging

An X-ray may demonstrate widening of the medial epicondylar apophysis in comparison to the contralateral elbow.

Given the complexity and various ages of closure of the multiple different physes about the elbow, comparison films of the contralateral elbow should be obtained in all skeletally immature patients with elbow pain.

Treatment

Nonoperative

- *First 4–6 weeks:* Rest from throwing activities. Apply ice, use NSAIDs, and work on range of movement.
- *After 4–6 weeks:* Once a full, painless range of movement is attained, begin a stretching and strengthening program. Avoid any exercises that elicit pain. A gradual throwing program may be commenced only if the patient is pain free.

Ulnar collateral ligament injury

History

In acute UCL injury, individuals often note a sudden onset of medial elbow pain. This may be associated with a popping sensation and generally occurs as a result of throwing or falling.

In chronic UCL injury, individuals often note a history of repeated bouts of inner elbow pain during and after throwing. They report that the pain initially responded to conservative treatment but returns when activity is resumed. Given the chronicity of the instability, the athlete may also complain of ulnar nerve irritation (due to stretching of the nerve with the increased valgus laxity), symptoms of medial epicondylosis (due to attempts at muscular stabilization), or catching and locking (from loose bodies and arthritic changes).

This injury is most often the result of repetitive microtrauma from overuse.

Examination

Evaluate for swelling, local UCL tenderness (located 2 cm distal to the medial epicondyle), and instability to valgus stress testing.

Flexion contractures and cubitus valgus deformities are common in throwers. Posteromedial osteophytes may be palpable.

In chronic injuries, olecranon tenderness may also be elicited by bringing the arm into valgus and extension.

Imaging

Plain X-rays may be normal. In chronic cases there may be ectopic bone formation in the UCL, posteromedial osteophyte formation at the olecranon and coronoid, and loose bodies.

Stress films may confirm medial instability.

MRI allows assessment of the UCL.

Treatment

Nonoperative

- *First 8 weeks:* Aim to settle the acute symptoms and to restore normal range of motion with relative rest, ice, analgesics, and NSAIDs. The patient should begin range of motion and a gentle strengthening regime and avoid exercises that cause pain.
- *8–16 weeks:* Throwing activities are resumed if the patient demonstrates a full range of motion and has no pain. The throwing program should be slowly advanced with the goal of returning to sport at 4–6 months following injury.

Operative

Surgery is considered when patients continue to have pain despite this program and in conditions of chronic instability and impairment. For acute instability, repair may be performed. In chronic cases, reconstruction using a tendon graft is often employed.

Prevention of the condition is important through adequate conditioning, warm-up, stretching, and appropriate technique.

Osteochondritis dissecans and osteochondrosis

History

Osteochondritis dissecans (OCD) is a spontaneous osteonecrosis. When it occurs in the elbow, it most commonly affects the capitellum or radial head.

Osteochondrosis (Panner's disease) is necrosis, fragmentation, and regeneration of the capitellar growth plate. These may occur in association with repetitive valgus stress in skeletally immature individuals. It is often seen in gymnastics, racket sports, and throwing sports and most commonly affects the dominant arm.

Patients often complain of pain in the lateral elbow that is exacerbated by throwing or upper-limb weight bearing.

Examination

Tenderness is localized to the capitellum or radial head. Patients may present with a flexion contracture.

The active radiocapitellar compression test is positive; forearm pronation and supination with the elbow in full extension results in pain if OCD is present.

Patients may describe a locking sensation secondary to loose body formation.

Imaging

In early stages it may be necessary to X-ray the other side for comparison to detect subtle changes. X-rays may show fragmentation of an island of subchondral bone in the radial head or capitellum.

X-rays may be normal. If OCD is suspected, further imaging, usually using an MRI, is necessary. MRI allows for evaluation of the overlying articular cartilage.

Treatment

This is often based on MRI findings.

Nonoperative

For lesions in which the overlying articular cartilage is intact, treatment includes relative rest, followed by range-of-motion and strengthening exercises. The athlete is restricted from throwing and other heavy activities until there is radiographic evidence of healing.

If pain and flexion contracture persist beyond 6 weeks, surgical intervention is considered.

Operative

For lesions in which the overlying articular cartilage is not intact, treatment depends on the size of the fragments.

Small fragments are commonly excised. Large fragments are often repaired. Large defects may require allograft reconstruction.

Prevention

Guidelines regarding pitch limits should not be exceeded and activity should stop if symptoms recur.

Lateral epicondylosis (tennis elbow)

History

This is a chronic, noninflammatory condition of the wrist extensor muscles, most commonly the extensor carpi radialis brevis (ECRB).

Patients complain of dull lateral elbow pain. This is usually associated with a repetitive flexion–extension or pronation–supination activity. Pain may occur during sports (tennis backhand stroke) or during normal daily activities (turning a doorknob, opening a jar, or typing on a computer).

Examination

There is tenderness over the ECRB origin at the lateral epicondyle. The tenderness may be diffuse, over the origins of the extensor digitorum communis (EDC) and/or ECRL.

Pain may be reproduced with passive wrist flexion or with active resisted wrist extension or resisted supination.

Grasping or pinching with the wrist extended usually reproduces pain at the point of maximal tenderness (frequently, 1–2 cm distal to the lateral epicondyle).

Examine the equipment and assess technique. Factors associated with tennis elbow include: heavier, stiffer, more tightly strung rackets; incorrect grip size; metal rackets; inexperienced players; and bad backhand technique.

Diagnosis

Imaging studies are not routinely performed. X-ray may demonstrate a spur at the lateral epicondyle or calcification of the common extensor tendon.

Ultrasound shows decreased echogenicity, inhomogeneity, and thickening of the tendon, and a local fluid collection may be seen.

MRI may demonstrate an increased signal intensity of the extensor tendons close to their origin on the lateral epicondyle.

Treatment

The key to treatment is making patients aware that this is an overuse syndrome.

Nonoperative

Relative rest, ice (10–20 minutes every 2 hours in the acute stages), compression, and NSAIDs (topical NSAIDs such as voltaren gel are preferable) are indicated.

Compression straps or counterforce braces applied distally to the bulk of the extensor mass may help. The brace is tightened to a comfortable degree of tension with the forearm muscles relaxed, so that a maximum contraction is limited. The brace may be worn for the entirety of a tennis match or may be tightened just prior to a golf swing. Constant use of the brace is not advised.

If these conservative measures fail, an injection of lidocaine and corticosteroid may be considered. A combination of 2 mL of bupivicaine and 1 mL of 40 mg/mL depomedrol is used.

Only one injection shoul be given over the course of therapy. Repeated injections may result in tendon compromise and other complications. Following the injection, a comprehensive rehabilitation program is initiated and the patient is reminded that continuing rehabilitation exercises and proper mechanics are important for prevention of recurrence.

If the injury is related to athletics, patients should be encouraged to seek professional instruction to identify biomechanical errors in form.

Operative

Surgery is reserved for those patients with disabling symptoms who fail to respond to all nonoperative measures over the course of 1 year.

Multiple surgical options exist for the treatment of lateral epicondylosis. We prefer excision of the damaged tendon and local drilling of the subchondral bone of the lateral epicondyle, followed by repair of the extensor origin.

Posterolateral rotatory instability

History

Posterolateral rotatory instability (PLRI) is a rotatory subluxation of the radius and ulna relative to the distal humerus. This occurs as a result of injury to the ulnar portion of the lateral collateral ligament complex (ULCL).

Patients typically report elbow discomfort associated with a painful clicking, snapping, clunking, locking, or giving-way sensation.

Symptoms are often produced when the patient extends their elbow with the forearm supinated—for example, when using their hands to get out of a chair with their forearms maximally supinated.

Examination

Strength and range of motion are often normal. Patients typically demonstrate apprehension or guarding during the pivot shift examination.

Imaging

Plain X-rays are often normal unless there is an LCL avulsion off the lateral epicondyle.

Stress radiographs can be helpful and may demonstrate posterolateral radial head dislocation with widening of the ulnohumeral joint. MRI is helpful in confirming the diagnosis.

Treatment

Nonoperative

Activity should be modified and a hinged brace with forearm pronation and an extension block worn. As these injuries are most often chronic, symptoms recur when the patient is out of the brace.

Operative

Repair may be attempted if local tissues are adequate; otherwise, reconstruction of the lateral collateral ligament complex using a free tendon graft is necessary.

Acute injuries

Rupture of the biceps

History

This may occur with trauma, usually with the elbow in 90° flexion, or as a result of an eccentric load to the bicep. There is a sudden tearing pain in the antecubital fossa followed by a deep aching discomfort. It is more common with anabolic steroid use.

Examination

There is a palpable gap, a bulbous swelling in the arm, and weakness of elbow flexion and supination. A partial rupture of the tendon produces pain and local crepitus on supination and flexion.

Imaging

MRI will confirm tendon rupture.

Treatment

Management is early (within 3 weeks) surgical repair. Chronic injuries may require allograft reconstruction or augmentation.

Triceps rupture

History

Triceps rupture is usually an avulsion injury at the tendo-osseous junction. Patients may describe a sudden tear or pop, pain, swelling, and weakness of elbow extension. Partial ruptures, usually in the central third of the tendon, can also occur. Other injuries may occur simultaneously, including fracture of the radial head.

The injury usually occurs after a fall onto the outstretched hand, but can occur after a direct blow. If there is spontaneous rupture, consider anabolic steroid use.

Examination

There is swelling and tenderness near the triceps insertion to the olecranon, a palpable gap, and weakness of elbow extension.

Imaging

X-rays will often show flecks of avulsed bone proximal to the olecranon. It is also important to exclude a fracture of the head of the radius. MRI will confirm tendon rupture.

Treatment

In acute ruptures, tendon reattachment is usually possible. In chronic cases these injuries may require allograft reconstruction or augmentation.

Elbow dislocation

History

These may be complicated (with fracture) or simple (without). Displacement is usually posterior or posterolateral and there is considerable soft tissue injury. They usually occur after a fall onto the outstretched hand with the elbow in extension.

Examination

There is pain, swelling, and deformity. It is important to assess neurovascular status.

Imaging

X-rays may show fractures of the radial head, coronoid, and olecranon process. Fracture indicates a complicated dislocation.

Treatment

Closed reduction is performed. Apply longitudinal traction with one hand and with the other, apply pressure to relocate the olecranon back onto the trochlea. Assess neurovascular status and elbow stability (extent of soft tissue damage) afterward.

In patients with a radial head fracture, look especially at the coronoid process. Fractures here, including small "avulsion" fractures, may be the only radiographic indication of the "terrible triad" elbow dislocation. These injuries result in significant instability unless addressed operatively.

Supracondylar fractures

History

These fractures occur most commonly in children as a result of a fall onto outstretched hand with the elbow pushed into extension.

Examination

On examination there is pain, swelling, and an S-deformity of the elbow. It is essential to check neurovascular status. (Vascular injuries occur in 2%–3% of displaced fractures and 10% have a neurological injury.)

Evaluate for an associated compartment syndrome. An increasing narcotic requirement, pain out of proportion to physical examination, and pain with passive extension of the fingers should alert the examiner to the possibility of this surgical emergency. Forearm compartment pressure testing may be required to make the diagnosis.

Imaging

Use X-rays to confirm and characterize the fracture.

Treatment

For extension-type fractures, a line is drawn down the anterior humerus on the lateral X-ray. If this line intersects the capitellum, the fracture is generally considered stable. If this line fails to intersect the capitellum, the fracture is considered unstable.

An exception to this rule is when the AP radiograph identifies impaction with varus deformity of >5°, or valgus >10°. These fractures are considered unstable regardless of the appearance of the lateral X-ray.

Stable fractures can be treated nonoperatively. The patient is placed in a posterior splint at 90° for 3 weeks. Monitor radiographs serially to assess for displacement. Motion is allowed to recover naturally.

Unstable fractures are treated operatively, most often with closed reduction and percutaneus pinning. Complex fractures, or those associated with neurovascular injury, may require open reduction and fixation. Adults with this type of fracture generally require open reduction and fixation.

Lateral condylar fractures

History

These fractures often result from a fall onto the outstretched hand. Separation can occur at the growth plate, especially in patients 4–10 years old. This may cause long-term growth plate damage and deformity.

Patients describe lateral elbow pain, swelling, and dysfunction.

Examination

Tenderness, swelling, and occasional crepitus at the lateral condyle are evident.

Imaging

Confirm the diagnosis on X-ray; obtain a 45° internal oblique view to assess displacement.

Treatment

Place a stable fracture (<2 mm maximal displacement on any X-ray) into a posterior splint at 90°. If it is unstable (displaced >2 mm), reduction and fixation are necessary.

Radial head and neck fractures

History

Radial head fractures usually occur in adults and radial neck injuries in children. They occur after a fall onto an outstretched hand, with the elbow pushed into valgus.

Examination

There is tenderness and swelling in the area of the radial head. There may be limitation in supination and pronation.

Imaging

X-rays are used for diagnosis.

Treatment

In adults, an undisplaced fracture of the radial head is treated in a posterior splint. A displaced fracture requires open reduction and fixation or if comminuted, radial head replacement may be necessary.

In children, where the fracture is of the radial neck, closed or open, reduction is needed if there is beyond 30° of radial tilt.

Monteggia fractures (ulna fracture with radial head dislocation, in children)

History

This usually occurs after a fall onto an outstretched hand. Patients complain of diffuse elbow pain and swelling.

Examination

There is tenderness to palpation and crepitus at the ulna fracture site. Elbow range of movement is limited in flexion, extension, pronation, and supination.

Imaging

On X-rays, a line drawn through the center of the radial head should bisect the capitellum on all views.

These injuries are commonly misdiagnosed as simple ulna fractures and may lead to long-term disability as a result of the radial head dislocation.

Treatment

These injuries are treated with closed reduction and immobilization. Monitor for displacement on serial X-ray.

Chronic elbow injuries

For anatomy of the superficial and deep flexor and extensor muscles of the arm and forearm, see Figures 4.2 and 4.3.

Distal biceps tendinopathy

History

Tendinosis of the distal end of biceps brachii can occur with repetitive supination and flexion activities.

Examination

Pain is felt in the antecubital fossa, and local swelling and tenderness may be noted. Pain is worse with resisted supination.

Imaging

MRI may demonstrate thickening of the distal bicep insertion.

Treatment

Treatment includes relative rest, ice, NSAIDs, and modification of activities. Failure to address the problem can result in rupture.

Ulnar neuropathy

History

The ulnar nerve is vulnerable along its path through the cubital tunnel posterior to the medial epicondyle. Those who perform repetitive throwing or flexion activities are particularly vulnerable to dislocation or subluxation of the nerve. The nerve is at risk of direct trauma and compression (see Table 4.1).

Common sites of ulnar nerve compression about the elbow include the medial intramuscular septum, the arcade of Struthers, the medial epicondyle, the cubital retinaculum, Osborne's ligament, and the flexor carpi ulnaris muscle.

Patients may report a sharp or burning, deep, aching pain at the medial elbow and proximal forearm. This may radiate proximally or distally.

Paraesthesias, dysaesthesias, and anesthesia in the ulnar one and a half digits may be noted. Patients may report clumsiness with their hands.

Recurrent dislocation or subluxation of the nerve can cause a popping or snapping sensation with elbow flexion and extension.

Examination

Look for valgus deformity of the elbow, a mild flexion contracture, medial collateral ligament (MCL) instability, and soft tissue swelling at the ulnar groove.

Patients may have tenderness and thickening of the nerve. There may be wasting of the small muscles of the hand and hypothenar eminence. Sensation may be decreased in the ulnar one and a half digits.

Elbow flexion (Phalen's test at the elbow) and percussion of the nerve along its course (Tinel's test) may elicit symptoms.

Those with ulnar nerve subluxation may be able to demonstrate the phenomenon. It may be possible to dislocate the nerve from the groove.

(a)

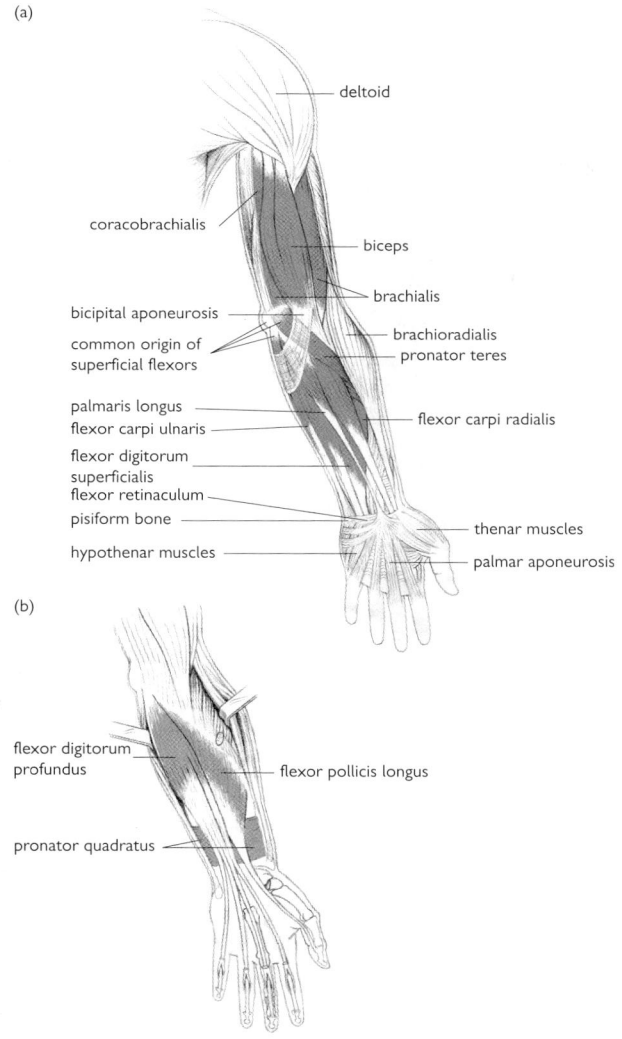

deltoid

coracobrachialis

biceps

brachialis

bicipital aponeurosis

common origin of
superficial flexors

brachioradialis
pronator teres

palmaris longus
flexor carpi ulnaris

flexor carpi radialis

flexor digitorum
superficialis
flexor retinaculum
pisiform bone

thenar muscles

hypothenar muscles

palmar aponeurosis

(b)

flexor digitorum
profundus

flexor pollicis longus

pronator quadratus

Figure 4.2 (a) Superficial flexor muscles of the arm and forearm. (b) Deep flexor muscles of the forearm. Reproduced with permission from MacKinnon P, Morris J (2005). *Oxford Textbook of Functional Anatomy*, Vol. 1. Oxford: Oxford University Press, ©2005.

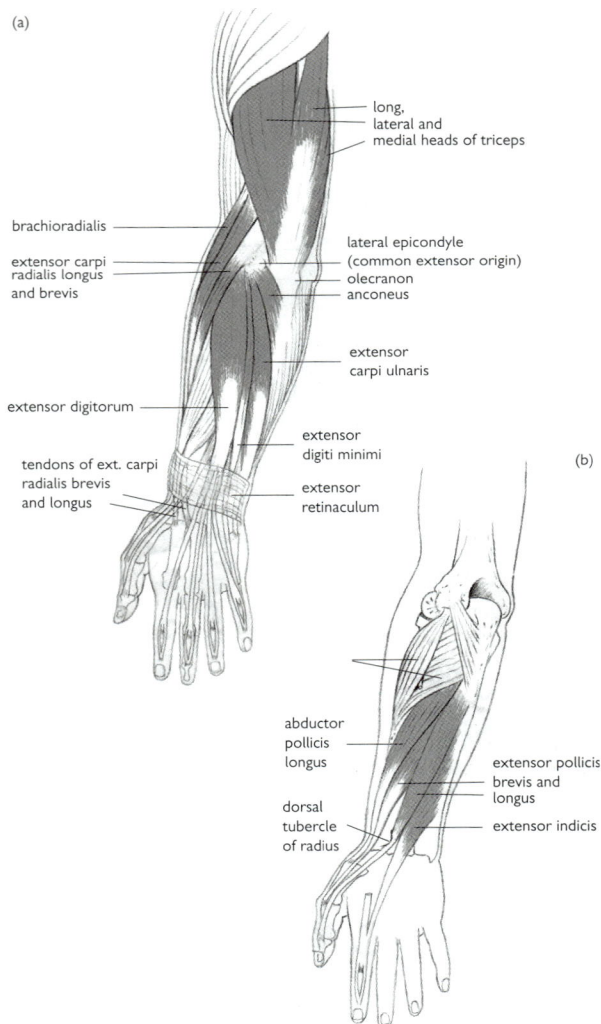

(a)

long,
lateral and
medial heads of triceps

brachioradialis

extensor carpi
radialis longus
and brevis

lateral epicondyle
(common extensor origin)
olecranon
anconeus

extensor
carpi ulnaris

extensor digitorum

extensor
digiti minimi

(b)

tendons of ext. carpi
radialis brevis
and longus

extensor
retinaculum

abductor
pollicis
longus

extensor pollicis
brevis and
longus

dorsal
tubercle
of radius

extensor indicis

Figure 4.3 (a) Superficial extensor muscles of the arm and forearm. (b) Deep extensor muscles of the forearm. Reproduced with permission from MacKinnon P, Morris J (2005). *Oxford Textbook of Functional Anatomy*, Vol. 1. Oxford, UK: Oxford University Press. ©2005.

Table 4.1 Radioulnar and wrist joint: movements, principal muscles, and their innervation[1]

Movement	Principal muscles	Peripheral nerve	Spinal root origin
Supination	Biceps	Musculocutaneous nerve	C 5, 6
	Supinator	Radial nerve (deep branch)	C 5, 6, 7
Pronation	Pronator teres	Median nerve	C 5, 6, 7
	Pronator quadratus	Median nerve	C 5, 6, 7, 8
Flexion	*Common flexor origin muscles*		
	Flexor carpi radialis	Median nerve	C 5, 6, 7
	Flexor carpi ulnaris	Ulnar nerve	C 5, 6, 7, 8
	(Palmaris longus)	Median nerve	C 5, 6, 7
	Long digital flexors	Median and ulnar nerves	C 5, 6, 7
Extension	*Common extensor origin muscles*		
	Extensor carpi radialis longus and brevis	Radial nerve (trunk and deep branch*)	C 5, 6, 7
	Extensor carpi ulnaris	Radial nerve (deep branch*)	C 5, 6, 7, 8
	Long digital extensors		
Abduction	Flexor carpi radialis	Median nerve	C 5, 6, 7
	Extensor carpi radialis longus and brevis	Radial nerve	C 5, 6, 7
	Abductor pollicis longus and brevis	Radial nerve (deep branch*)	C 5, 6, 7, 8
Adduction	Flexor carpi ulnaris	Ulnar nerve	C 5, 6, 7, 8
	Extensor carpi ulnaris	Radial nerve (deep branch*)	C 5, 6, 7, 8

* The deep branch of the radial nerve is also called the posterior interosseous nerve from its position in the extensor compartment posterior to the interosseous membrane.

1 Reproduced with permission from MacKinnon P, Morris J (2005). *Oxford Textbook of Functional Anatomy*, Vol 1. Oxford: Oxford University Press. © 2005.

A Martin Gruber anastamosis, where there is communication between the median and ulnar nerves in the forearm, occurs in 15% of people and may confuse clinical findings.

Imaging and diagnostic tests

Nerve conduction studies may show reduced conduction velocity by more than 33% across the site of compression compared to the unaffected arm. An X-ray may show osteophytes but is generally negative.

Treatment

Nonoperative

Relative rest and protection, and splinting the elbow at 30° of flexion may provide symptomatic relief. Ice, NSAIDs, and simple analgesics are often unhelpful. Gentle range-of-motion exercises are started as soon as tolerated.

Return to normal activities can begin after full strength is regained with a progressive strengthening regime of forearm musculature and correction of faulty technique or instability, where appropriate.

Operative

Surgical decompression, transposition, and correction of instability or other pathology may be necessary if symptoms persist despite nonoperative treatment.

All potential sources of compression of the nerve should be explored, even when a specific site of compression has been indicated by electrodiagnostic studies, since more than one site of compression can exist.

Pronator syndrome

History

Median nerve compression at the elbow and proximal forearm is known as pronator syndrome. It causes a vague aching pain at the proximal, volar surface of the forearm.

There is often a history of repetitive strenuous use of the forearm. Patients may report dysaesthesias in the distribution of the median nerve in the hand.

Sites of compression include the supracondylar process and ligament of Struthers, the lacertus fibrosis, the pronator teres, and the flexor digitorum superficialis.

Imaging and diagnostic tests

Electrodiagnostic studies help to confirm median nerve latency. X-rays are generally normal but may identify a large supracondylar process.

Treatment

Nonoperative

Passive stretching of the forearm musculature, NSAIDs, and elbow splinting in neutral rotation are indicated. Symptoms may take 2–3 months to improve.

Operative

Surgical intervention may be necessary if symptoms fail to resolve despite appropriate nonoperative treatment.

Surgery involves exploration and decompression of the nerve from 5 cm proximal to the elbow to the forearm, at all potential sites of compression.

Anterior interosseous syndrome

History
Compression of the anterior interosseous nerve results in a pure motor paralysis of flexor pollicus longus and the index flexor digitorum profundus.

Patients report a loss of dexterity or weakness of pinch. They often recall a deep, unremitting pain in the proximal forearm that preceded the onset of symptoms.

Examination
There is weakness of pinch grip. During attempted pinch, the index finger extends at the distal interphalangeal joint with compensatory increased flexion of the proximal interphalangeal joint. The thumb hyperextends at the interphalangeal joint and increases flexion at the metacarpophalangeal joint.

Diagnosis
After 2–3 weeks, electromyographic (EMG) studies will show signs of denervation of affected muscles.

Treatment
NSAIDs and relative rest for 8–12 weeks are indicated. Those who remain symptomatic are considered for surgery, which involves a similar approach to that for pronator syndrome.

Posterior interosseus nerve (PIN) syndrome

History
Sites of PIN entrapment include the fibrous bands anterior to the radial head, the leash of Henry, the tendinous origin of ECRB, the arcade of Frohse, and distal edge of the supinator.

Nerve compression can also occur from synovitis at the radiocapitellar joint, fractures, ganglia tumors, vascular anomalies, or other local masses.

The superficial radial nerve can be entrapped alone or in combination with the posterior interosseous branch. The radial nerve can also be entrapped above the level of the elbow, due to a lateral intermuscular septum, although this is rare.

Patients often report aching pain in the belly of the extensor muscle that is worse with forearm pronation and passive wrist flexion. Pain may be more diffuse over the extensor forearm and there may be exacerbation after exertion and pain at night.

This syndrome is often misdiagnosed as refractory tennis elbow.

The injury is associated with repetitive rotary movements, e.g., discus throwing and racquet sports.

Examination
There is tenderness to palpation over the course of the PIN, deep to the extensor muscle belly and just distal to the radial head.

Pain may be reproduced with resisted extension of the middle finger with the elbow extended, and on resisted supination of the extended forearm.

Imaging and diagnostic tests

Neurophysiology studies are frequently normal. There may be a decrease in motor conduction velocity in the radial nerve across the entrapment site, and changes in the muscles innervated distal to the entrapment site.

Treatment

Relative rest, stretching, and activity modification are the usual treatment.

In resistant cases, exploration of the nerve is necessary. Surgical procedures used in the treatment of lateral epicondylitis may be followed.

Olecranon bursitis

History

Patients often report a direct blow to the olecranon followed by significant swelling and pain. It may present acutely or chronically and can be septic or aseptic.

Examination

There is swelling at the posterior elbow, representing a thickened bursa and/or bursal fluid. There is often exquisite tenderness to palpation of the olecranon

In sepsis or crystal-induced bursitis, the patient may be systemically ill with a fever, cellulitis, and local lymphadenopathy.

Imaging and diagnostic tests

Inflammatory markers (ESR, CRP) and white blood cell count may be elevated in systemic sepsis and crystal-induced bursitis. If sepsis is suspected, blood cultures and sterile aspiration of the bursal fluid, plus analysis by Gram stain and culture and crystals, are warranted.

X-rays are not performed routinely; calcification and olecranon spurs may be evident but may be coincidental.

Treatment

Most uncomplicated cases are managed symptomatically with regular ice, NSAIDs, and local protection by an elbow pad or dressing. Aspiration without injection can help to relieve pain and allows bursal fluid to be obtained for examination, though at the risk of possible infection.

Injection of hydrocortisone 10 mg is rarely necessary but may benefit persisting bursitis, especially with an inflammatory arthritis or crystals. Relative rest for 5 days after aspiration is recommended. Septic bursitis is a contraindication to steroid injection.

Return to contact activities is permitted once the patient is asymptomatic, but a protective elbow pad should be worn initially.

When sepsis is confirmed in those who are systemically well and with little cellulitis, aspiration of the bursa is followed by oral broad-spectrum antibiotics. Progress should be monitored and intravenous antibiotics commenced in those who fail to respond and in those with systemic symptoms. Open drainage and lavage may be necessary.

Wrist and hand

Epidemiology

Overall, wrist and hand injuries account for between 3% and 9% of all sports injuries. Incidence varies among sports, with up to 87% of gymnasts reported to experience wrist pain during their career, since the wrist is a weight-bearing joint in many of the activities of this sport.

Hand injuries account for 44% of all injuries in rock climbing.

Injuries to the hand and wrist are common in tennis and golf (especially the left hand in right-handed golfers).

The majority of injuries are soft tissue, but a diagnosis of "wrist sprain" should only be made by exclusion of other more serious injuries.

Hand and wrist injuries are more common in children and may involve the epiphyseal plates with the potential for growth disturbance.

Wrist biomechanics

For anatomy of the hands and wrist, see Figures 5.1 and 5.2.

Normal daily activities require 30° of extension, 5° flexion, 10° radial deviation, and 15° of ulnar deviation. Most activities of daily living (ADLs) are performed in extension and ulnar deviation.

Throwing requires a similar degree of extension and radioulnar deviation, but flexion is increased to 80–90° at the end of the acceleration phase prior to ball release.

Studies of the golf swing have shown a flexion–extension arc of 103° in the right wrist compared with 71° in the left wrist for right-handed players (advanced players show less movement at the left wrist but more at the right).

In extension, 66% of the force is borne radiocarpally and 34% mid-carpally. In flexion, 40% is radiocarpal and 60% is mid-carpal.

With an intact triangular fibrocartilage complex (TFCC), the radius bears 82% and the ulna 18% of the force during axial loading of the wrist. This pattern of force transmission can be altered in sports such as gymnastics, where a significant load can be applied to the ulnar side of the wrist. Excision of the TFCC increases the load on the radius to 94%.

Ulnar shortening (negative ulnar variance) of 2.5 mm reduces the ulnar load bearing to 4%, while lengthening by 2.5 mm increases it to 42%.

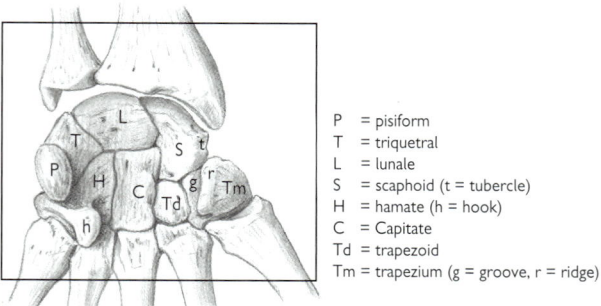

P = pisiform
T = triquetral
L = lunale
S = scaphoid (t = tubercle)
H = hamate (h = hook)
C = Capitate
Td = trapezoid
Tm = trapezium (g = groove, r = ridge)

Figure 5.1 Carpal bones, anterior view. Reproduced with permission from MacKinnon P, Morris J (2005). *Oxford Textbook of Functional Anatomy*, Vol. 1. Oxford, UK: Oxford University Press. ©2005.

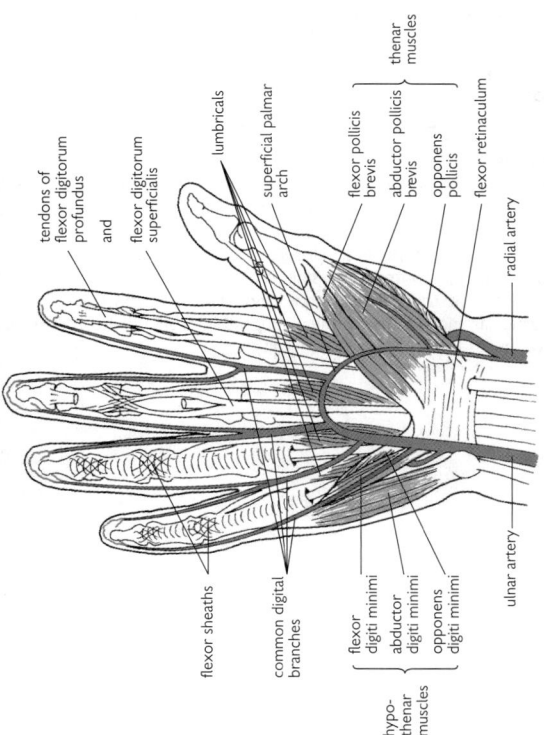

Figure 5.2 Superficial aspect of the palm. Reproduced with permission from MacKinnon P, Morris J (2005). *Oxford Textbook of Functional Anatomy*, Vol. 1. Oxford, UK: Oxford University Press. ©2005.

Fracture of the distal radius

History and examination

Fracture of the distal radius is common in the elderly athlete (approximately 7% of all Colles' fractures occur during sport) and are caused by a fall on the outstretched hand.

Dorsal angulation and impaction lead to the classic "dinner fork" deformity. Injury may involve the epiphyseal plate in children (especially distal radius) and careful follow-up is required to ensure that premature growth arrest does not occur (see also Radial epiphysitis (gymnast's wrist), p. 194).

Diagnosis

Diagnosis is confirmed by X-ray (see Fig. 5.3).

Treatment

Accurate closed reduction and cast immobilization are required for 6–8 weeks, with weekly X-ray checks for the first 3 weeks to ensure that a satisfactory position is being maintained.

Acceptable parameters after closed reduction include radial length within 5 mm of the contralateral side, radial inclination >15°, sagittal tilt <10° dorsal and up to 20° volar, and <1 mm articular incongruity.

Intra-articular incongruity in the young athlete should be treated by operative means to restore joint congruity.

(a)

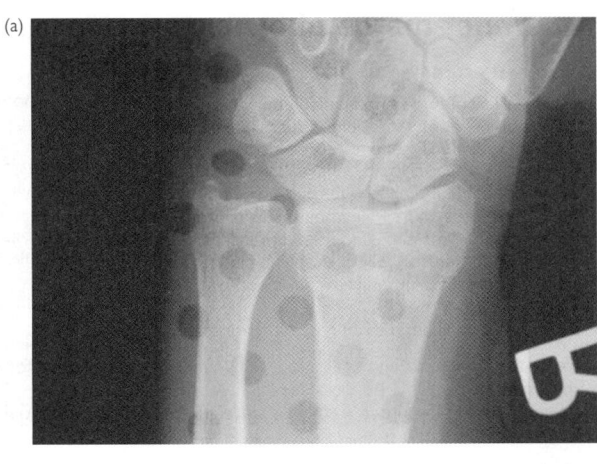

(b)

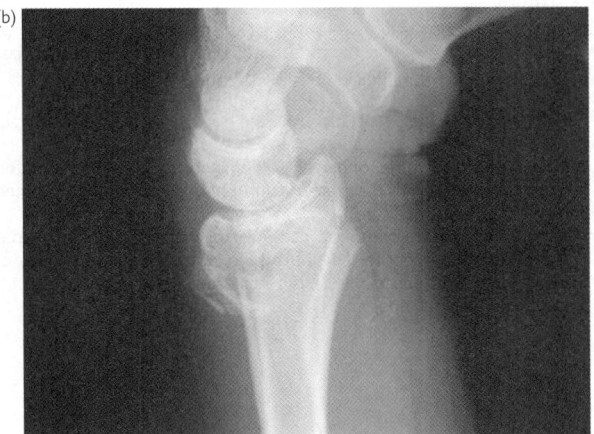

Figure 5.3 Anteroposterior and lateral radiographs of a distal radius fracture.

Fracture of the scaphoid

History and examination

This is caused by a fall onto the outstretched hand and is thus common in football, basketball, hockey, and rugby. These injuries may also occur in boxing.

Clinical findings include tenderness in the anatomical snuff box (always compare with the uninjured side) and over the palmar scaphoid. There will be pain when an axial load is applied to the first metacarpal.

These fractures are common in sports and are important not to miss, as they have the potential for delayed or nonunion, with subsequent avascular necrosis and long-term disability.

Diagnosis

Plain X-rays may initially be normal. Therefore if fracture is suspected, initial treatment should be immobilization in a thumb spica splint/cast followed by repeat X-ray in 7–10 days (see Fig. 5.4).

MRI scanning is very useful in making an early diagnosis of scaphoid fracture.

Treatment

Fractures with a good potential to heal include incomplete, nondisplaced fractures and those involving the distal scaphoid. Treatment is immobilization in a short- or long-arm thumb spica cast for a period of 8–12 weeks (average time to union is $9^{1}/_{2}$ weeks).

Those requiring surgery include displaced fractures, proximal pole fractures, comminuted fractures, and those with >10° of angulation.

Nonunion occurs in approximately 10%–15% of cases. This complication is preventable by early recognition and appropriate treatment as detailed above.

A diagnosis of a "sprained wrist" can only be made by exclusion, and it is much better to err on the side of caution and immobilize all cases of suspected scaphoid fracture, even if the initial X-rays are negative.

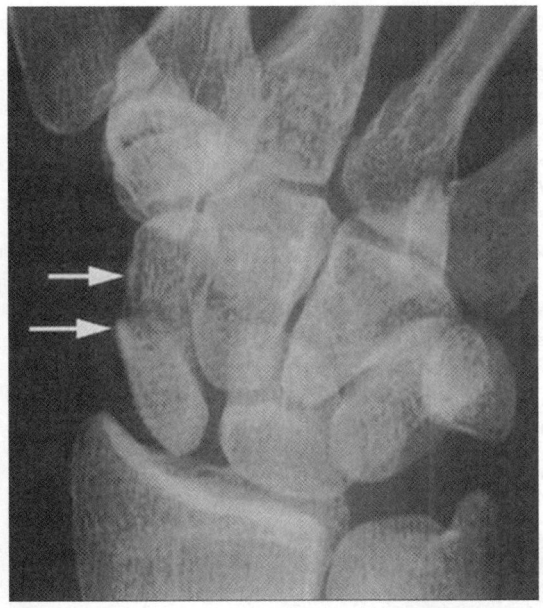

Figure 5.4 Anteroposterior radiograph of a displaced scaphoid fracture.

Fracture of the hamate

History and examination

These fractures occur in racquet sports, golf, and baseball and are caused by the butt of the racquet, golf club, or baseball bat forcibly impacting on the hypothenar eminence and hamate hook (see Fig. 5.5). In golf it may be due to the club being gripped too close to the butt.

Fractures of the hook of the hamate comprise 2%–4% of all carpal fractures. Injury to the ulnar nerve may occur in this area and cause the patient to present with numbness and paresthesias, or weakness of the ulnar innervated muscles. The patient will also have pain and tenderness to direct palpation.

Diagnosis

Diagnosis is confirmed on CT scan—fractures of the hamate are difficult to see on plain X-rays.

Treatment

Acute fractures are treated conservatively with cast immobilization for 4–6 weeks. Unrecognized fractures typically go on to nonunion and require open reduction and internal fixation, or excision of the fractured hook.

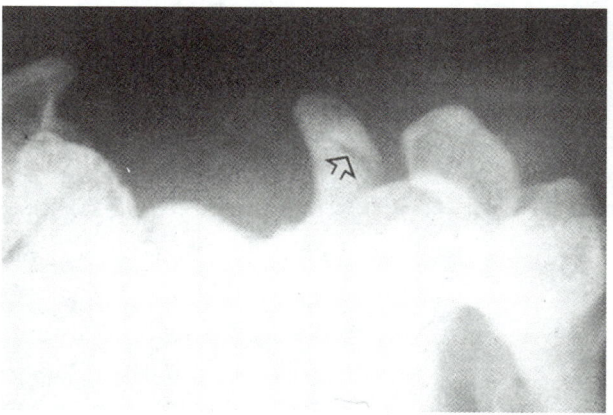

Figure 5.5 Carpal tunnel profile view radiograph of a fracture of the hook of the hamate.

Fracture of the pisiform

History and examination

The pisiform may occasionally be fractured by a direct blow.

Treatment

Treatment is with cast immobilization in ulnar deviation and 30° of flexion.

Excision with preservation of the flexor carpi ulnaris tendon can be performed if symptomatic nonunion occurs or if symptomatic pisotriquetral degeneration develops.

Fracture of the fifth metacarpal neck (boxer's fracture)

History and examination

Fractures of the neck of the fifth metacarpal are common in combat sports (hence the term "boxer's fracture").

Diagnosis

- X-ray (see Fig. 5.6).
- It is important to check for malrotation (best observed by asking the patient to make a clenched fist).

Treatment

Angulation is common, but if >40° the fracture should be closed reduced.

Most fractures can be treated conservatively with cast immobilization in the functional position (metacarpophalangeals flexed 70° with the interphalangeals extended). Unstable fractures should be managed surgically.

Shortening may occur and percutaneous pinning should be considered in the competitive boxer.

Open fractures should be presumed to be the result of a human bite and treated with aggressive irrigation and debridement in addition to antibiotics.

Return to sport depends on the need for hand function, but can be expected after approximately 2 weeks in stable, nondisplaced fractures.

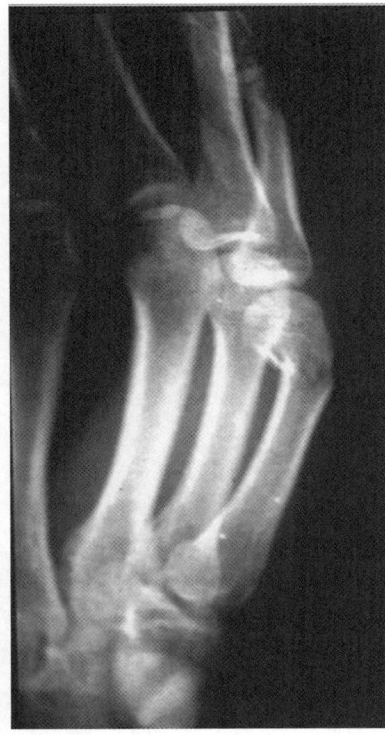

Figure 5.6 Oblique radiograph of a fifth metacarpal neck (boxer's) fracture.

Fracture–dislocation of the first metacarpal base (Bennett's or Rolando's fracture)

- The mechanism involves an axial load on a partially flexed thumb.
- The pull of abductor pollicis longus causes displacement of the metacarpal shaft.
- Treatment is by closed or open reduction and pinning, followed by 4–6 weeks cast immobilization.
- A further period of splinting is necessary on return to sport.

Phalangeal shaft fractures

It is very important to check for malrotation (most common in spiral fractures of the proximal phalanx)—ask the patient to make a clenched fist and any rotational deformity should become obvious. Also assess for any tendon or volar plate injury.

Stable fractures can be managed conservatively by casting or "buddy taping" for 3–4 weeks, but careful follow-up of all injuries is advised to ensure return of full function.

Unstable fractures should be treated operatively.

Dislocation of the carpal bones

History and examination

Perilunate dislocations may occur after a fall (see Fig. 5.7). The capitate can dislocate dorsally or, more severely, the lunate can dislocate volarly and may cause compression of the median nerve.

More common than an acute dislocation is the development of scapholunate dissociation following a tear of the scapholunate ligament.

There is tenderness over the radial side of the lunate and Watson's test will be positive (pressure over the scaphoid tuberosity as the wrist is moved from ulnar to radial deviation will result in the scaphoid being felt to sublux dorsally).

Diagnosis

Careful scrutiny of a lateral view will demonstrate perilunate dislocations.

A clenched-fist posteroanterior X-ray will demonstrate a gap between the scaphoid and the lunate in cases of scapholunate dissociation (the "Terry Thomas" sign).

Treatment

Treatment of perilunate dislocation is by open reduction and repair of the torn ligaments along with 8 weeks cast immobilization.

Treatment of scapholunate dissociation following an acute tear is surgical with open reduction and repair of the damaged ligament.

(a)

(b)

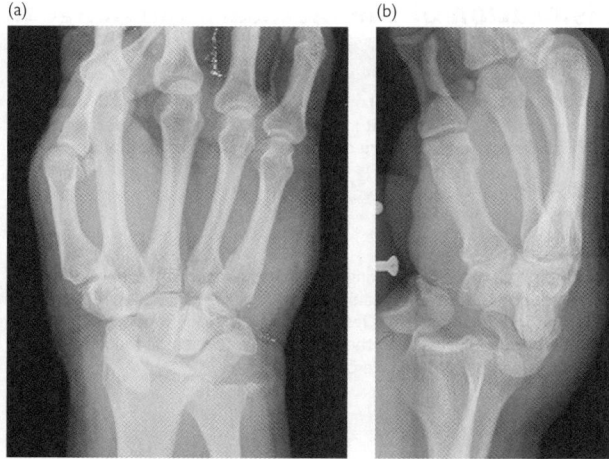

Figure 5.7 Anteroposterior and lateral radiographs of a perilunate dislocation.

Dislocation of the metacarpophalangeal (MCP) joints

History and examination

- These are less common that interphalangeal (IP) joint dislocations.
- Dorsal dislocations are more common than volar dislocations.

Diagnosis

- X-ray

Treatment

Simple dislocations have striking deformity (almost 90° hyperextension), can be reduced with gentle manipulation, and are stable after reduction.

Complex dislocations have less deformity (bayonet apposition of joint surfaces; MC head palpable in the palm), are irreducible secondary to volar plate interposition, and require open reduction.

Dislocation of the interphalangeal (IP) joints

History and examination

- Dislocations of the distal IP (DIP) joints are often caused by a ball hitting the tip of the finger.
- Dislocations of the proximal IP (PIP) joints are extremely common in sports and may be reduced on the field of play.
- Dorsal dislocations are more common than volar dislocations for DIP and PIP dislocations.

Diagnosis

X-rays should be performed to exclude complicating fractures.

Treatment

It is important not to undertreat these injuries as residual deformity and disability can result. Treatment depends on the direction of dislocation, post-reduction stability, and presence of fracture.

The typical dorsal PIP dislocation that is stable after reduction can be treated with splinting in slight flexion for 2–3 days followed by initiation of active motion.

Mallet finger

History and examination

- Rupture of the terminal extensor tendon at or near its attachment to the distal phalanx results in an inability to actively extend the tip of the finger.
- It commonly occurs when the tip of the finger is struck by a ball, e.g., in attempting to catch a basketball or football.

Diagnosis

- X-ray (see Fig. 5.8)

Treatment

Occasionally a small avulsion fracture may be evident on X-ray and consideration should be given to surgical fixation if there is DIP joint subluxation. Otherwise, treatment is with a splint that holds the DIP joint in extension for a period of 6 weeks.

It is very important that the splint be worn continuously, even in bed at night. If removed, e.g., for washing, then care should be taken to ensure that the distal phalanx is held in full extension at all times.

Splinting is effective even in injuries up to 3 months old.

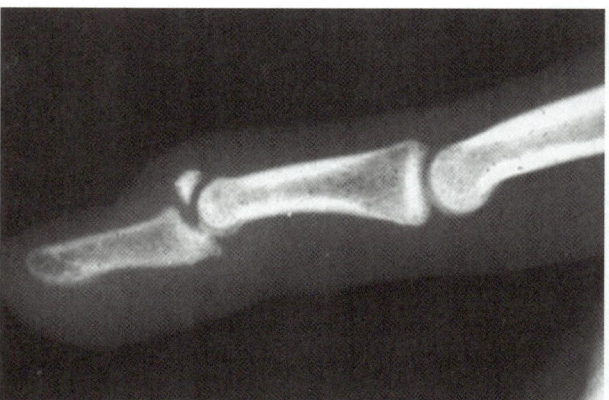

Figure 5.8 Lateral radiograph demonstrating a bony mallet injury with volar subluxation of the distal phalanx at the DIP joint.

Jersey finger

History and examination

- Avulsion of the flexor digitorum profundus tendon at its attachment to the distal phalanx results in an inability to actively flex the tip of the finger.
- As the name suggests, it is usually caused when a player tries to grab the jersey of an opponent and the finger is forcibly extended.
- The ring finger is most often involved.
- When examining for this injury, the PIP joint should be fixed in extension and the patient asked to actively flex the DIP joint.

Diagnosis

- X-ray

Treatment

Treatment is by early surgical intervention to reattach the avulsed fragment followed by a period of immobilization in a splint.

Boutonniere deformity

History and examination

Disruption of the central slip of the extensor digitorum communis tendon at the PIP joint may result in development of a fixed flexion deformity at the PIP joint with subsequent hyperextension at the DIP joint—the so-called Boutonniere deformity.

Diagnosis

- X-ray

Treatment

Inability to actively extend the PIP joint or the presence of an extensor lag in an acute injury should result in the finger being splinted to hold the PIP joint in full extension for a period of 6 weeks with the DIP joint free.

Treatment in established cases is very difficult and prevention is the best policy.

Sagittal band rupture (boxer's knuckle)

- Direct trauma, due either to single or repetitive blows, can cause a longitudinal tear in the sagittal bands over the MCP joints in the boxer.
- The radial sagittal band of the third MCP joint is most commonly affected.
- Examination reveals a lag in active extension at the MCP joint.
- Treatment of acute injuries is immobilization with the MCP joint in extension and the IP joints free for 6 weeks.

Ulnar collateral ligament injuries of the thumb MCP joint (skier's thumb)

History and examination

Injury to the ulnar collateral ligament (UCL) of the thumb MCP joint is common in skiers and results from a fall on the outstretched hand, forcing the thumb into abduction and extension against the ski pole (see Fig. 5.9).

On examination there will be tenderness to palpation at the ulnar side of the thumb at the level of the MCP joint. There will be excessive (>30° compared to the uninjured side in a complete tear) laxity when the thumb is stressed into abduction.

Diagnosis

• X-ray to exclude an avulsion fracture

Treatment

Partial tears of the UCL (10–20° of laxity with a definite end point) can be treated conservatively with splint immobilization for a period of 6 weeks.

Complete tears should be repaired surgically, as there is a significant chance of the adductor aponeurosis becoming interposed between the torn ligament and its distal attachment (the so-called Stener lesion), preventing healing of the ligament and resulting in chronic instability and disability. Following surgery, the thumb is immobilized for 6 weeks and should be protected with strapping for another 8 weeks on return to sports.

The term "gamekeeper's thumb" is used to describe a chronic injury of the UCL because of the gradual attenuation of the ligament over years caused by breaking rabbits' necks.

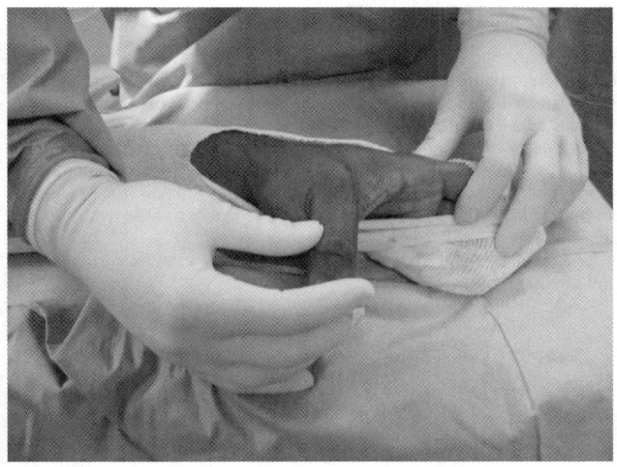

Figure 5.9 Clinical photograph demonstrating laxity to valgus stress in a patient with an ulnar collateral ligament injury of the thumb MCP joint.

Other collateral ligament injuries

Injuries to the radial collateral ligament of the thumb may also occur. These can generally be treated conservatively with cast immobilization as the risk of soft tissue interposition is less and good results can be expected.

Tears of the collateral ligaments of the PIP joint can occur at any of the fingers, e.g., when attempting to catch a ball or falling onto the finger.

Injuries with <20° of lateral instability are managed with a short period of immobilization (1–3 weeks) followed by "buddy taping" for 3–4 weeks. Injuries with >20° of lateral instability are often treated with surgical repair.

Collateral ligament sprains can result in many months of discomfort and swelling.

Carpal tunnel syndrome

History and examination

This syndrome is due to compression of the median nerve within the carpal tunnel at the wrist joint. It may occur in athletes secondary to flexor tenosynovitis. It is more common in pregnant patients and those with diabetes and hypothyroidism; it can occur with repetitive overuse.

The patient presents with pain or tingling in the distribution of the median nerve in the hand (thumb, index, middle, and radial half of the ring finger). Symptoms are often worse at night and in chronic cases can lead to muscle wasting of the thenar eminence.

Tinel's sign may be positive over the median nerve at the wrist. Phalen's test is positive if numbness is elicited by holding the wrist in hyperflexion for 30 seconds.

The differential diagnosis includes cervical radiculopathy, and a thorough examination of the cervical spine should be performed.

Diagnosis

The clinical diagnosis may be confirmed by nerve conduction studies.

Treatment

Milder cases can be treated by corticosteroid injection, while more severe cases will require surgical decompression. Splinting of the wrist and NSAIDs may be helpful.

Ulnar nerve compression

History and examination

Compression of the ulnar nerve at the wrist can occur as the nerve passes through Guyon's canal between the pisiform and the hamate. This is common in cyclists and is due to pressure of the hands against the handlebars.

Symptoms can be motor (weakness of finger abduction), sensory (numbness or tingling in the ulnar $1^{1}/_{2}$ digits), or mixed, depending on the branch of the nerve affected.

Diagnosis

The clinical diagnosis may be confirmed by nerve conduction studies.

Treatment

Treatment includes the use of cycling gloves or handlebar padding and changes to the position of the hands when cycling, anti-inflammatory medication, or, in severe or chronic cases, surgical decompression.

Other nerve injury syndromes

Direct compression of the posterior interosseous nerve (PIN syndrome or radial tunnel syndrome) can occur in gymnasts from hyperextension of the wrist and in athletes who repetitively supinate and pronate their forearms (in racquet sports or golf). It can mimic lateral epicondylitis of the elbow, although the site of tenderness is distal to the common extensor origin.

PIN syndrome causes motor symptoms with weakness in MCP joint extension.

Radial tunnel syndrome is a pain syndrome and can cause aching pain in the dorsoradial forearm that radiates from the lateral elbow to the dorsal aspect of the wrist.

Treatment of both syndromes is activity modification and splinting of the wrist.

De Quervain's tenosynovitis

History and examination

Inflammation of the tendons of extensor pollicis brevis (EPB) and abductor pollicis longus (APL) can occur as they pass through a tight fibrous tunnel at the level of the radial styloid. It is common in racquet sports and rowers as well as in certain occupations, e.g., carpenters.

In the acute stage there will be swelling, tenderness, and occasionally palpable crepitus at the base of the thumb with pain on resisted testing.

Finkelstein's test is performed by adducting the thumb across the palm of the hand and then placing the wrist into ulnar deviation—this maneuver will cause pain in affected individuals.

Diagnosis

None is required—this is a clinical diagnosis.

Treatment

Treatment may include avoidance of aggravating activities, a short period of immobilization in a splint, and corticosteroid injection to the tendon sheath. Response to corticosteroid injection is variable, with one-third of patients requiring more than one injection.

In chronic cases the tendon sheath may become thickened and stenosed, requiring surgical decompression.

Pain may arise more proximally at the site where the tendons of APL and EPB cross over the wrist extensors. This condition is known as intersection syndrome, is most common in weight lifters and rowers, and occurs approximately 4 cm proximal to the wrist.

Treatment is similar to that used for De Quervain's tenosynovitis. Surgery is occasionally necessary.

Other tendinopathies

All tendons that cross the wrist are subject to overuse and can become painful—extensor carpi ulnaris (ECU), flexor carpi ulnaris (FCU), and flexor carpi radialis (FCR) are particularly prone to developing problems.

ECU tendinopathy is associated with the double-handed backhand technique in tennis.

These tendinopathies are treated with activity modification, splinting, NSAIDs, and corticosteroid injections. Operative treatment (tenosynovectomy with sheath release) is considered if conservative treatment fails.

Acute subluxation of ECU can occur in sports such as tennis, golf, and weight lifting.

If identified acutely, immobilization in pronation and radial deviation is generally successful. Surgical stabilization is necessary in recurrent or chronic cases.

Stenosing tenosynovitis can affect any of the flexor tendons of the hand at the level of the MCP joint, causing a triggering effect (*trigger finger*). A tender thickening or nodule is felt at this level.

A single steroid injection to the affected tendon sheath is often curative. Surgery is occasionally necessary.

Ganglion

History and examination

A *ganglion* is a degenerative cyst of either a joint capsule or a tendon sheath. They are very common at the wrist, especially at the scapholunate joint.

Treatment

Often asymptomatic, larger ganglions may be treated by aspiration and corticosteroid injection.

However, recurrence is very common—the only definitive treatment is complete surgical excision.

Impaction syndromes

History and examination

Several impingement or impaction syndromes can occur at the wrist joint—these are especially common in gymnasts.

Entities described include the ulnar-triquetral, scaphoid, and triquetro-lunate impaction syndrome.

Soft tissue impingement (capsulitis) may also occur (diagnosed by excluding other causes of dorsal wrist pain, e.g., ganglion).

Diagnosis

- X-rays to assess ulnar variance and carpal alignment
- MRI scans may be helpful in showing bone stress and in excluding other causes of wrist pain

Treatment

These conditions require rest from the impact activities that cause pain, until symptoms resolve.

Radial epiphysitis (gymnast's wrist)

- Stress reaction at the distal radial epiphysis
- Occurs secondary to overloading

History and examination

- Most commonly seen in gymnasts secondary to upper-limb weight bearing
- Insidious onset of unilateral or bilateral dorsal wrist pain with or without swelling
- Pain is exacerbated by upper-limb weight bearing, e.g., hand stands, bench presses, or use of parallel or uneven bars
- Limitation of wrist extension often present
- Focal tenderness over the distal radial epiphysis
- Forced extension of the wrist reproduces the pain

Diagnosis

- Affected epiphysis appears widened, sclerotic, and irregular on X-ray.
- Imaging of the asymptomatic side may be required to detect subtle changes.

Treatment

As with other stress reactions, management involves unloading the injured area (i.e., avoiding upper-limb weight bearing) until the pain resolves.

Physical therapy is aimed at restoring full range of motion and strengthening the wrist flexors.

If the distal radial epiphysis appears to be closing prematurely, specialist referral is warranted.

Prognosis

If untreated, radial epiphysitis can cause premature closure of the distal radial epiphysis.

Radial epiphysitis may be associated with positive ulnar variance (a relative overgrowth of the ulna), which is a common finding in gymnasts.

Triangular fibrocartilage complex (TFCC) tears

The TFCC is composed of triangular fibrocartilage and ligaments on the ulnar side of the wrist between the ulna and the carpus.

There is a cartilage disc that covers the ulnar head and blends with the dorsal and palmar radioulnar ligaments. It contributes to the stability of the ulnar side of the wrist joint.

The TFCC can be injured as the result of a fall, or tears may occur with repetitive overuse (e.g., in gymnasts) or degeneration.

History and examination

- Can be torn with activities involving wrist extension and ulnar deviation, e.g., gymnastics and tennis
- Ulnar wrist pain and swelling exacerbated by wrist extension and ulnar deviation
- May be tender to palpation in this region
- Compression and ulnar deviation of the wrist may elicit pain
- A clicking sensation may be present
- Grip strength is commonly reduced

Diagnosis

Plain X-rays are generally unhelpful, although positive ulnar variance may be seen. MRI is diagnostic.

Treatment

Conservative treatment involves rest from provocative activities and splinting or taping to prevent excessive wrist extension and ulnar deviation. If symptoms do not settle with conservative treatment, orthopedic referral is required.

Surgical treatment includes wrist arthroscopy, debridement or repair of the injured tissue (peripheral tears are within the vascular zone and may be repaired), and sometimes an ulnar-shortening osteotomy to correct positive ulnar variance.

Symptoms are likely to recur when associated with positive ulnar variance and when provocative activities are continued.

Kienbock's disease

This is an avascular necrosis affecting the lunate of unknown etiology, affecting mostly young males aged 20–40 years.

It is often associated with repeated minor wrist trauma.

History and examination

Kienbock's disease commonly presents in adolescence or later with restricted range of motion in the wrist and loss of grip strength. Dorsal wrist pain is exacerbated by loading the wrist in extension.

Often there is a history of recurrent loading of the wrist, e.g., gymnastics, racquet sports, repetitive falls.

This condition is often associated with a short ulna—normally 80% of forces are directed through the scapholunate/distal radius articulation. If the ulna is short (negative ulnar variance), then even more force is transmitted through the lunate.

Diagnosis

X-ray may be normal in the early phases but later demonstrates sclerosis and flattening of the lunate (see Fig. 5.10). It may also show negative ulnar variance.

Bone scan and MRI will be positive in the early stages.

Treatment

Treatment depends on the staging of the process, with stages 1 and 2 responding to rest and radial shortening if negative ulnar variance is present.

If diagnosed in the early stages before significant X-ray changes have occurred, rest from exacerbating activities and bracing or cast immobilization may prevent lunate collapse.

More advanced cases with lunate collapse, changes in carpal alignment, and/or wrist arthrosis require intercarpal arthrodeses, proximal row carpectomy (PRC), or wrist arthrodesis.

Long-term disability is common after compressive changes have occurred.

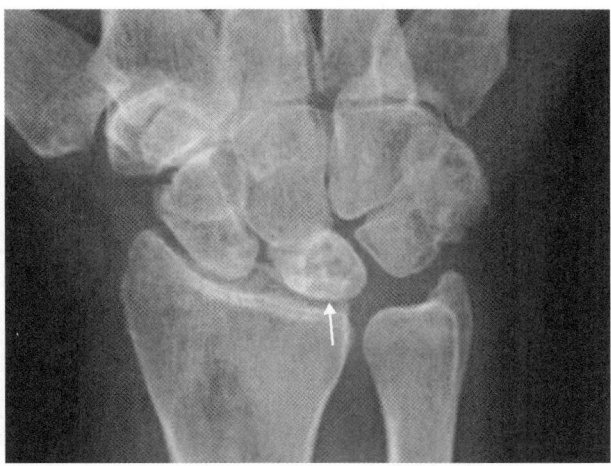

Figure 5.10 Anteroposterior radiograph demonstrating sclerosis of the lunate in a patient with Kienbock's disease.

Spine

History

Most episodes of back pain in sports are gradual in onset because of repeated stresses, although pain may present as a specific event. Understand the demands of sport, exercise, and occupation.

Pain
- Chief complaint: back pain vs. lower extremity pain
- Character
- Location and radiation with pattern of radiation
- Relationship to exercise or activity
- Exacerbating and alleviating factors

Neurological symptoms
- Numbness, tingling, pins and needles
- Weakness
- Bowel or bladder complaints

Past history
- Spinal problems
- Orthopedic problems

Family history
- Spinal problems

Be sure to note any medical or rheumatological symptoms (insidious and persistent, morning pain or stiffness), mechanical abnormalities (intermittent and associated with activity), disc herniation and nerve impingement (radiates to lower leg or foot), or tumor (night pain). Also note if there is relief with aspirin (osteoid osteoma).

Problems that show familial predisposition include disc disease, ankylosing spondylitis, Reiter's syndrome, and other spondylolarthropathies.

Red flags in history of a patient with back pain
- Less than 10 years of age
- First episode of back pain and over 60 years old
- Unexplained weight loss
- Chronic cough
- Night pain
- Intermenstrual bleeding
- Altered bowel function
- Altered bladder control
- Visual disturbance, balance problems, upper-limb dysesthesias
- Past history of cancer or corticosteroid use
- Bilateral weakness of lower extremities

Examination

Inspection

With patient standing:
- *From behind*: check level of shoulders, lateral curvature or scoliosis, lumbar list, lengths of lower limbs (level of posterior superior iliac spines), or hair tufts over spine
- *From side*: check increased kyphosis, decreased lordosis

Lumbar list (painful scoliosis) may be due to unilateral muscle spasm, or nerve root irritation may be due to disc herniation.

Palpation

Palpate each spinous process for possible step-off, posterior superior iliac crest (PSIS)/sacroiliac region, facet joints for tenderness and paraspinal muscles for tenderness or spasm, and gluteal muscle/sciatic notch for tenderness. See Figures 6.1, 6.2, and 6.3.

Active and passive movement

Restriction of spinal movement may be due to muscle spasm as a result of pathology in one or more functional unit. Note pain during any of the movements tested.

Lumbar flexion (normal is 40–60°) occurs by reversing the lordosis. During re-extension the lumbar lordosis is regained in the final 45°.

Toe touching with straight legs is influenced by hip mobility, and hamstring tightness so is not useful for assessment. However, lumbar flexion may be assessed by measuring the increased distance between marked points over the spinous processes with flexion (Schober's test). Inability to touch the toes because of hamstring tightness is a classic finding in spondylolisthesis.

Lumbar extension (normal is 20–30°) is painful with facet joint or pars interarticularis pathology; this is called "posterior element pain." It can be due to posterior disc pathology or closing of the foramen on nerve roots.

Lumbar lateral flexion (normal is 20°) is painful with ipsilateral facet joint pathology or lateral disc protrusion (radicular pain), but is often a non-specific sign.

Lumbar rotation occurs with thoracic rotation (normal is 90°) and is assessed with pelvis and hips fixed (held by examiner or sitting).

Neurological examination

- *Sensory*: light touch over back and abdomen, legs, perianal sensation
- *Lower limb reflexes (L4 knee, S1 ankle), superficial anal reflex*: touching perianal skin causes contraction of sphincter and external anal muscles (S2, S3, and S4)
- *Motor*: squat and return to standing, walk on heels (weak ankle dorsiflexors—L4) and then toes (weak gastrocsoleus—S1); muscle strength testing for nerve root assessment (L1—hip flexion, L2—hip flexion, L3—knee extension, L4—foot dorsiflexion, L5—great toe extension, foot inversion, S1—knee flexion and foot plantar flexion and eversion); sphincter tone and contractility

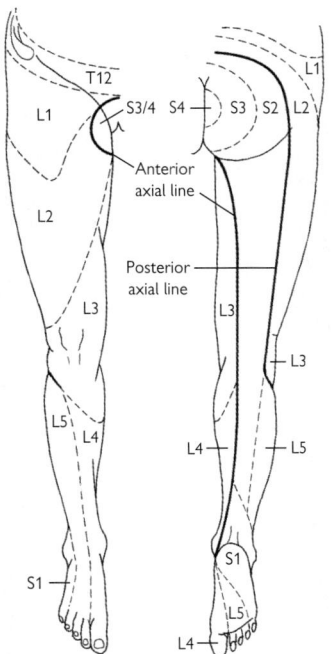

Figure 6.1 Dermatomes of lower limb; note the axial lines. Reproduced with permission from Mackinnon P, Morris J (2005). *Oxford Textbook of Functional Anatomy*, Vol. 1. Oxford, UK: Oxford University Press. ©2005.

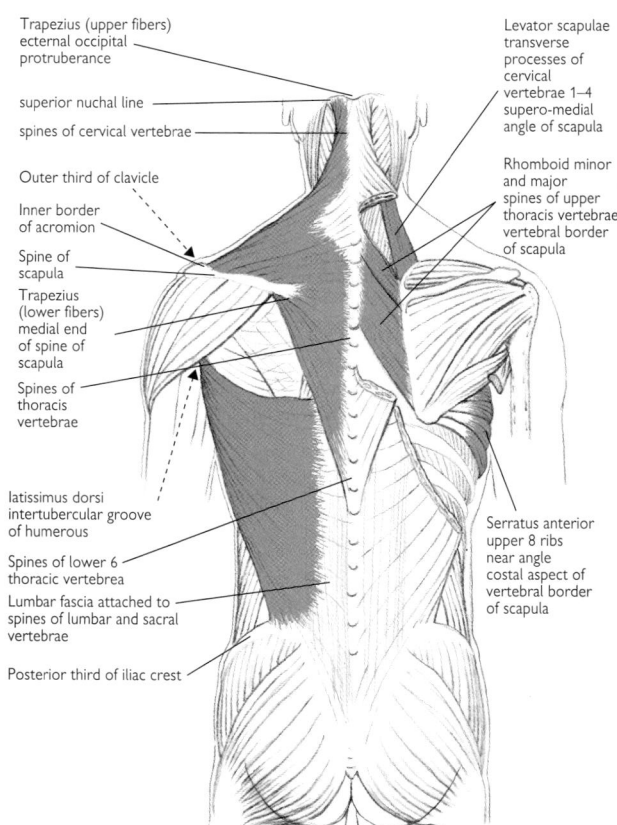

Trapezius (upper fibers)
ecternal occipital
protruberance

superior nuchal line

spines of cervical vertebrae

Outer third of clavicle

Inner border
of acromion

Spine of
scapula

Trapezius
(lower fibers)
medial end
of spine of
scapula

Spines of
thoracis
vertebrae

latissimus dorsi
intertubercular groove
of humerous

Spines of lower 6
thoracic vertebrea

Lumbar fascia attached to
spines of lumbar and sacral
vertebrae

Posterior third of iliac crest

Levator scapulae
transverse
processes of
cervical
vertebrae 1–4
supero-medial
angle of scapula

Rhomboid minor
and major
spines of upper
thoracis vertebrae
vertebral border
of scapula

Serratus anterior
upper 8 ribs
near angle
costal aspect of
vertebral border
of scapula

Figure 6.2 Superficial muscles of the shoulder girdle and back. Reproduced with permission from MacKinnon P, Morris J (2005). *Oxford Textbook of Functional Anatomy*, Vol. 1. Oxford, UK: Oxford University Press. ©2005.

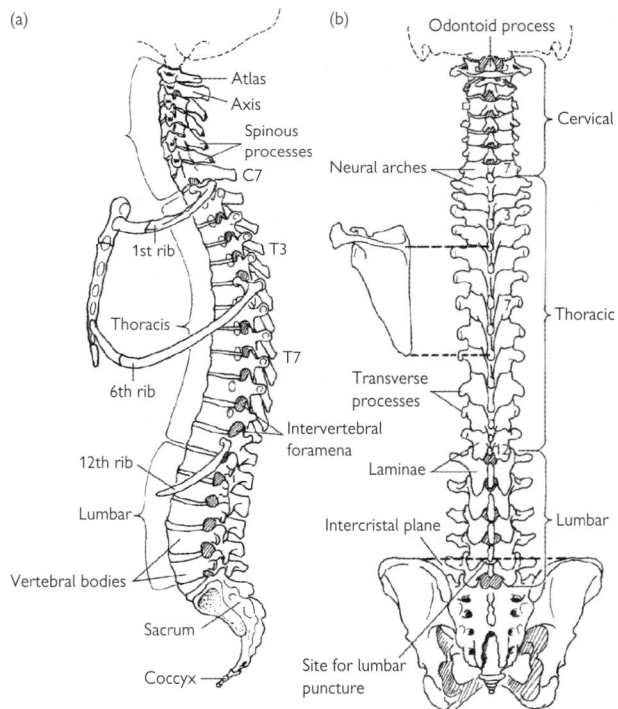

Figure 6.3 Vertebral column. (a) Lateral view; (b) posterior view. Reproduced with permission from MacKinnon P, Morris J (2005). *Oxford Textbook of Functional Anatomy*, Vol. 1. Oxford, UK: Oxford University Press. ©2005.

Special tests

Sciatic and femoral nerve tension tests

The principle test is stretching the dura and nerve root to produce leg pain. A positive test will reproduce the patient's radicular symptoms.

Sciatic nerve tests
- Straight-leg raise (Fig. 6.4a)
- *Contralateral straight-leg raise*: reproduction of radiating lower extremity pain with straight-leg raise of the contralateral limb; extremely sensitive and specific for herniated nucleus pulposus
- *Leseaque test*: patient supine with hips flexed to 90°; knee slowly extended
- *Bowstring sign*: examiner presses in popliteal fossa and causes increased pain in leg
- *Slump test*: patient sits "slumped"; progressive increase in tension by flexing neck, extending knee, and dorsiflexing foot

Ankle dorsiflexion and neck flexion should aggravate radicular pain or decrease the angle of straight-leg raise.

A false-positive result is pain with <30° or >70° of straight-leg raise, production of back pain with no leg pain.

Femoral nerve test (Fig. 6.4b)
For lateral decubitus, extend the hip then flex the knee to 90°. A positive test is recorded if there is pain in the thigh with this maneuver. Repeat on the opposite side.

(a)

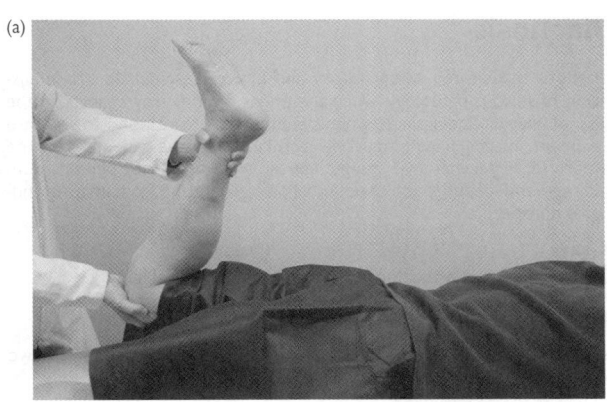

(b)

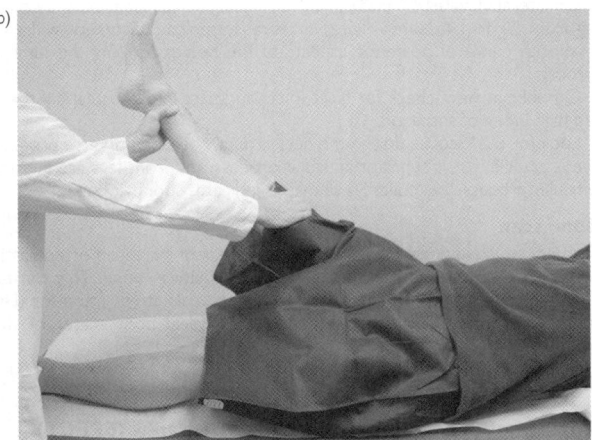

Figure 6.4 (a) Straight-leg raise test and (b) femoral nerve stretch text.

Diagnosis

Diagnosis is indicated when history and physical examination raise suspicion of serious pathology, when treatment options may change on the basis of imaging findings, and when symptoms fail to respond to standard treatment. Imaging findings must be correlated with the patient's signs and symptoms, as degenerative changes appear in asymptomatic persons from early age, and identification of potential pain generators from imaging findings is nonspecific.

X-rays

Obtain routine anteroposterior (AP) and lateral views (Fig. 6.5).
- *Advantages*: cheap, low radiation dose, define bones
- *Disadvantage*: do not define soft tissues

On AP view, check spinous process and two transverse processes, two pedicles, two laminae, and two facet joints (vertical in lumbar spine) at each level; assess alignment.

On lateral view, assess bodies of the vertebrae and disc spacing increasing from L1 to L4. Lumbar intervertebral foraminae alignment will give a smooth curve of posterior aspects of the bodies forming the lumbar lordosis.

On oblique view, check for facet joints and pars interarticularis if there is a high index of suspicion.

Look for the "Scottie dog"—the neck is pars, nose is transverse process, eye is pedicle, ear is superior articular process, and front legs are inferior articular process. If a "collar" is seen, this indicates spondylolysis.

Bone scan

Technetium-labeled injection is taken up in areas of increased osteoblastic activity, demonstrating increased metabolic activity in bone. This can be detected by a gamma camera. A bone scan reveals stress fractures (i.e., spondylolysis) but also epiphyses and metaphyseal bone plates of the young.
- *Advantage*: high sensitivity
- *Disadvantage*: low specificity, radiation dose

Single photon emission computed tomography (SPECT)

SPECT gives a more precise anatomical localization of a "hot spot" than bone scan. It is the imaging modality of choice to identify spondylolysis.

Computed tomography (CT)

CT is the imaging modality of choice for visualization of bone and bony abnormalities.
- *Advantage*: good to detect fractures and impingement of spinal canal, evaluate spinal tumors
- *Disadvantages*: radiation dose, slices may miss pathology

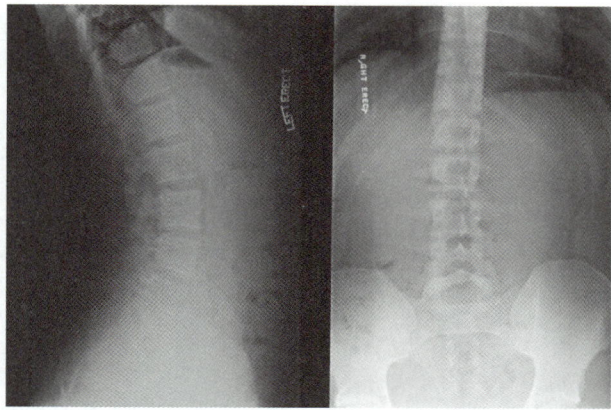

Figure 6.5 Anteroposterior and lateral X-ray and normal lumbar spine.

Myelography

Injecting radio-opaque dye into the spinal canal outlines the spinal cord and nerve roots on subsequent plain X-rays. This can reveal nerve root compression, though not its cause (i.e., prolapsed disc, osteophyte, or tumor).

CT myelography

Myelography is combined with CT technology for even greater detail.

Magnetic resonance imaging (MRI)

MRI provides excellent visualization of soft tissues, including discs (see Fig. 6.6). It can be used to assess impingement of nerve roots and may indicate hemorrhage from ligamentous injury. MRI can be used to detect atrophy in paraspinal muscles and changes in the spinal cord, such as syringomyelia. In most cases it has superseded myelography.

- *Advantage*: no radiation
- *Disadvantage*: cost, metallic artifact

Discography

This involves injection of radio-opaque dye into the disc space under pressure, while monitoring for leakage of intradiscal fluid and annular distension and assessing pain response. Reproduction of the patient's typical low back pain suggests a positive test. The reliability of this procedure in identifying the specific source of pain is debated. The use of this procedure in the young athlete has not been studied and is not routinely recommended in this population.

(a)   (b)

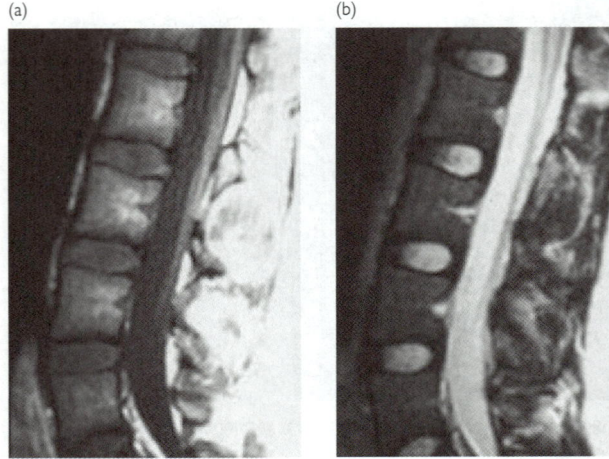

Figure 6.6 (a) Normal lumbar spine T1MRI saggital view. (b) Normal lumbar spine T2MRI sagittal view.

Acute spinal injury

History and examination

Awareness of possible catastrophic injury is most important when an athlete goes down on the field. Question the athlete and witnesses of the injury.

Primary survey on the field in acute injury should include evaluation of unconsciousness, airway, breathing, and circulation to identify life-threatening injuries. Neurological screening can then be done to assess associated head trauma and injuries that could produce instability of the spine and threaten neurological structures.

Cervical spine injury and potential instability should be presumed in anyone who is unconscious after head injury.

When to immobilize?
- An unconscious athlete
- Pain in the spine secondary to high-velocity injury
- Any neurological signs or complaint of numbness, weakness, or paralysis

Transportation should be on a spinal board by trained personnel to ensure immobilization in the position in which the athlete was found. In general, equipment such as helmets should not be removed unless airway access is required.

The cervical spine will need assessment by cervical spine X-ray and clearance by appropriate professionals on the basis of signs, symptoms, and clinical condition.

Acute injuries of the back in sports

- Muscular strain and ligament sprain
- Degenerative disc disease
- Isthmic spondylolysis
- Isthmic spondylolisthesis
- Compression or stress fractures of the vertebral bodies, unless trauma was extreme, are usually pathological (osteoporosis in elderly athletes or the young female with the female athletic triad of disordered eating, amenorrhea, and osteoporosis)
- Fracture dislocations: high-energy injuries (e.g., diving, car racing) with a high risk of spinal cord injury

Low back pain is a symptom, not a diagnosis. It is often not associated with any identifiable anatomical abnormality. Back pain episodes are common in the general nonathletic population, and athletes may or may not be at higher risk according to their sport of preference.

Management of musculoligamentous injuries of the back

- Sprains and strains of the back are thought to be common and self-limited. Radiological imaging is not indicated unless clinical findings suggest other causes. Offending activities should be avoided early on. Ice can be applied in 20-minute sessions and muscle spasm may also be controlled by anti-spasmodic medication.

Rehabilitation programs aim to restore normal core muscle strength and muscle firing patterns. Return to sport can be initiated when the athlete is pain-free with nearly normal mobility, strength, and endurance.

Disc disease

Disc disease is a continuum from degeneration to herniation. Sports participation may be a risk factor for development of disc degeneration but not necessarily back pain.

As the disc loses water content with age, more stress is transferred to the annulus fibrosis, which may develop radial tears. These tears may cause local back pain, but have the potential to allow herniation of the nucleus through annulus and consequent nerve root pain.

Diagnosis

Loss of disc space height on plain radiographs and disc dessication (loss of water content) on MRI indicate degenerative disc changes. These findings, which are consistent with normal aging, have been variably associated with the likelihood of back pain in athletes, but the high rate of these findings in asymptomatic individuals limits a cause-and-effect connection.

Treatment

Treatment of presumed acute discogenic back pain involves adequate analgesia and antispasmodics if needed and then rehabilitation to improve core muscle strength and firing pattern to decrease the load on the disc. Treatment then focuses progressively on sport-specific postures and activities.

Disc herniation

Disc herniation is most common in the fifth decade of life, although up to 2% of cases occur in those under 18 years. In disc herniation, the nucleus pulposus extrudes through a tear in the annulus fibrosis (Fig. 6.7). The herniation may press on the nerve root, causing leg pain, numbness, and weakness. Chemical mediators may also cause a component of radicular pain.

Classically, the history may suggest symptoms of disc degeneration prior to more acute intense back pain, after which, over the next 48 hours, buttock and leg pain develops. If bilateral leg numbness or weakness is present, consider the possibility of "cauda equina syndrome" and ask about loss of visceral function (e.g., bladder and bowel, fecal or urinary incontinence or retention) and saddle anesthesia.

Appropriate treatment of cauda equina is urgent spinal decompression.

Examination

With acute disc herniation, the patient may stand with a list away from the side of the leg pain and flex asymmetrically away from that side as well. Muscle weakness, sensory loss, and reflex changes in the lower limbs may give an indication of the level of the herniation. Sciatic or femoral nerve tension signs may be positive.

In cauda equina syndrome, perianal and scrotal sensation and sphincter tone may be lost. MRI is the diagnosis of choice but is not necessary acutely unless cauda equina syndrome is suspected.

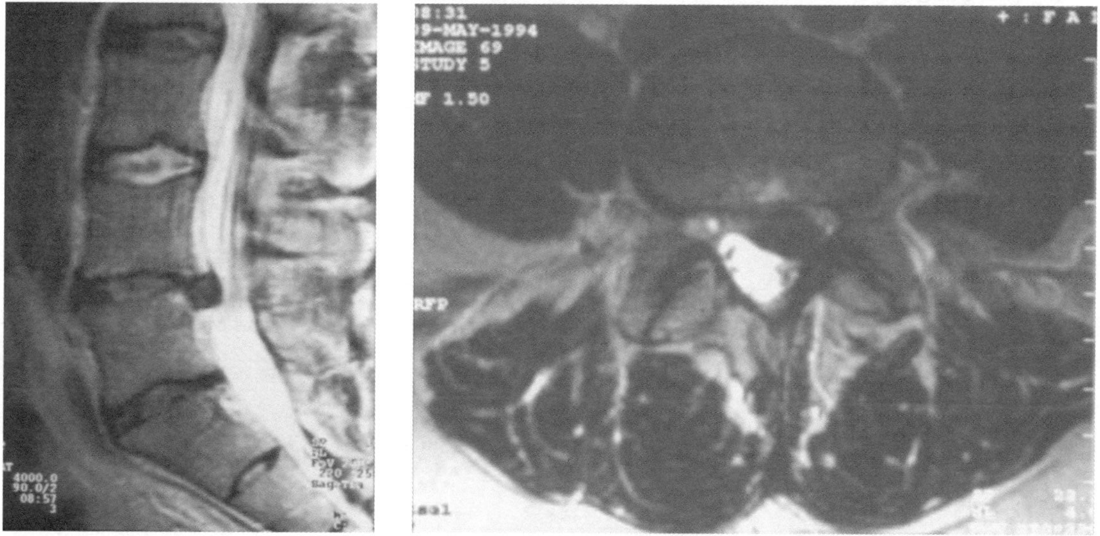

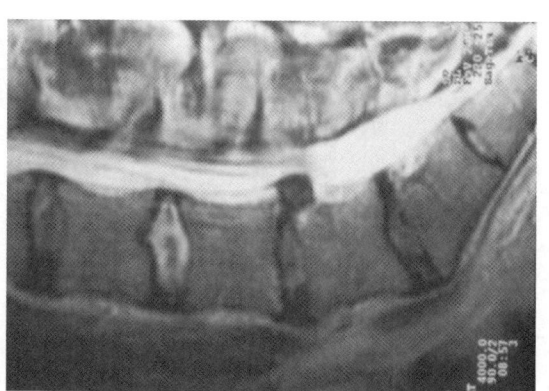

Figure 6.7 (a) Lumbar herniated nucleus pulposus (HNP) sagittal view. (b) Lumbar HNP axial view.

Treatment

Treatment of disc herniation involves analgesia and antispasmodics and limited bed rest if there is severe pain on movement. However, activity should be encouraged as soon as the patient can cope with it. Back extension exercises may be useful. An epidural injection may be effective in reducing pain, but may not improve neurological deficit.

In persistent cases (e.g., 6 weeks with no response) microdiscectomy may be performed, although studies suggest the long-term results after 2 years are no better than with continued conservative management. Rehabilitation to maximize core strength and optimize spinal flexibility may allow progressive return to sport.

Cauda equina syndrome requires emergent surgical decompression.

Pars interarticularis and spondylolysis

Definition

Pars interarticularis is the narrowest section of the lamina, bridge of bone between the inferior and superior articular process of the vertebra (also called "isthmus").

Spondylolysis is fracture of the pars interarticularis.

Asymptomatic spondylolysis is present in about 5% of the skeletally mature general population. It is not present in the newborn, but has been seen in 6-year-olds.

The pars interarticularis is vulnerable to stress fracture in those engaging in repeated hyperextension of the spine. This occurs in many sports but particularly in gymnasts and offensive linemen because of the nature of their sports.

Some children may also have a genetic weakness in the pars interarticularis that predisposes them to this condition. These cases occur most commonly at L5 (85%–95%) and L4 (5%–15%) but occasionally they occur at a higher level and can be unilateral or bilateral.

Imaging with bone scan and CT reveals a continuum of mild stress reaction to complete fracture with potential for nonunion. The lower three lumbar vertebrae are most at risk.

The term *spondylolysis* covers defects in the pars interarticularis, but defects have also been described in the pedicle and other posterior elements of the spine from sporting activities.

Posterior-element pain is generally characterized by pain on extension and particularly a positive one-legged hyperextension test (stork test). Pain usually occurs when the foot of the ipsilateral side to the pars lesion is on the ground. Adding rotation toward the affected side is more sensitive for a stress lesion (Fitch test). The reliability and specificity of these tests is questionable.

Diagnosis

Plain X-ray with oblique view (Fig. 6.8), which may show a "collar" on the Scottie dog, is the recommended initial imaging modality. However, pain radiography lacks sensitivity. Therefore, if there is high clinical suspicion, triple-phase bone scanning with SPECT is the optimal next study. "Hot spots" in the posterior elements indicate possible sites of spondylolysis, which can then be identified with a CT scan.

Unfortunately, MRI, which does not pose radiation risks to the patient, poorly delineates bony structures and may only be positive acutely with bone stress presenting as edema.

Treatment

Increased uptake on bone scan or SPECT indicates bone stress. Treatment should include rest from pain-provoking activities, which usually is sport. A lumbosacral orthosis molded in 10–15° of flexion may be used to prevent hyperextension.

For those with early bone stress reaction, 6 weeks' rest may be sufficient, but 12 weeks may be required to allow healing of established stress fractures. When patients are pain free, thorough rehabilitation of the spinal and abdominal musculature is necessary. Return to sports should be gradual and depend on symptoms. Imaging is not useful in predicting the time to return to sports.

Established spondylolysis with wide sclerotic bone margins and negative bone scan is unlikely to heal, even with rest and bracing. Management is designed to allow pain to settle. Then rehabilitation is started to provide dynamic stability though exercises and an earlier (less cautious) attempt to return to sports.

Persistent pain despite activity modification and rehabilitation may respond to a period of bracing. Pain preventing successful return to sports could be treated by surgical stabilization, by either pars bone grafting or fusion, although patients must be counseled that outcomes are not always favorable. A local anesthetic "lysis" block may give useful information regarding the potential benefit of treating the lysis surgically.

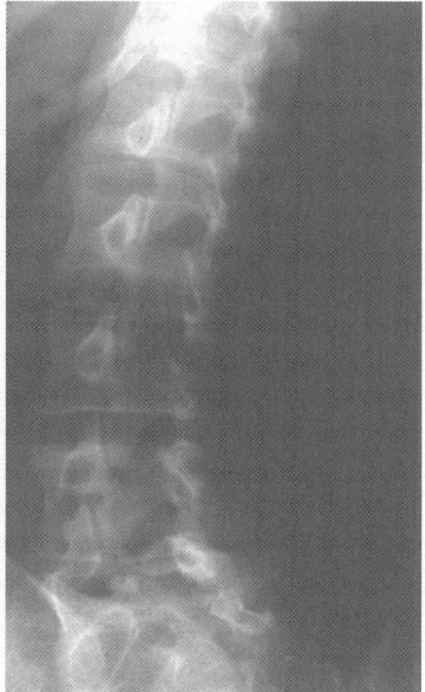

Figure 6.8 Pars defect oblique view.

Spondylolisthesis

Definition
Spondylolisthesis: anterior displacement of one vertebral body on another

Classification of spondylolisthesis (Wiltse, 1976)
- Dysplastic
- Isthmic (lytic or elongated)
- Degenerative
- Traumatic (fractures)
- Pathological

Grading of spondylolisthesis (Meyerding, 1932)
Grading is based on displacement of the vertebral body relative to the lower vertebral body anteroposterior diameter.
- Grade 1 = 0%–25%
- Grade 2 = 26%–50%
- Grade 3 = 51%–75%
- Grade 4 = 76%–100%
- Grade 5 >100% (spondyloptosis)

Spondylolisthesis in the young athlete
- If there are bilateral pars defects, spondylolisthesis can occur.
- Progression of spondylolisthesis is uncommon but is most likely to occur during the time of peak height velocity.

Examination may reveal the step-off in the spine and hamstrings are often tight, requiring clinical differentiation from sciatic nerve tension. Lateral plain X-rays will demonstrate nearly all spondylolistheses, but MRI may be useful to assess nerve root foramina and disc quality, which may be compromised in spondylolisthesis.

Spondylolisthesis may progress in the skeletally immature. However, sporting involvement does not appear to be a risk factor; thus there is no evidence to exclude an athlete from participation. Nevertheless, it may be wise to avoid gymnastics and weight lifting if the patient is at stage 2 or 3. Surgery may be considered for those at stage 3 or those with nerve root entrapment.

History and examination
- May be asymptomatic. Do not assume that back pain is due to a radiologically proven spondylolysis or spondylolisthesis unless the clinical picture is consistent.
- Symptomatic pars stress fractures present with an insidious onset of unilateral or bilateral pain in the lumbar region (most commonly at the level of the belt), which may then radiate to the buttocks and leg.
- Pain often is worse with activities requiring lumbar extension.
- Clinical findings: may have increased lumbar lordosis and tenderness around the facet joint region at the affected level.

- Pain is reproduced by lumbar extension, which is often worse when standing on the leg of the affected side.
- There are no neurological signs in the lower limbs.

Diagnosis
- X-ray including oblique view. This gives the classic "Scottie dog" appearance when a pars defect is present.
- Lateral view is also useful to determine whether a spondylolisthesis exists and its severity (Fig. 6.9).
- Spondylolisthesis is graded 1–4 according to the degree of slip: grade 1: 25%, grade 2: 25%–50%, grade 3: 50%–75%, grade 4 >75%
- With recent symptom onset the X-ray is often normal.
- A bone scan including SPECT views is very sensitive for recent stress fractures. A hot spot at the site of the defect suggests that the fracture is recent and active. If no hot spot (i.e., no osteoblastic reaction) is seen, active remodeling is not occurring.
- Bone-scan changes often remain positive for many months and are not useful as a means of timing return to sports.
- CT scanning is useful for staging fractures.

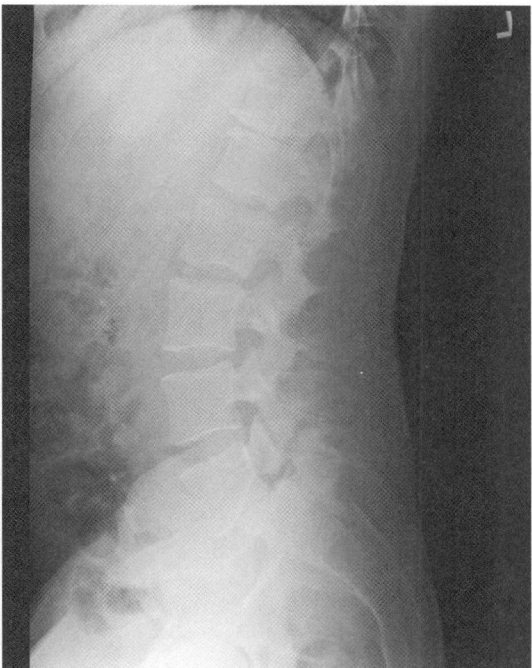

Figure 6.9 Lumbar spondylolisthesis.

Treatment

- Avoid lumbar extension activities.
- Some clinicians recommend the use of a brace to prevent lumbar extension (e.g., modified Boston brace), especially if the athlete has pain with activities of daily living.
- Use of a brace has not been shown to increase the rate of fracture healing.
- Physiotherapy should include an abdominal strengthening program and postural retraining to address excessive lumbar lordosis and anterior pelvic tilt.
- A flexibility program to improve hamstring and gluteal flexibility should also be included.
- Return to sports, which usually occurs within 3–6 months, should be based on symptom resolution, absence of clinical signs, and good core trunk strength.
- Monitor for slip progression during the growing years, as progression may (rarely) require surgical stabilization.
- If there is persistent pain despite appropriate rehabilitation and in those with a grade 3 or 4 spondylolisthesis (>50% slip) or when the slip is progressing, referral to a specialist is indicated. These children should avoid sports requiring lumbar extension and contact.

Prognosis

- Fractures treated in the early phase appear to have a good prognosis, especially if they are unilateral.
- Early- and progressive-stage fractures have a 40–80% chance of fracture healing.
- Terminal-stage fractures rarely unite.
- Excellent clinical outcomes can be achieved in the absence of fracture healing.
- Bone stimulator use has not been shown to change the rate of healing.

Further reading

Morita T, et al. (1995) Lumbar spondylolysis in children and adolescents. *J Bone Joint Surg* (Br) **77B**: 620–625.

Scheuermann's disease

Scheuermann's kyphosis is manifested by vertebral body wedging, vertebral end plate irregularities, diminished anterior vertebral growth, and premature disc degeneration. Compressive forces cause wedging deformity of the vertebral bodies, resulting in a thoracic kyphosis.

The etiology is unknown but it is considered an osteochondrosis affecting growth plates (ring epiphysis) of vertebral bodies. It affects the thoracic spine predominantly but can occur in the lumbar spine or at the thoracolumbar junction.

It occurs in adolescents with onset just before puberty and is the most common cause of hyperkyphosis in adolescence. Incidence is between 1% and 8% of the general population. There appears to be an increased familial incidence of the condition. Scheuermann's kyphosis may be a coincidental radiographic diagnosis and may or may not be a cause of nonspecific low back pain in the adolescent or young adult.

History and examination
- Commonly presents in the active adolescent
- May have mid-thoracic pain with activity
- May present as a painless thoracic kyphosis in the late teenage years or 20s with concerns about "poor posture"
- Tightness of hamstrings and thoracolumbar fascia is common
- Excessive lumbar lordosis often present

Diagnosis
- Wedging of >5° in three or more consecutive vertebrae on lateral X-ray is diagnostic.
- Disc degeneration on MRI has been shown in 50% of patients compared to 10% of asymptomatic controls, but it is unclear if this is primary or due to abnormal mechanical loading of the kyphotic spine.
- Schmorl's nodes (irregularities in the cartilage end plate causing irregular ossification) are commonly present.

Treatment
- Persistent pain and/or progression of kyphosis is not inevitable.
- Aim to resolve pain and stop progression of deformity.
- Avoid offending activities until symptoms resolve.
- Hamstrings and thoracolumbar fascia stretches
- Abdominal core-muscle strengthening program
- If kyphosis is >50° at presentation, an extension brace (e.g., a Milwaukee or DuPont brace) should be used in addition to exercises.
- Rarely, if kyphosis is >70° and bracing and exercises have failed or pain is severe despite treatment, surgery may be warranted.

Prognosis
- Exercises will reduce symptoms but will not correct the existing deformity.
- Use of a brace before skeletal maturity may improve kyphosis.
- Pain is usually self-limiting and resolves with skeletal maturity unless kyphosis is severe.

Sacroiliac joint

Sacroiliac joint motion is small, not more than 2–3° in the transverse or longitudinal plane. No muscles directly cross the joint. Pain may come from trauma or perhaps overuse-type injuries. Sacroiliac joint pain may be greater in sports requiring unilateral loading such as kicking and throwing but has been reported in cross country skiers and rowers.

Sacroillitis is an early manifestation of seronegative arthritities, such as ankylosing spondylitis or Reiter's syndrome.

Factors predisposing to overuse injury of sacroiliac joint

- Ligamentous laxity due to hormonal changes of pregnancy
- Leg-length discrepancy
- Gait abnormality
- Prolonged vigorous exercise
- Scoliosis
- Running on uneven terrain or a cambered road

History and examination

History or physical examination findings do not identify the sacroiliac joint as the pain generator. Pain in the low back, sacrum, pelvis, gluteal region, and groin has been ascribed to an origin in the sacroiliac joint.

Unilateral pain is more common than bilateral by a 4:1 ratio. The presentation most consistent with sacroiliac joint pain is unilateral pain localized below the L5 spinous process.

Clinical findings

- Local pain over joint line (posterior inferior iliac spine)
- Pain on compression or distraction of the iliac crests
- Pain on FABER leverage test (flexion abduction external rotation)

Diagnosis

Imaging may help rule out other sources of pain but is generally helpful in evaluating sacroiliac joint pain.

Plain radiographs, a bone scan, and MRI may be helpful in identifying sacral fractures, tumors, sacroiliitis, and ankylosing spondylitis.

HLA_{B27} may be positive in those with ankylosing spondylitis.

Treatment

Address biomechanical factors, such as pelvic mobility, leg-length discrepancy, hip rotation, footwear, and training factors. Treat with analgesia, NSAIDs, and ice and consider use of a sacroiliac belt.

Second-line treatment might include corticosteroid injections into the localized painful area or intra-articularly as a diagnostic and therapeutic approach.

Hip and pelvis

Examination of the hip

For anatomy of the hip and lower limbs, see Figures 7.1, 7.2, and 7.3.

History

The usual complaints are as follows:

- Pain
- Limp
- Decreased walking or running distances
- Snapping or clicking sensation of the hip
- Stiffness
- Deformity

Look for evidence of asymmetry or biomechanical abnormality.

Inspection

- Scars
- Sinuses
- Swellings
- Muscle wasting

Apparent limb-length discrepancy is noted by measuring the distance from umbilicus to medial malleolus.

Real limb-length discrepancy is noted by measuring the distance from anterior superior iliac spine (ASIS) (or any ipsilateral fixed bony point) to medial malleolus after squaring the pelvis (unmask the fixed abduction or adduction deformity of the affected limb so that both ASIS and medial malleolus are leveled, and place the normal limb in a similar position).

Examine gait, usually before the above sequence.

Palpation

- Skin temperature
- Tenderness over the femoral head and greater trochanter
- Palpate swellings if present

Active and passive movements

The pelvis must be squared and stabilized before hip movements are measured (see Table 7.1).

A normal hip has the following:

- Flexion range of 0–130°
- Extension of 0–10°
- Abduction of 0–45°
- Adduction of 0–40°
- Internal rotation of 0–30°
- External rotation of 0–60°

Note pain at extremes of movements and restriction. In early osteoarthritis, internal rotation is restricted. In advanced osteoarthritis, there is fixed flexion deformity with absent extension, decreased abduction, adduction, and external and internal rotation. All movements are associated with pain (see Table 7.2).

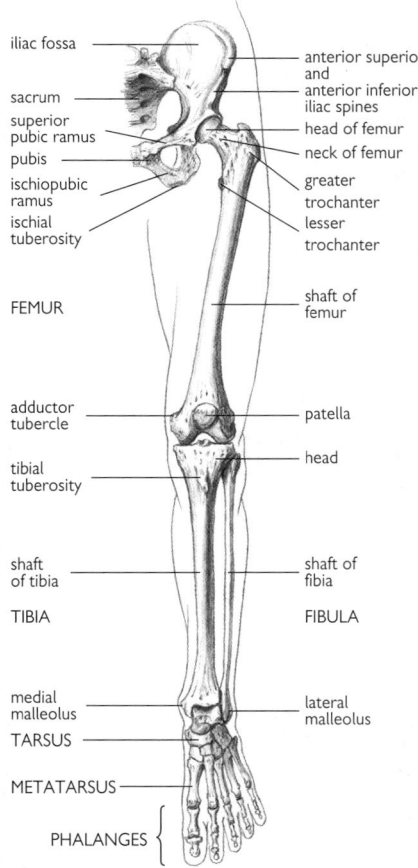

Figure 7.1 Bones of the lower limb and pelvic girdle, anterior view. Reproduced with permission from Mackinnon P, Morris J (2005). *Oxford Textbook of Functional Anatomy*, Vol. 1. Oxford, UK: Oxford University Press. ©2005.

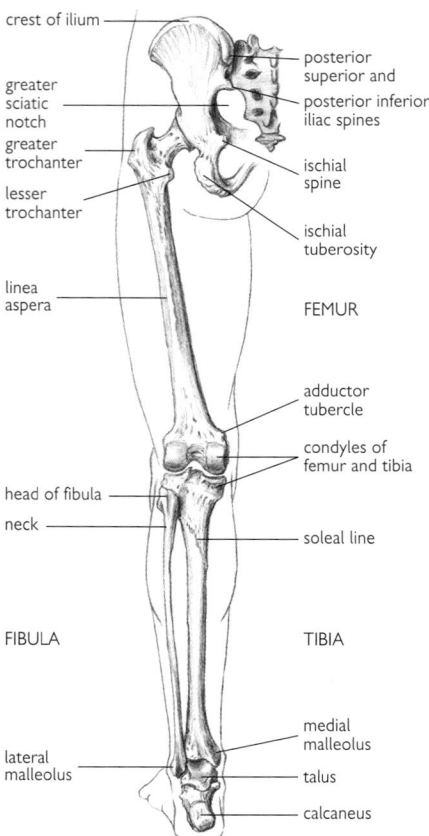

crest of ilium

posterior superior and

posterior inferior iliac spines

greater sciatic notch

ischial spine

greater trochanter

lesser trochanter

ischial tuberosity

linea aspera

FEMUR

adductor tubercle

condyles of femur and tibia

head of fibula

neck

soleal line

FIBULA

TIBIA

medial malleolus

lateral malleolus

talus

calcaneus

Figure 7.2 Bones of the lower limb and pelvic girdle, posterior view. Reproduced with permission from Mackinnon P, Morris J (2005). *Oxford Textbook of Functional Anatomy*, Vol. 1. Oxford, UK: Oxford University Press. ©2005.

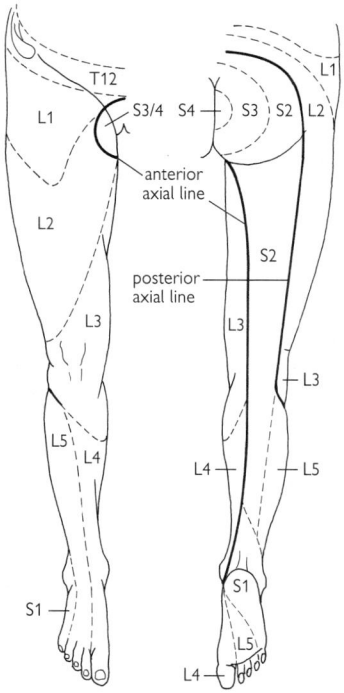

Figure 7.3 Dermatomes of lower limb; note the axial lines. Reproduced with permission from Mackinnon P, Morris J (2005). *Oxford Textbook of Functional Anatomy,* Vol. 1. Oxford, UK: Oxford University Press. ©2005.

Table 7.1 Hip joint: movements, principal muscles, and innervation

Movement	Principal muscles	Peripheral nerve	Spinal root origin
Flexion	Psoas major	Ventral rami of lumbar nerves	L1, 2, 3
	Iliacus	Femoral nerve	L2, 3
	Rectus femoris	Femoral nerve	L2, 3, 4
	Pectineus	Femoral nerve	L2, 3, 4
Extension	Gluteus maximus	Inferior gluteal nerve	L5, S1, 2
	Hamstrings	Sciatic nerve (tibial component)	L5, S1, 2
Adduction	Adductors longus, brevis, magnus, and gracilis	Obturator nerve	L2, 3, 4
Abduction	Gluteus medius and minimus	Superior gluteal nerve	L4, 5, S1
	Tensor fasciae latae	Superior gluteal nerve	L4, 5, S1
Medial rotation	Tensor fasciae latae	Superior gluteal nerve	L4, 5, S1
	Gluteus medius and minimus	Superior gluteal nerve	L4, 5, S1
	Adductor longus	Obturator nerve	L2, 3, 4
Lateral rotation	Obturator externus	Obturator nerve	L2, 3, 4
	Sartorius	Femoral nerve	L2, 3, 4
	Quadratus femoris	Sacral plexus	L4, 5, S1
	Obturator internus	Sacral plexus	L5, S1, 2
	Gluteus maximus	Inferior gluteal nerve	L5, S1, 2

Table 7.2 Main spinal nerve root supplying movements of lower limb

	Movement	Main nerve roots
Hip	Flexion, adduction	L2, 3, 4
Knee	Extension, abduction	L4, 5, S1
	Extension	L3, 4
Ankle	Flexion	L5, S1
	Flexion (plantar flexion)	L4, 5
Subtalar joint	Extension (dorsiflexion)	L5, S1
	Inversion	L5
Toes (long muscles)	Eversion	L5, S1
	Flexion (plantar flexion)	L5, S1, 2
Toes (small muscles of foot)	Extension (dorsiflexion)	L 1, 2, 3 S1, 2, 3

Because of the rotation of the lower limb, extension of the knee is supplied by higher segments.

Reproduced with permission from Mackinnon P, Morris J (2005). *Oxford Textbook of Functional Anatomy*, Vol. 1. Oxford, UK: Oxford University Press. ©2005.

Special tests

Trendelenburg test

This test helps in assessing the integrity of the abductor mechanism of the hip. Patients are asked to stand on one leg, and the position of the pelvis is noted. If the pelvis drops and patients sway to the loaded leg, the test is positive.

Pain on weight bearing, weakness of hip abductors, shortening of femoral neck, and dislocation or subluxation of the hip joint result in a Trendelenburg positive test.

Thomas' test

Fixed flexion deformity of the hip can be masked by the pelvic tilt and exaggerate the lumbar lordosis. This test helps unmask the fixed flexion deformity of the hip and measure the true range of hip flexion.

In supine position, both hips are flexed until the lumbar lordosis is obliterated (confirmed by examiner's hand). The normal (or contralateral) hip is kept flexed, and the affected hip is lowered to the maximum possible extent. The angle between the examination table and the lower limb is the fixed flexion deformity angle.

Tests for suspected labral tears

- Pain on flexion, adduction, and internal rotation of the hip joint occurs with anterior superior tears.
- Pain on passive hyperextension, abduction, and external rotation occurs with posterior tears.
- Pain when moving the hip from a position of full flexion of the hip with external rotation and full abduction to extension, abduction, and internal rotation occurs with anterior tears.
- Pain when moving the hip from extension, abduction, and external rotation to flexion, adduction, and internal rotation occurs with posterior tears.

These maneuvers may also be accompanied by clicking and locking sensations. Hip examination is completed by performing neurovascular examination of the lower limb and examining the contralateral hip and ipsilateral knee, joint, and spine.

Diagnosis

Plain radiographs to investigate the bony architecture, CT scan to obtain further bony detail or better define a fracture pattern, MR scan to investigate the soft tissues (labrum, tendons, ligaments, and articular cartilage), bone scan to rule out infection or occult fracture, and arthroscopy are helpful to confirm clinical diagnoses.

Femur: acute injury

Femoral shaft fractures follow a high-energy injury, and associated injuries must be ruled out. Follow advanced trauma life support (ATLS) guidelines (airway with cervical spine control, breathing, circulation, disability assessment, and exposure) when managing such injuries.

On secondary survey associated injuries can be identified. Fractures are usually closed, and if open, they are often associated with other injuries to the extremity.

The mechanism of injury is usually a torsional stress causing a spiral fracture that may extend into the proximal or distal metaphysis. A direct force causes transverse or oblique fractures. Severe trauma results in comminuted or segmental fractures.

History and examination

- There is severe pain, with obvious swelling and deformity.
- The patient is unable to move the limb.
- Beware of hypovolemic shock; up to 1.5 liters of blood may be lost into the thigh.
- Check and document the presence of distal pulses and the neurological status of the affected limb.

Diagnosis

- Radiographs to include both hip and knee joints. The incidence of ipsilateral femoral shaft and femoral neck fractures is 3%.

Treatment

- Manage shock:
  - Two wide-bore venous cannulae (brown or gray)
  - Hartmann's/lactated Ringers solution is preferred.
  - Urinary catheterization
  - Cross-match 2–4 units of blood
- Analgesia
- Adequate splint (Thomas splint)
- The gold standard is early closed intramedullary nailing for closed fractures (<24 hours)
- Fix the femoral neck first, if injury is present
- Open fractures need emergency debridement and stabilization

Although pediatric femoral shaft fractures can be managed with traction, they can also be managed with spica casting or flexible nails, depending on the age of the child.

Complications

- Fat embolism
- Infection
- Delayed union requiring dynamization of interlocking nail
- Nonunion may require reamed exchange nailing
- Malunion (may need corrective surgery)

Growth plate injury

The growth plate (physis) can be injured in many ways. The most common cause of growth plate injury is trauma. Other causes, although less common, include disuse, infection, tumor, vascular impairment, neural involvement, metabolic abnormalities, radiation, laser injury, electrical injury, burns, frostbite, chronic stress, and iatrogenic or surgical insults.[1]

Physeal fractures

The physis is the weakest structure near a pediatric joint. These fractures occur at a male-to-female ratio of 2:1. In males, the peak incidence is at 14 years, and in females it is at 11–12 years.

The most common sites of injury are the phalanges of fingers (37%), followed by the distal radius (18%). Children present with pain, inability to use the limb, and a possible deformity.

Anteroposterior (AP) and lateral radiographs of the affected part will usually confirm the diagnosis. Occasionally, stress views, tomograms, CT scans, MR scan, or ultrasound scan can help detect growth plate injury.

Classification

The Salter–Harris classification of the physeal injuries is widely used.
1. Separation of the epiphysis from the metaphysis with disruption of the complete physis. Distal fibula is a common site.
2. Separation of part of the physis, with a portion of metaphysis attached to the epiphysis (Thurston–Holland sign). Finger phalanges and distal radius are common sites.
3. Fracture of the epiphysis extending into the physis. Finger phalanges and the distal tibia are common sites.
4. The fracture traverses metaphysis, physis, epiphysis, and the articular cartilage. Lateral condyle of humerus, finger phalanges, and the distal tibia are common sites.
5. This injury is end-on crush of the physis. Diagnosis is retrospective as radiographs are normal at initial presentation.

Treatment

Immediate anatomical reduction by either gentle closed or open methods and adequate fixation by conservative or surgical methods will favor restoration of function and normal growth.

Complications

If the entire physis is affected, bone length is retarded. If a part of physis is affected, angular deformity may result.

1 Peterson HA (2001). Physeal injuries and growth arrest. In Beaty JH, Kasser JR (eds.), *Fracture in Children*. Philadelphia: Lippincott Williams & Wilkins, pp. 91–138.

Femoral neck stress fracture

Stress fractures occur when bone cannot adapt quickly enough in response to the repeated traumatic strain from exercise. Long-distance runners and dancers (especially females) are prone to femoral neck stress fractures.

Predisposing factors include changes in the training program with increase in intensity, frequency, and duration; changes in shoes; running on a different surface; and nutritional deficiency. Female athletes with abnormal menstrual cycles and hormonal imbalance due to relative osteoporosis are also at risk.

History and examination

- Deep, aching pain in the groin that may radiate to the knee
- Pain is progressive, occurs with activity, and resolves with rest.
- Pain becomes constant if activities are continued without modification.
- It may present with a limp.
- There may be no specific site of point tenderness.
- Range of motion (ROM) of the hip, particularly internal rotation, may be limited because of pain.
- Walking, static running, or hopping on the affected extremity often reproduces the pain.

The differential diagnosis includes infection, tumor, compartment syndrome, arthritis, ligamentous, or soft tissue injuries.

Diagnosis

- Plain radiographs may be negative.
- MRI is more sensitive, specific, and accurate than a bone scan in identifying a femoral neck stress fracture.
- Femoral neck stress fractures are classified by Fullerton and Snowdy[1] as tension (type I—superior aspect of the femoral neck), compression (type II—inferior aspect of the femoral neck), or displaced (type III).

Treatment

- Tension (type I) and displaced (type III) fractures should be internally fixed and referred urgently to orthopedic surgeons.
- Compression (type II) fractures can be managed conservatively with non- or partial weight bearing depending on pain and analgesia. Nonimpact activities are initiated once the patient has become pain-free.
- Internal fixation in athletes with stress fractures of the femoral neck aids early rehabilitation and return to sports.

Complications

- Avascular necrosis
- Nonunion (with conservative management)
- Varus deformity (with conservative management)
- Displacement (with conservative management)

Prognosis

Any of the mentioned complications may lead to inability to return to pre-injury performance levels.

Prevention

A gradual progression in the intensity and duration of all conditioning activities is crucial in the prevention of stress fractures. A useful rule of thumb is that an increase in training volume (distance) or intensity should not exceed 10% per week.

1 Fullerton LRJ, Snowdy HA. (1988). Femoral neck stress fractures. *Am J Sports Med*, **16**(11): 365–377.

Trochanteric bursitis

Trochanteric bursitis is inflammation of the greater trochanteric bursa. This bursa minimizes the friction between the greater trochanter and the iliotibial band, which passes over the bursa.

Predisposing factors include a broad pelvis (female runners), training on banked surfaces or roads with a slope, and a recent increase in mileage, duration, or intensity of training.

History and examination
- Lateral hip pain, occasionally radiating along the distal lateral thigh
- May be associated with snapping or clicking sensation
- Point tenderness over the greater trochanter may be associated with crepitus on hip flexion and extension
- Provocative positions include external rotation and adduction

The differential diagnosis includes the following:
- Stress fractures
- Gluteus medius tendinopathy (dancers)
- Lumbosacral radiculopathy
- Avascular necrosis
- Osteoarthritis

Diagnosis

Diagnosis is usually made by clinical examination. Radiographs may help rule out other conditions.

The role of ultrasound and MRI is unclear and usually not required for diagnosis.

Treatment

Most patients improve with conservative management:
- Rest
- Iliotibial band and tensor fascia lata stretching
- Gluteal muscle strengthening
- Anti-inflammatory drugs
- Iontophoresis
- Ultrasound
- Injection of local anesthetic (5 mL of 1% lidocaine 10 mg/mL) into the point of maximal tenderness

Surgical management may be offered following failed conservative management. The iliotibial band is released by a cruciform incision with or without debridement of the trochanteric bursa. The iliotibial band may also be Z-lengthened or an ellipse of tissue can be excised.

Iliotibial band friction syndrome

The iliotibial band friction syndrome (ITBFS), an overuse injury, is characterized by pain on the outer aspect of the knee due to irritation and inflammation of the distal portion of the iliotibial band as it crosses the lateral femoral epicondyle. This is seen in long-distance runners, cyclists, and other endurance athletes.

Friction (or impingement) occurs predominantly in the stance phase, between the posterior edge of the iliotibial band and the underlying lateral femoral epicondyle. Downhill running predisposes the runner to ITBFS because the knee flexion angle at footstrike is reduced.

There is a higher incidence where long-distance running is in vogue, or where the climate is cool and running surfaces are slippery.

History and examination

Pain is usually poorly localized over the lateral aspect of the knee, is aggravated by running long distances or excessive striding, and is more severe running downhill. Pain may be relieved by walking with a stiff or a straight knee.

Point tenderness is about 2 cm above the joint line when the knee is flexed at 30° and palpated over the lateral femoral epicondyle.

Flexion and extension of the knee may produce a crepitus.

Pain is worse during weight-bearing flexion and extension. Pain is typically worse at the 30° while flexion is occurring.

The differential diagnosis includes knee pathologies such as meniscal tears, ligament injuries, and loose bodies.

Diagnosis

Diagnosis is usually clinical and diagnosis including radiographs and MRI scan help in ruling out other pathologies but cannot positively confirm ITBFS.

Treatment

Conservative treatment is effective in most cases and includes the following:

- Reduction of activity
- Oral anti-inflammatories
- Ice, heat, ultrasound, and/or electrical stimulation
- Stretching exercises to address any excessive ITB tightness; hip flexion tightness or contracture will need to be stretched before the ITB can be adequately stretched

Physical therapy in combination with analgesic/anti-inflammatory medication is the optimum combination. Some clinicians recommend injections of local anesthetic and corticosteroid.

Surgery may be offered to patients who are resistant to conservative management. It is performed with the knee held in 30° of flexion and consists of cruciform incision of the iliotibial band or a limited resection of a small triangular piece at the posterior part of the iliotibial band covering the lateral femoral epicondyle. Prognosis is good with low morbidity and quick return to sports.

Thigh contusion

For anatomy of thigh muscles see Figure 7.4.

Proximal thigh contusions are common athletic injuries, particularly in contact sports, as a result of direct trauma. The muscle is compressed between the external force and the subjacent femur. Severe injuries result in large hematomas that limit range of motion (ROM).

There is often significant hemorrhage and swelling.

History and examination

Classification[1] (ROM assessed at 12–24 hours after the event):
- *Mild thigh contusions:* active ROM of the knee >90°
- *Moderate thigh contusions:* active ROM of the knee 45–90°
- *Severe thigh contusions:* active ROM of the knee <45°

Treatment

Initial management for an anterior thigh contusion involves rest, immobilization with the knee in flexion, ice, and compression to maintain motion and minimize hematoma formation.
- Weight bearing is limited until the patient regains good quadriceps muscle control and 90° of pain-free knee motion.
- Functional rehabilitation and nonimpact sports are allowed when ROM has reached 120° and there is no residual muscle atrophy.
- Return to full activity: normal strength and ROM (3 weeks). More severe injuries may have a longer recovery time.

Average disability time is 13 days for mild contusions, 19 days for moderate contusions, and 21 days for severe contusions.

If there is a major hematoma and if an athlete struggles to regain motion, refer to an orthopedic surgeon or a radiologist for evacuation or aspiration of the hematoma. MRI or ultrasound scan will demonstrate the size and location of the hematoma. The aspiration can be performed under ultrasound guidance with aseptic technique.

Protect the involved area with padding to avoid repeat injury.

Complications

Development of myositis ossificans depends on the severity of the initial injury. It is more likely with repeated trauma. This process may appear histologically similar to that of osteosarcoma, but the history is usually distinct and the periphery of a myositis ossificans lesion is mature (see Myositis ossificans, p. 242).

Loss of ROM and loss of functional outcome can occur.

Indomethacin may be useful for prevention of myositis.

☛ Monitor closely high-energy contusions for thigh and gluteal compartment syndromes in acute stages. Emergency fasciotomy may be rarely required, but serial examinations are an absolute requirement.

---

1 Ryan JB, Wheeler JH, Hopkinson WJ, et al. (1991) Quadriceps contusions. West Point update. *AM J Sports Med* **19**(3), 299–304.

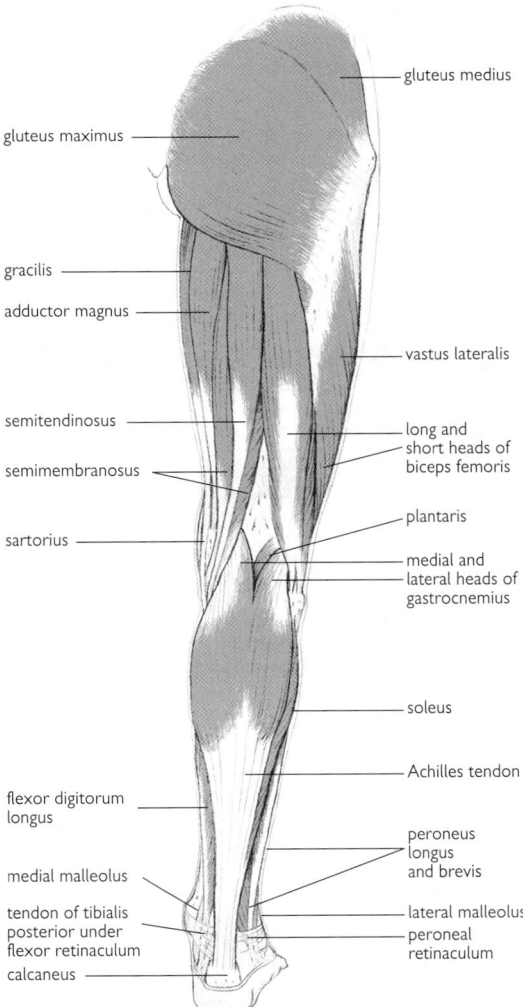

Figure 7.4 Muscles at the back of the lower limb. Reproduced with permission from Mackinnon P, Morris J (2005). *Oxford Textbook of Functional Anatomy*, Vol. 1. Oxford, UK: Oxford University Press. ©2005.

Myositis ossificans

This is usually a self-limiting condition in which a mass of heterotopic bone forms within the soft tissues. The term is a misnomer, as the muscle is not inflamed, and the process is not limited to the muscle. Other descriptive terms include heterotopic bone formation, pseudomalignant osseous tumor of the soft tissue, extraosseous localized non-neoplastic bone and cartilage formation, myositis ossificans circumscripta, and pseudomalignant myositis ossificans.

The condition develops within 1–2 weeks of direct trauma to the area or unusual muscular exertion. A history of trauma cannot be elicited in 50% of patients. It is more common in adolescents and young males.

Typical sites include the thigh (quadriceps femoris and adductor muscles), elbow (flexor muscles), buttocks (gluteal muscles), shoulder, and calf. The proximal portion of the extremity is more frequently affected than the distal part.

The pathological process includes muscle necrosis and hemorrhage after trauma. Histologically, there is marked proliferation of spindle cells with a well-recognized zoning phenomenon.

- The least differentiated tissue lies in the central zone.
- In the middle or intermediate zone, the osteoid is more organized and separated by a loose cellular stroma.
- The outer zone is the most mature, consisting of well-formed bone that may form a shell around the entire lesion. Cartilage formation may also be present.

Soft tissue or bone sarcomas do not exhibit a similar zonal phenomenon.

History and examination

There is usually pain, swelling, and stiffness of the surrounding joints. On examination, there is often a red, warm swelling, soft tissue tenderness and, in later stages, a hard mass is palpable.

Diagnosis

In the early stages, plain radiographs may be unremarkable except for nonspecific soft tissue swelling. A periosteal reaction may be seen if the lesion is juxtacortical. By 3–6 weeks there is faint calcification and at 6–8 weeks, a lacy pattern of new bone forms around the periphery of the mass. Complete maturation is usual in 6–12 months.

A bone scan is highly sensitive because of the profuse osteoblastic activity and bone formation, and is nonspecific, as soft tissue and bone tumors also show increased activity. The MRI findings vary according to the stage of the disease.

The differential diagnosis includes soft tissue sarcoma and osteogenic sarcoma.

Treatment

The extremity should be placed in flexion with a compression wrap for the first 24 hours to help decrease hematoma formation. Ice should also be applied in 20- to 30-minute intervals 3 to 4 times a day for the first 48 hours.

Initiation of oral anti-inflammatories (especially indomethacin 25–50 mg three times a day) should be instituted promptly for at least 1 week after injury as well. Gentle active movements may begin once pain improves.

Oral bisphosphonates, potent inhibitors of calcification, are effective in modifying the process of heterotopic ossification but should be used cautiously in females of child-bearing age because these agents' long half-life and teratogenic potential.

The area should be padded if the player returns to sports prior to maturation of the lesion. Players in contact sports should wear appropriate padding for myositis ossificans prevention as well.

Surgical resection is appropriate if the mass causes functional impairment and is best performed when the lesion has matured. Rapid recurrence occurs after resection of an immature lesion. If left alone, the mass may reduce in size with time and, in some instances, disappear.

Osteoarthritis (OA) of the hip

Osteoarthritis is a progressive, degenerative joint disease of the hip. The more correct terminology is *coxarthrosis*: *coxa* is hip, and *arthrosis* is degeneration of a joint. *Osteoarthritis* is a misnomer as inflammation is not the primary pathological process.

Overall, OA affects 13.9% of adults aged 25 and older and 33.6% (12.4 million) of those 65+, an estimated 26.9 million US adults in 2005, up from 21 million in 1990 (believed to be conservative estimate).[1]

In one study, ex-professional soccer players had a significantly higher prevalence of OA of the hip than an age-matched group of radiographic controls.[2] A Finnish study of international competing athletes showed increased risk of OA of the hip for all athletes, but those involved in endurance sports (long-distance running, cross-country skiing) were admitted to hospital care for OA at a later age than those involved in power sports (boxing, weight lifting, wrestling, throwing) or mixed sports (soccer, hockey, basketball, track).

Regular cyclical loading of joints is required to maintain normal articular cartilage composition, structure, and function. Prolonged static loading, repeated sudden excessive loading, or the absence of loading may, however, cause degradation of articular cartilage.

Repetitive joint use, under abnormal loading conditions, is a risk factor for OA. This includes the following:
- Participation in heavy physical activity before 50 years of age
- An elite level in high joint-loading sports
- Combination of heavy recreational physical activity with heavy occupational workload
- Continued use of the joint after injury in sporting activity

History and examination

Symptoms usually include pain, stiffness, deformity (late stages), and loss of mobility.

Clinical findings
- Muscle wasting
- Tenderness
- Deformity
- Reduced ROM (loss of internal rotation seen in early OA, normal range is 0–40°)
- Crepitus
- Alteration of gait

1 Lawrence RC, Felson DT, Helmick CG, et al. (2008). Estimates of the prevalence of arthritis and other rheumatic conditions in the United States. Part II. *Arthritis Rheu* **58**(1):26–35.

2 GJ Shepard, AJ Banks, WG Ryan (2003). Ex-professional association footballers have an increased prevalence of osteoarthritis of the hip despite not having sustained notable hip injuries compared with age matched controls. *Br J Sports Med* **37**: 80–81.

Diagnosis

Plain radiographs demonstrate the following features:

- Loss of joint space
- Osteophyte formation
- Subchondral cyst formation
- Subchondral sclerosis
- Erosion of bones, loose bodies, and subluxed joint are characteristic of advanced OA.

Treatment

- Analgesia
- NSAIDs
- Physical therapy: Strengthening exercises, ROM exercises, and functional training are beneficial.
- Oral chondroitin sulfate and glucosamine sulfate may help to alleviate pain in early OA of the hip.
- Osteotomy, total hip replacement, and hip resurfacing are the surgical options.

Osteotomy, if performed in the early stages, can delay the progression of OA of the hip through redistribution of load on the articular cartilage. Eventually, patients who undergo osteotomy may require total hip replacement.

Metal-on-metal hip resurfacing has allowed many young patients, usually younger than 65 years with OA of the hip, to return to recreational sports like cycling, rowing, swimming, jogging, and surfing. Competitive sports such as sprints and gymnastics are not recommended.

Hip resurfacing has inherent stability, which decreases the risk of postoperative dislocation of the hip.

Osteitis pubis

Osteitis pubis is a degenerative condition of the pubic symphysis and surrounding muscle insertions. It is usually secondary to overuse or trauma. It occurs typically in sports with sprinting, kicking, and sudden changes of direction, such as running, basketball, soccer, ice hockey, soccer, rugby, and tennis. Pelvic surgery and childbirth also predispose to osteitis pubis.

It occurs in almost any patient population, is self-limiting, and usually improves within 1 year. It is recurrent in 25% of athletes.

History and examination
- Exercise-induced pain or pubic tenderness
- Pain may also occur while walking, radiating to the peroneal, testicular, suprapubic, or inguinal region, and can also develop in the scrotum after ejaculation.
- Clicking may indicate vertical instability.

Clinical findings
- Tenderness over pubic symphysis, aggravated by pelvic compression
- Painful hip abduction
- Wide-based gait

The differential diagnosis includes adductor sprains, a hernia, and prostatitis in men. Sexually acquired reactive arthritis (SARA) can manifest as osteitis pubis.

Osteomyelitis of the symphysis pubis can occur concomitantly with osteitis pubis. A biopsy and culture of the affected area is necessary to rule out osteomyelitis.

Diagnosis

Radiographs are negative in the early stages. They may reveal widening of symphysis pubis, irregular contour of articular surfaces, and periarticular sclerosis in late stages. Flamingo views help demonstrate vertical instability of the symphysis.

MRI, CT scan, and bone scintigraphy can confirm osteitis pubis early.

Blood diagnosis such as white blood cells (WBC), erythrocyte sedimentation rate (ESR), and C-reactive protein (CRP) may be abnormal and raised. Blood cultures are necessary to rule out infection.

Treatment
- Rest
- Avoidance of pain-producing activity
- Analgesics
- Adductor stretching and eccentric strengthening after symptomatic improvement of pain

Stretching is performed at least daily, with flexibility being the main focus of therapy. Aquatic conditioning may be started at this time with the exception of frog-kicking, which uses the adductors extensively.

Sports-specific activities are added late in this phase, with offending motions added last.

Rarely, vertical instability of symphysis pubis can complicate osteitis pubis. This is surgically managed by arthrodesis with compression plating and bone grafting.[1]

Prognosis is good if tackled early. In chronic cases, injection of the symphysis pubis under image intensifier guidance with an injection of corticosteroid and local anesthetic may be of some value before proceeding to surgery.

1 Williams PR, Thomas DP, Downes EM (2000). Osteitis pubis and instability of the pubic symphysis. When nonoperative measures fail. *Am J Sports Med* **28**(3):350–355.

Sports hernia (Gilmore's groin)

Sports hernia (Gilmore's groin) is an overuse syndrome common in athletes participating in sports that require repetitive twisting and turning at high speeds, e.g., field hockey, ice hockey, soccer, and tennis.

Hip abduction, adduction, and flexion–extension with the resultant pelvic motion produce a shearing force across the pubic symphysis, leading to stress on the inguinal wall musculature perpendicular to the fibers of the fascia and muscle. Pull from the adductor musculature against a fixed lower extremity can cause significant shear forces across the hemipelvis. Subsequent attenuation or tearing of the transversalis fascia or conjoined tendon can be the source of pain.

Abnormalities at the insertion of the rectus abdominis muscle or avulsions of part of the internal oblique muscle fibers at the pubic tubercle, abnormalities in the external oblique muscle and aponeurosis, and entrapment of the genital branches of the ilioinguinal or genitofemoral nerves have been suggested as sources of pain.

History and examination

Unilateral groin pain of insidious onset that occurs with exercise and is aggravated by coughing and sneezing may radiate laterally, across the midline, into the adductor region, scrotum, and testicles. Occasionally, athletes report a sudden tearing sensation.

Clinical findings

- Local tenderness over the conjoined tendon, pubic tubercle, and midinguinal region, or a tender, dilated superficial inguinal ring
- Pain with resisted adduction, resisted sit-up, and reproducible with Valsalva maneuver

The differential diagnosis includes osteitis pubis, adductor tendinopathy, symphyseal instability, osteoarthritis, and tumor.

Diagnosis

Plain radiographs and bone scan can help rule out the above conditions. MRI may be useful to detect abnormalities within the muscles or pubic symphysis.

Treatment

Conservative management is occasionally effective for groin injuries, but results in a protracted clinical course. Surgery can be considered if conservative management fails after 6–8 weeks.

Conventional or laparoscopic herniorrhaphy may be successful, but recurrence of pain may occur depending on area of injury. Mesh reinforcement is often performed during these repairs.

Return to sports can occur within 6–12 weeks after specific rehabilitation targeted at abdominal strengthening, adductor muscle flexibility, and a graduated return to activity.

If adductor muscle pain is present preoperatively, adductor muscle release or recession is combined with herniorrhaphy.

Groin pain

Groin pain is a nonspecific descriptive syndrome that is difficult to diagnose because of the complex anatomy and the possibility of coexisting injuries.

The overall incidence of injuries causing groin pain varies but it is prevalent (2%–5%) in athletes participating in ice hockey, fencing, handball, cross-country skiing, hurdling, high jumping, and soccer (5%–7% of all soccer injuries). These sports involve side-to-side cutting, quick accelerations and decelerations, and sudden directional changes.

The diagnosis may be unclear in up to 30% of cases.

History and examination

Acute onset of groin pain may be due to muscle contusion, sprain, or bony injury including fractures and dislocation of the hip joint. In muscle contusions and sprain, the athletes suffer swelling of the affected part, which may show bruising. In complete muscle tears, a gap may be palpable between the ruptured ends. In athletes with bony injuries, there is pain, swelling, deformity, and inability to bear weight on the affected limb.

In patients with chronic groin pain, a careful history including the onset, inciting event, and aggravating and relieving factors should be obtained. It is important to consider the age of the athlete, as different conditions affect the groin and hip in adolescents and children compared to those in adults (see Tables 7.3 and 7.4).

Children and adolescents presenting with groin pain and pain on weight bearing of the affected limb should be evaluated to exclude septic arthritis, avascular necrosis of the hip, Legg–Calvé–Perthes disease, and slipped capital femoral epiphysis. Apophyseal avulsion fractures may present with acute groin or hip pain after an injury.

Tendon lesions are rare in children and adolescents.

Clinical examination

- Adequate exposure of the groin and hip
- Inspection of the symmetry and anatomic irregularity
- Palpation of the affected area for tenderness
- Assessment of the ROM of the joints
- Measurement for discrepancy of leg length (see Examination of the hip, p. 226).
- Evaluation of gait, including the performance of sprints, jumps, and activities that exacerbate the athlete's pain
- Neurological examination may reveal areas of numbness and motor weakness

Diagnosis

Plain radiographs may show fractures, avulsion fractures in adolescents, established osteitis pubis, later stages of stress fracture and osteomyelitis, slipped femoral epiphysis, or osteoarthritis.

A bone scan can help demonstrate osteitis pubis, stress fracture, osteomyelitis, synovitis, avascular necrosis, sacroiliitis, tendoperiosteal lesion, or muscle tear.

Ultrasound may show a muscle tear, hematoma, inguinal hernia, or bursitis. Nerve conduction studies may demonstrate ilioinguinal neuropathy or obturator neuropathy.

CT scans and MRIs may show disc pathology, radicular lesions, osteitis pubis, and other bone and soft tissue disorders.

Table 7.3 Common disorders producing groin pain in adults

Acute onset

- Muscle strains
- Contusions (hip pointer)
- Acetabular labral tears and loose bodies
- Proximal femur fractures

Insidious onset

- Sports hernias and athletic pubalgia
- Osteitis pubis
- Bursitis
- Snapping hip syndrome
- Stress fractures
- Osteoarthritis

Other disorders

- Lumbar spine abnormalities
- Compression neuropathies

Table 7.4 Disorders producing groin pain in children and adolescents

Acute onset

- Contusions (hip pointer)
- Avulsions and apophyseal injuries
- Proximal femur fractures

Insidious onset

- Avascular necrosis of the hip
- Legg–Calvé–Perthes disease
- Slipped capital femoral epiphysis

Avulsions around the ilium

The relative weakness of the growth plate at the apophysis of skeletally immature athletes predisposes them to a variety of avulsion fractures. Usually, they result from a violent eccentric muscle contraction.

Avulsion fractures of the ASIS are usually due to the following:
- Avulsion of the sartorius origin
- Avulsion of the tensor fascia lata origin

Avulsion of sartorius usually results from sprinting. The fragment is smaller and displaced anteriorly. Tensor fascia lata avulsion is due to twisting injury. The fragment is much larger and displaced laterally.

Avulsion of anterior inferior iliac spine results from forceful flexion of the hip by the rectus femoris. Avulsion of the ischial tuberosity results from forceful contraction of the hamstrings.

History and examination
- Severe, sudden-onset, and well-localized pain over ASIS
- Localized tenderness, swelling, and eventual ecchymosis
- Posture that reduces tension on the involved muscle
- Resisted contraction or stretching of the involved muscle worsens the pain.

Diagnosis
Plain radiographs, including comparison views, can usually identify the injury if the fragment is visible.

Treatment
Conservative
- Rest
- Analgesia
- Comfortable positioning with protected weight-bearing and gradual return to activity
- Strengthening is begun after full, pain-free ROM is achieved.

The periosteum and surrounding fascia often limit severe displacement. Reported disadvantages include a reduction in strength, and function, and, in some patients, the formation of a painful callus.

Surgery
Surgery is preferred to conservative management if:
- The size of the fragment is large enough to hold metal work.
- Displacement of the fracture fragment is ≥2 cm.

Return to play
Patients should not return to competition until full strength and motion are restored.

Piriformis syndrome

The sciatic nerve exits the pelvis below the piriformis muscle and above the short external rotators. Entrapment of the nerve at this point causes piriformis syndrome.[1] In piriformis syndrome, patients usually describe cramping or aching in the buttock and/or hamstrings. The causative factors include an abnormal tenseness or spasticity of the piriformis due to either trauma and overuse or muscle and nerve anomaly. In 6.2% of the population, the sciatic nerve passes through the piriformis muscle.

Tumors, vascular anomalies, and changes of gluteal muscles and nerves can predispose to piriformis syndrome. Post-traumatic piriformis syndrome may occur secondary to a contusion in the gluteal area. It occurs in middle-aged recreational athletes playing tennis, running, and cross-country skiing.

History and examination
- Pain is located maximally at the middle–upper part of the buttock during and after physical exercise.
- Pain radiates to the posterior thigh, calf, outer leg, ankle, and heel. There may be night pain.
- The leg may be held in semiflexion and in external rotation.

The differential diagnosis includes entrapment of the gluteal nerves, hamstring pain from entrapment of the posterior cutaneous nerve of the thigh, and sciatica.

Clinical findings
- Pinpoint tenderness on palpation at the upper middle gluteus; resisted internal–external rotation tests with straight leg may be positive.
- Straight-leg raise (SLR) test is negative.
- Reflexes, motor functions, and sensations are usually normal.
- Piriformis stretching is positive.
- Local anesthetic infiltration test is positive when the pain disappears.

Diagnosis
MR scan demonstrates the size and thickness of piriformis muscles, side difference, and anomalies.

Electromyography (EMG) examination may demonstrate distal radiculopathy or changes of proximal but not lumbar nerve roots. H-reflex (a monosynaptic reflex elicited by stimulating a nerve) may be delayed in piriformis syndrome when measured with hip in flexion, abduction, and internal rotation.

1 Yeoman W (1928). The relationship of arthritis of the sacro-iliac joint to sciatica. *Lancet*, ii, 1119–1122.

Treatment

Conservative management
- Muscle relaxation
- Stretching every 2–3 hours in either a supine or standing position with the involved hip flexed and passively adducted/internally rotated
- Pelvic posture correction, core stabilization, hip and sacroiliac joint mobilization, strengthening of the gluteal and pelvic musculature
- Refer to orthopedic surgeon or pain specialist; local anesthetic and a steroid injection into the piriformis muscle can be useful if physical therapy fails; it is important to avoid injecting the sciatic nerve
- Injection and physical therapy may be as effective as surgical treatment

Surgical management
- Offered after failure of conservative management
- Piriformis muscle is divided and sciatic nerve is released
- Light training in 1 month; intensive training in 2 months
- The results are good or excellent in 50%–85% of cases

Technique of injection of piriformis
This injection should only be undertaken by a specialist. The description of the technique is given only to help the reader understand the anatomy. The painful piriformis muscle can be identified by palpating the buttocks or by palpating transrectally in males and transvaginally in females.

A spinal needle or 25-gauge 1.5-inch needle is directly aimed at the examining finger. The location is usually through the sciatic notch and inferior to the bony margin; the most common trigger point is 1 inch lateral and caudal to the midpoint of the lateral border of the sacrum.

Snapping hip syndrome

In this syndrome there is an audible "snap" or "click" upon flexion and extension of the hip (*coxa saltans*—*coxa* is Latin for "hip," and *saltans* means "jumping"—a term to describe the feeling of the popping or snapping hip).

External causes include snapping of the iliotibial band or gluteus maximus over the greater trochanter. Internal causes are snapping of the iliopsoas tendon over the iliopectineal eminence, over the femoral head, or over the lesser trochanter.

Intra-articular causes include acetabular labral tear and intra-articular loose body.

External

History and examination

External causes are more common than other causes of snapping hip and occur more often in females.

An audible, painless snapping occurs with a sensation of the hip jumping out of place or giving way. The thickened posterior border of iliotibial band or anterior border of gluteus maximus muscle near its insertion catches the superior margin of the greater trochanter as the hip is flexed, adducted, or internally rotated, causing snapping.

The snapping is reproducible by passive hip flexion in an adducted position with the knee in extension.

Treatment

Reassure the patient that the hip joint is not subluxing or dislocating. Conservative management with rest, analgesics, NSAIDs, ice, ultrasound, and iontophoresis is usually successful. Stretching and strengthening exercises of iliotibial band are also useful.

Refer to orthopedic surgeon for surgical release or Z-plasty of iliotibial band if conservative management fails.

Internal

History and examination

A less common cause of snapping hip is internal. A snapping sensation is localized to the anterior part of the groin.

The snapping may be reproduced by extending and adducting the hip from a flexed and abducted position. The iliopsoas tendon shifts from lateral to medial over the iliopectineal eminence and/or the femoral head when the hip is brought from flexion into extension.

Diagnosis

Ultrasonography during hip motion may demonstrate the tendon subluxation. An MRI scan will help demonstrate a thickened tendon and fluid in the iliopsoas bursa.

Bursography may reproduce the symptoms associated with abnormal movement of the iliopsoas tendon and is diagnostic of internal snapping hip syndrome, but is invasive.

Local anesthetic injection (5 mL of 1% lidocaine 10 mg/mL) into the iliopsoas bursa and/or around the tendon may be diagnostic.

Treatment

Conservative management with rest, analgesics, NSAIDs, ice, ultrasound, and iontophoresisis is usually successful.

Physical therapy includes stretching of the hip flexors and rotators, then strengthening and gradual return to sports.

Symptoms refractory to physical therapy may be relieved by surgical lengthening of the iliopsoas tendon.

Intra-articular

History and examination

Trauma or synovial chondromatosis may predispose to intra-articular loose bodies.

Labral tears may cause groin pain. Incidence is high in patients with dysplastic hips.

Diagnosis

Plain radiographs help rule out bony pathology. MR arthrography can help confirm the diagnosis.

Arthroscopy of the hip joint may be both diagnostic and therapeutic in these patients and is considered the gold standard.

Hamstring injury

The hamstring muscle group is prone to strains, which mostly occur near the proximal musculotendinous junction. Hamstring injuries account for 30%–40% of lower limb injuries sustained in sports. The recurrence of hamstring strain is 33%.

Such injuries occur commonly in sports that require rapid active knee extension (e.g., sprinting, track and field, jumping, football, soccer, rugby) and in sports where there is muscle contraction at a position of maximal muscle lengthening (e.g., martial arts, dance, water-skiing).

The mechanism of injury is usually a passive stretch or a protective eccentric action (muscle develops tension while lengthening) to the hamstring muscles decelerating the lower leg.

Predisposing factors for hamstring injuries include the following:

Extrinsic factors
- Warm-up
- Fatigue
- Fitness level and training modalities

Intrinsic factors
- Eccentric strength deficits (muscle unable to develop tension)
- Flexibility
- Age
- Joint dysfunction
- Immobilization and rehabilitation of injured muscle

History and examination

There may be sudden onset of sharp posterior thigh pain. This may be associated with an audible "pop," resulting in immediate disability.

On examination, there may be bruising on the posterior thigh localized to the site of injury, or it may be more diffuse. There is tenderness on palpation and muscle spasm over the hamstring musculature. In complete proximal ruptures, a palpable defect is present proximally, and the muscle belly is prominent distally.

Diagnosis

- *Plain radiograph:* to exclude bony avulsion from ischial tuberosity
- *Ultrasound scan:* dynamic method, useful for diagnosis and follow-up
- *MRI:* better details

Treatment

Conservative
- Rest the limb to prevent further injury.
- Ice: apply as soon as possible as it helps prevent further bleeding and swelling and alleviates pain. Apply ice for ≤20 minutes for every 2 hours for the first 48–72 hours.
  Avoid direct contact of ice with skin to prevent ice burns. Crushed ice in a plastic bag, commercial cold packs, wrapping the ice in a damp towel, or bags of frozen peas are different suggested modes of applying ice.

- Compression
- Elevation helps reduce hematoma formation and limits tissue damage.
- Active ROM exercises within limits of pain tolerance after 1–5 days depending on the severity of injury
- Mobilize the patient with crutches until pain free.

Inflammation is essential for the process of healing, but some authors feel the body may overshoot the inflammatory response to injury. NSAIDs, by their anti-inflammatory effect, may or may not delay healing. No additive effect on healing of acute hamstring injuries was found when diclofenac was added to standard physiotherapeutic modalities in a double-blind placebo controlled trial.[1] Therefore, NSAIDs may be of limited benefit in these injuries.

Corticosteroid injections have also been used immediately after injury, but their use remains controversial.

Physical therapy

Early immobilization is suggested to accelerate the formation of a granulation tissue matrix and can hasten healing. Prolonged complete immobilization will result in muscle atrophy, loss of strength and length, and inelastic scar formation (to be avoided).

In the first 4 weeks following injury, physical therapy is focused on strengthening, improving ROM, and flexibility:

- Passive static stretching is begun.
- Warm up the muscle tissues prior to stretching and exercising.
- Strengthening exercises are to be initiated by an expert therapist, within the available pain-free ROM.
- Later, concentric exercises with resistance, increasing gradually as tolerated, should be started.
- The next stage is the inclusion of high-speed, low-resistance isokinetic exercises.
- Resistance is increased gradually, while exercise speed is decreased.
- The patient then progresses from concentric to eccentric strengthening exercises.

After 4 weeks, stretching and strengthening exercises are continued to maintain flexibility and an adequate hamstring-to-quadriceps strength ratio. Strength testing can be performed using isokinetic exercise equipment.

A rehabilitation program consisting of progressive agility and trunk stabilization exercises is more effective than a program emphasizing isolated hamstring stretching and strengthening for promoting return to sports and preventing injury recurrence in athletes suffering an acute hamstring strain.[2]

1 Reynolds JF, Noakes TD, Schwellnus MP, et al. (1995). Non-steroidal anti-inflammatory drugs fail to enhance healing of acute hamstring injuries treated with physiotherapy. *S Afr Med J*, **85**(6):517–522.
2 Sherry MA, Best TM (2004). A comparison of 2 rehabilitation programs in the treatment of acute hamstring strains. *J Orthop Sports Phys Ther*, **34**(3):116–125.

Surgical management

The indication for surgery in an acute hamstring strain is a complete rupture at or near the origin from the ischial tuberosity, or distally at its insertion. These should be identified clinically by a large defect or from an ischial tuberosity bone avulsion with displacement by 2 cm on radiographs. In such cases, reattachment is indicated.

In chronic cases, tendinopathy results from scarring and abnormal healing. The diagnosis is clinical and confirmed by imaging (MRI). Surgical management is by longitudinal tenotomy of the injured hamstring tendon close to the insertion. The surgical results are usually good.

Return to play

The patient can return to play when the strength of the injured hamstring reaches 90% of the strength of the unaffected hamstring and when the patient has a full ROM. At least a 50%–60% hamstring-to-quadriceps ratio is desired.

Prior to return to play, sports-specific training maximizes recovery and minimizes chances for additional injury.

Return to competition can be allowed after 20 ± 7 days for grade I lesions, after 36 ± 15 days for grade II lesions, and after 45 ± 14 days for grade III lesions.[3]

Prevention

- Pre-exercise stretching
- Adequate warm-up
- Avoid block drills too early in the training season
- Thermal pants may help reduce risk of recurrent hamstring injury[4]

Identification of factors leading to injury and the development of appropriate preventative strategy to avoid re-injury are crucial.

Preseason screening may help identify athletes at risk according to deficits in skills, aerobic and anaerobic capability, general health, or musculoskeletal function, as these factors may predispose individuals to hamstring injuries.

3 Creta D, Nanni G, Vincentelli F (2004). Injuries of the hamstrings. The Rehabilitation of Sport Muscle and Tendon Injuries—International Congress 2004. Available at: http://www.isokinetic. com/ pdf_attivita/2004/2004_02.pdf
4 Upton PA, Noakes TD, Juritz JM (1996). Thermal pants may reduce the risk of recurrent hamstring injuries in rugby players. *Br J Sports Med* **30**(1):57–60.

Obturator nerve entrapment

History and examination

The obturator nerve (L2–4) is formed in the psoas muscle and descends within the muscle, emerging from the medial border at the brim of the pelvis. The obturator nerve divides at the obturator notch into anterior and posterior divisions in the obturator foramen.

The anterior division supplies the hip joint and adductor longus, brevis, and gracilis, with a sensory branch to the medial thigh. The posterior division supplies the obturator internus and adductor magnus.

Entrapment of the nerve may occur within the fascia as it leaves the pelvis, or by an obturator hernia or intrapelvic mass. There is usually pain and dysesthesia in the medial thigh, together with weakness of the adductor group, worsened by activity.

Examination is often normal, although there may be reduced cutaneous sensation over an area of skin along the middle of the medial thigh and/or weakness of adductors.

Diagnosis

Specialized neurophysiological tests or nerve blockade may confirm the diagnosis.

Treatment

Surgical release of the fascia overlying the nerve in the obturator foramen will release the entrapment. Neurolysis along the length of the nerve from the obturator foramen to the fascia between pectineus and adductor longus is required to ensure release.

Dislocation and subluxation of the hip joint

History and examination

Dislocation of the hip occurs only with considerable trauma, but subluxation may occur in adolescents with congenital hyperlaxity syndrome (or more rarely in those with significant neuromuscular impairment). Patients may describe a clunking, snapping, or popping in the groin followed by aching.

Athletes who report pain out of proportion to their injury should be evaluated for possible subluxation as blood accumulates in the joint but the capsule is intact and so pain continues to increase from time of injury.

Examination may be normal, although usually there is hypermobility and poor pelvic girdle muscle strength.

Imaging

Standard X-ray series (pre- and post-reduction if necessary) may be followed by MRI, which may demonstrate the characteristic triad of findings: hemarthrosis, a posterior acetabular lip fracture or posterior labral tear, and an iliofemoral ligament disruption.

The presence of a significant hemarthrosis may warrant aspiration under fluoroscopy to decrease intracapsular pressure to in turn decrease the risk of avascular necrosis.

Treatment

Relocation (if dislocated) followed by strengthening and stability exercises is usually successful in treating dislocations.

Surgical intervention may be required to address labral pathology, loose bodies, and/or joint stabilization. Surgery should be delayed if possible for at least 6 weeks so repeat MRI can be performed to rule out early avascular necrosis prior to placing the hip in traction.

Femoroacetabular impingement (FAI)

History and examination

FAI is becoming a more commonly recognized entity in athletics. Athletes may have predisposing factors in childhood such as slipped capital femoral epiphysis or Perthes disease. Impingement can occur as a result of femoral-sided impingement (cam impingement), acetabular rim impingement (pincer impingement), or a combination of both.

Patients commonly have a component of both in producing FAI. Labral tears with or without mechanical symptoms may accompany FAI. Patients usually present with atraumatic anterior hip pain with activity of gradual onset. There is usually no history of recent trauma, although remote trauma may be of significance.

Examination may reveal pain upon internal rotation of the hip and decreased ROM if impingement is moderate to severe. Mechanical symptoms may be reproduced if labral pathology is present. Gluteus weakness is also common.

Imaging

X-ray may reveal spurring, decreased joint space, and sclerosis. MRI arthography is helpful to evaluate bony edema and labral pathology.

Treatment

Mild impingement may be treated with NSAIDs and physical therapy and gradual return to activity. Labral tears may need arthroscopic debridement. Open surgical femoral neck decompression may be needed in more advanced cases to restore motion and function in cam impingement whereas arthroscopic acetabular resection is needed to reduce pincer impingement.

Patients can return to a previous level of activity in 4–6 months depending on severity of surgical intervention.

Stress fractures of the pubic rami

History and examination

Pelvic stress fractures, most frequently involving the pubic rami, account for 1%–2% of stress fractures and can be serious. They may arise from overuse (fatigue fractures) or subnormal bone strength (insufficiency fractures).

Patients usually describe a severe, deeply felt pain in the groin, and possibly the perineum, of gradual onset. The symptoms may follow an increase in training load or, occasionally, with minimal or no trauma during a long-distance race in an osteoporotic individual.

Weight bearing is painful, and pain occurs at rest and at night. A sudden worsening may indicate a completion of the fracture. The patient must be advised to rest and have the problem investigated urgently.

Diagnosis

The most common stress fracture is of the pubic rami. As with all stress fractures, the diagnosis can be made by plain X-ray after 3 weeks, but earlier on technetium bone scan or MRI scan.

Management

Rest is essential, in the expectation that the fracture will heal without complication. Patients should be non–weight bearing with crutches while symptoms persist. Athletes can participate in non–weight-bearing sports when the stress fracture has settled sufficiently to allow walking.

The usual course of treatment is 6–12 weeks.

Consideration of bone density testing may be done in females with repeated stress injuries of the pelvis or proximal femur.

Calcific tendinopathy of the hip

History and examination

Calcification at the site of origin of one or more muscles of the thigh, most commonly the rectus femoris, gluteus maximus, or vastus lateralis, is rare.

There may be severe groin pain and limitation of movement (due to pain), without a history of trauma. On examination, there may be pain-induced global limitation of movement and/or pain on resisted testing of affected muscle groups.

Diagnosis

Confirmation is on X-ray or ultrasound.

Treatment

Treatment consists of relative rest, analgesics or NSAIDs, ultrasound, shock wave therapy, and, if necessary, image-guided local corticosteroid injection.

Acetabular labral tears

History and examination
The acetabular labrum is a thick rim of dense fibrous tissue that provides extra stability. The labrum can degenerate and tear, producing a flap that can interfere with the joint and give a deep, painful clunk during a range of activities.

There is an association between labral lesions and adjacent acetabular chondral damage, and labral disruption and degenerative joint disease are frequently part of a continuum of joint pathology.

On examination there may be impingement on internal rotation.

Diagnosis
Radiograph may show lateral marginal sclerosis in long-standing cases. MR arthrography of the hip may be helpful, particularly with lesions of the superior labrum.

Treatment
Arthroscopic trimming or repair is often successful. Corticosteroid injections have also been successful in alleviating symptoms in small tears without mechanical symptoms, although arthroscopy may still be warranted if symptoms persist.

Ischial (ischiogluteal) bursitis

History and examination
This may occur after a direct blow to the ischial tuberosity and cause localized pain and tenderness.

Diagnosis
It is confirmed with ultrasound.

Treatment
Relative rest, ice, anti-inflammatories, and cushioning are usually effective. A local guided injection of corticosteroid may be necessary. Surgical excision of the bursa is rarely necessary.

Sacroiliac joint (SIJ) disorders

History and examination

The SIJ is very stable with little joint movement. There is no single fixed axis of motion, with flexion–extension, translation, and rotation. While walking and running, the SIJs and ligaments absorb and dissipate stresses developed by twisting of the pelvis from flexion of one hip and extension of the other. Loss of mobility may cause stress fractures. There is debate as to whether the SIJ causes lower back and buttock pain in the absence of a true inflammatory sacroiliitis.

There may be joint strain or dysfunction following a direct blow to the joint, forceful torsion of the pelvis when rising from the crouched position, or sudden strong contraction of the hamstrings and/or abdominal muscles. But be careful in ascribing the cause, as "sacroiliac strains" are often subsequently found to be due to other pathologies. Forces on the sacroiliac ligaments are more likely to result in injury to the lumbosacral ligaments.

Pain may be felt in the buttock, groin, or thigh with activity and, in severe cases, at rest. Stress tests may exacerbate the pain.

Diagnosis

Radiographs of the SIJ are often normal in the absence of an inflammatory process. Bone scans can demonstrate sacroiliitis and stress fractures at the ridges of joint surfaces.

Where sacroiliitis is shown, it is important to look for the cause, including seronegative arthropathy or pyogenic infection.

Treatment

Muscle imbalance affecting the muscles of the thigh and abdomen and coexisting abnormalities in the lumbar spine should be addressed. Manipulation may help. A sacroiliac belt can provide some symptomatic relief.

If part of an inflammatory arthritis, sacroiliitis should be treated with analgesics, anti-inflammatories, physical therapy, other approaches indicated for the systemic condition, and, where necessary, image-guided local corticosteroid injection.

Injuries in children

Perthes disease

Etiology
- Avascular necrosis of the femoral head of unknown etiology

History and examination
- Presents at age 3–10, most commonly at 5–6 years
- Occurs more often in boys than in girls, at ratio of 4:1
- May have hip, groin, or sometimes knee pain, although pain is not a feature after the early stages
- May present with a painless limp

Diagnosis
- Radiograph changes depend on the stage of disease.
- In early stages, widening of the joint space may be the only sign. This is followed by patchy sclerosis, flattening, fragmentation, and collapse of the femoral capital epiphysis.
- Bone scanning is useful in early cases, when radiographs are normal.

Treatment
- Should be referred to a pediatric orthopedic surgeon for management
- Treatment varies according to the amount of the femoral head involved and age at presentation
- Includes modifying activity, use of braces, and, in severe cases, femoral osteotomy
- Bisphosphonates may be useful in early stages

Prognosis
- This depends on multiple factors, including age at presentation and amount of surface area involved.
- The younger the patient at presentation (<5 years of age), the better the prognosis.
- Risk of osteoarthritis depends on irregularity of joint surface.

Slipped upper capital femoral epiphysis

Posterior displacement of the upper femoral epiphysis on the femoral neck occurs in 1–3/100,000 Caucasian patients, two times more frequently in Afro-Americans, and four times more frequently in Polynesians. The male-to-female ratio is 2.5:1 and it occurs in girls at 11–13 years of age and in boys at 13–16 years of age.

It is bilateral in 20%–40% of patients and the contralateral slip occurs within 18 months of index slip. The predisposing factors include obesity, growth spurt, and endocrine abnormalities (hypothyroidism, renal rickets, pituitary deficiency, growth hormone deficiency).
- Displacement of the epiphysis before skeletal maturity
- Associated with delayed maturation and growth-plate stress (secondary to obesity)
- Hormonal factors may also play a role

Classification
Based on physeal stability
- *Stable*: able to weight bear with or without crutches
- *Unstable*: unable to weight bear, fracture-like symptoms

Based on duration
- *Acute*: <3 weeks (follows trauma)
- *Chronic*: >3 weeks
- Acute or chronic

Based on displacement
- Mild
- Moderate
- Severe

History and examination
There is sudden or insidious onset of pain and limp. At rest, the lower limb is held in external rotation. On further flexion, the lower limb goes into further external rotation. Internal rotation is restricted.
- Boys > girls (2:1)
- Overweight pubertal boy with pain and a limp
- Pain localized to the hip, groin, or knee
- Onset of pain usually gradual but may be acute
- Limitation of hip abduction, flexion, and internal rotation

Diagnosis
Radiographs demonstrate slip, which is graded 1–3. Obtain AP and frog leg lateral views. The severity of the slip is graded by the head–shaft angle on frog-leg lateral views. A mild slip is <30°, moderate is 30–60°, and severe is >60°. Subtle changes seen on radiographs before slip occurs include widening and irregularity of epiphysis.

CT scanning assesses the posterior displacement of the epiphysis and is useful for planning osteotomies.

MRI helps with early detection of avascular necrosis of the femoral epiphysis.

Treatment
Orthopedic referral for consideration of open reduction and stabilization is required.

The primary goal is to prevent further slip and promote closure of the physis. In situ pinning is used for mild and moderate slip. Osteotomy is for severe slip. Various techniques are described.

Complications
- Chondrolysis
- Avascular necrosis
- Subtrochanteric fracture
- Osteoarthritis

Prognosis
- Good if condition treated promptly with surgical stabilization
- If untreated, may result in avascular necrosis or premature osteoarthritis

Irritable hip

This is of unknown etiology but thought to be a transient synovitis, which may have a viral or autoimmune precipitant.

History and examination

- Child (usually aged 2–8) presents with pain or limp lasting from a few days to 1 week
- Restricted hip ROM due to pain
- Hip quadrant test (adduction, internal rotation, and compression with hip and knee flexed) is positive

Diagnosis

- Exclusion is diagnosed
- Radiographs, bone scans, and MRIs are normal.
- Labs are usually normal—may show mild elevation of WBC and ESR.
- It is important to exclude other more serious conditions such as Perthes disease, slipped upper capital femoral epiphysis, and septic arthritis.

Treatment and prognosis

- Rest and analgesia
- It may recur
- Prognosis is good, with no known long-term complications

Avulsion fractures

- Result of acute traction episode of the involved apophysis (by rectus femoris, hamstrings, or iliopsoas)
- The same injury mechanism in an adult would produce muscle tear

History and examination

There is history of a sudden onset of pain associated with rapid eccentric contraction of the involved muscle–tendon unit, for example, sprinting in the case of rectus femoris, or hurdling in the case of the hamstrings.

Diagnosis

Radiography of the involved apophysis is diagnostic.

Treatment

- Depends on amount of separation and the site involved
- Stretching and a graduated strengthening program combined with local physical therapy
- Graduated return to sports when symptoms have resolved
- Surgical reattachment is usually not necessary unless the bony fragment is displaced >2 cm
- There is good prognosis with adequate rehabilitation

Traction apophysitis of the ischial tuberosity

- The etiology is similar to that of other traction apophysitis.
- Repetitive traction of the hamstrings tendon at its origin at the ischial tuberosity

History and examination
This occurs in 12- to 16-year-old athletes who are involved in activities requiring forced hip flexion, such as dancing, soccer, hurdling, and the long jump.

Diagnosis
- Clinical
- No tests are required unless avulsion fracture is suspected

Treatment and prognosis
- Same management principles as traction apophysitis in other regions
- Prognosis is good

Knee

History

If acute
- Mechanism of injury
- Location and severity of pain
- Audible "pop" or "crack" at time of injury
- Ability to continue sport or activity
- Swelling
- Mechanical symptoms—locking, popping, or clicking
- Instability
- Past injury history
- Rule out acute infection

If chronic
- Duration of symptoms
- Association, if any, with prior trauma
- Effect on quality of life
- Previous treatments attempted
- Rule out systemic disease
- Rule out malignancy
- Rule out chronic infection

Examination

Inspection

Stance
- Limb alignment—normal is 5–7° of valgus
- Quadriceps atrophy
- Presence of effusion or ecchymosis
- Previous scars
- Presence or absence of foot arches
- Wear pattern of shoes

Gait
- *Antalgic gait pattern*: avoiding prolonged stance time on painful limb
- *Trendelenburg gait*: trunk lurches over limb with weak hip abductors
- *Steppage gait*: deep-knee flexion during swing to compensate for drop foot
- *Foot progression*: intoeing can be evidence of weak hip external rotators
- *Varus thrust*: on heel strike, tibia shifts laterally because of injury or attenuation of the posterolateral corner

Functional tests
- Inability to perform double leg squat can be due to patellofemoral pathology or quadriceps atrophy.
- Inability to perform single leg squat indicates poor core body strength.

Palpation

Anterior structures (see Fig. 8.1)
- Quadriceps insertion on patella
- Medial and lateral facets of patella
- Proximal, mid-, and distal portions of patella
- Bassett's sign: tenderness of the proximal patellar tendon in knee extension that is absent during deep-knee flexion suggests chronic patellar tendinosis
- Tibial tubercle
- Medial plicae

Medial structures
- Medial joint line
- Proximal, mid- and distal medial collateral ligament (MCL)
- Presence of abnormal meniscal cysts
- Pes anserinus tendons

Lateral structures
- Lateral joint line
- Biceps femoris
- Fibular head
- Iliotibial band, both over the lateral epicondyle and at Gerdy's tubercle

Posterior structures (see Fig. 8.2)
- Medial and lateral heads of gastrocnemius
- Presence of abnormal popliteal cyst

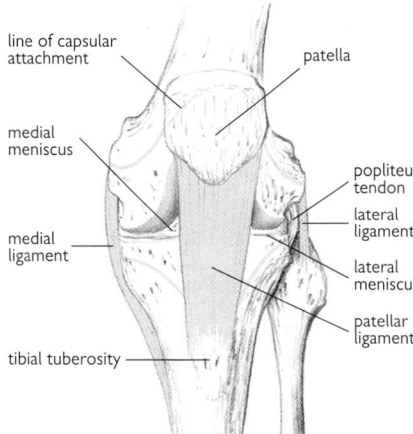

line of capsular attachment

patella

medial meniscus

popliteus tendon

lateral ligament

medial ligament

lateral meniscus

patellar ligament

tibial tuberosity

Figure 8.1 Knee joint: anterior view showing capsule attachments and ligaments. Reproduced with permission from MacKinnon P, Morris J (2005). *Oxford Textbook of Functional Anatomy*, Vol. 1. Oxford, UK: Oxford University Press. ©2005.

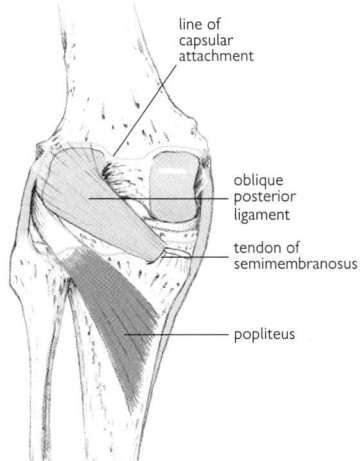

line of capsular attachment

oblique posterior ligament

tendon of semimembranosus

popliteus

Figure 8.2 Knee joint: posterior view showing oblique posterior ligament and attachment of popliteus. Reproduced with permission from MacKinnon P, Morris J (2005). *Oxford Textbook of Functional Anatomy*, Vol. 1. Oxford: Oxford University Press, ©2005.

Range of motion (ROM)
- Assess both passive and active ROM.
- Assess ROM of contralateral knee.
- Assess hamstring flexibility at 90° of hip and knee flexion.
- Assess the subject's hip joints and straight-leg raise to eliminate any possibility of referred pain, particularly in adolescents, where slipped upper femoral epiphysis should always be considered.
- If hyperextension of the knees is noted, consider checking for more generalized hypermobility syndrome.

Strength
- *Assess strength of quadriceps*: have patient resist flexion in both 0 and 90° of flexion.
- *Assess strength of hamstrings*: have patient resist extension in 90° of flexion.
- *Assess strength of hip abductors*: with hip abducted in the lateral decubitus position, attempt to adduct the leg. Prevent patient from opening hips, which recruits the powerful hip flexor muscles.
- *Assess strength of hip external rotators*: with hips and knees flexed to 90° in the seated position, attempt to prevent hip flexor influence.

Stability
Ligament injury grading
- *Grade 1*: pain felt on stressing ligament but no laxity.
- *Grade 2 (partial tear)*: pain and some laxity at site of injury, but a solid end-point at the limit of range.
- *Grade 3 (complete tear)*: pain and laxity with soft end-point at limit of range of movement. Clinically it may be difficult to distinguish between grades 2 and 3 because of pain-induced muscle spasm.

Anterior cruciate ligament (ACL)
- *Lachman's test*: with knee flexed 20°, an anterior load is applied to the tibia. The test can be performed in the prone position to help the patient relax their hamstrings.
- *Anterior drawer*: with knee flexed to 90°, the tibia is pulled anteriorly. Increased motion over that of the opposite side suggests ACL injury.
- *Pivot shift*: starting with the knee in full extension, valgus and internal rotation is applied while bringing the knee into flexion. Shifting occurs as a subluxated knee is reduced by this maneuver.

Posterior cruciate ligament (PCL)
- *Posterior sag*: resting position of tibia in the flexed knee is sagged posteriorly in the PCL deficient knee.
- *Posterior drawer*: with the knee flexed to 90°, the tibia is first pulled anteriorly to the normal resting position. Then a posterior force is applied to the tibia.
- *Dial test at 90°*: with patient in prone position and knees flexed to 90°, assess degree of external rotation compared to that of the contralateral limb. An increase of 15° or more suggests PCL injury.

MCL

- Instability to valgus stress at 30° of flexion suggests MCL injury.
- Instability to valgus stress in extension suggests injury to the posterior MCL, posterior oblique ligament, posteromedial capsule, and cruciate ligaments (see Fig. 8.3).

Lateral collateral ligament (LCL)

- Instability to varus stress at 30° of flexion suggests LCL injury.
- Instability to varus stress in extension suggests injury to the LCL and cruciate ligaments.

Posterolateral corner

- *Posterolateral drawer*: with knee flexed to 90°, apply posterior drawer combined with external rotation to the lateral tibial plateau. Increased motion compared to that of the contralateral side suggests posterolateral corner injury.
- *Dial test at 30°*: with patient in prone position and knees flexed to 30°, assess degree of external rotation compared to that of the contralateral limb. An increase of 15° or more suggests posterolateral corner injury.
- *Recurvatum test*: with knee extended and suspended by the great toe. Measure the degree of knee hyperextension and external rotation.

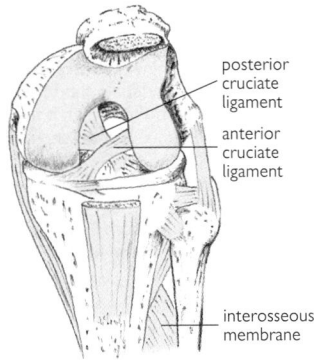

posterior cruciate ligament

anterior cruciate ligament

interosseous membrane

Figure 8.3 Cruciate ligaments, anterior view. Reproduced with permission from MacKinnon P, Morris J (2005). *Oxford Textbook of Functional Anatomy*, Vol. 1. Oxford, UK: Oxford University Press. ©2005.

Special tests

Menisci

Medial and lateral meniscal injuries are among the most common ortho-paedic injuries. History and physical examination are reliable for diagnosing acute injuries, although they are less reliable for degenerative tears.

McMurray's test

In this flexion–rotation test, the knee is flexed fully and extended, while internal and external rotation pressure is placed on it.

Positive tests are obtained with pain and/or palpable internal "clinking" felt by the examiner's hand on the joint line.

Apley's compression test

With the patient prone, the knee is flexed to 90°. A compressive load is applied as the knee is twisted in internal and external rotation.

Pain, clicking, or popping suggests meniscal injury.

Joint line tenderness

With the knee flexed to 90°, direct palpation along the joint line will elicit pain in the injured meniscus.

Iliotibial band (ITB)

A tight ITB can rub over and irritate the lateral epicondyle of the femur. Tightness can be assessed by Ober's test.

Ober's test

The subject lies on their side with the lower leg flexed at the hip. The upper leg is then extended at the hip with the examiner's hand resting on the pelvis to keep that neutral. The examiner then adducts the extended hip and the subject's knee should comfortably reach the couch. If the ITB is tight, the pelvis will move out of neutral or the knee will extend before it reaches the couch.

Tightness of the ITB can be confirmed on modified Thomas' test when the relaxed leg falls into external rotation at the hip.

ITB friction syndrome can be diagnosed by pressure from the examiner's thumb over the subject's lateral femoral condyle while the knee is repeatedly flexed and extended from 0 to 30°.

Diagnosis of knee injuries

Plain X-ray

Weight-bearing AP
- Look for joint space narrowing and osteophytes of the medial or lateral compartments.
- Look for tibial plateau fracture.
- Look for patellar fracture.
- Look for Segond fracture, an avulsion off the lateral tibial plateau that is pathognomonic for an ACL injury.
- If concerned about alignment, obtain full-length films of weight bearing.
- Stress views are indicated if there is suspicion for physeal injury.

Weight-bearing lateral
- Look for patellar fracture.
- Look for patella baja or infera.
Look for subluxation of the tibia, either anteriorly (ACL injury) or posteriorly (PCL injury).

Rosenberg views (weight bearing PA view with 45° of flexion)
- Look for osteochondral injuries, typically of the medial femoral condyle.
- Look for joint-space narrowing and osteophytes of the medial or lateral compartments (this view is often shows narrowing missed on AP).

Skyline view
- Look for joint-space narrowing of the patellofemoral compartment.
- Look for tilt or translation of the patella relative to the trochlea.

MRI scanning
MRI is used to assess soft tissue injury not seen on radiographs:
- Meniscal tears
- Ligament injury
- Chondral injury
- Patellar or quadriceps tendinopathy

Medial collateral ligament (MCL)

History and examination

The MCL is a strong, broad band of tissue on the medial aspect of the knee that resists valgus strain. It is often injured in football, rugby, and skiing.

The mechanism of injury is any forceful movement of the lower leg outward at the knee or a hard blow to the outside of the lower thigh, which causes the knee to buckle.

The MCL is closely associated with the medial meniscus, and the two structures are often injured in combination. Any forceful rotational element, in addition to a valgus strain, can rupture the MCL, medial meniscus, and anterior cruciate ligament—a severe injury described as O'Donoghue's triad.

Symptoms include pain, mild to moderate swelling on the medial aspect of the knee, joint effusion (not immediate), and feeling of instability (like a wobbly table leg). Injuries to the MCL are graded 1 to 3 according to severity (see Examination, p. 276).

Treatment

Most MCL injuries are treated by rehabilitation after initial PRICE management. Grade III MCL injuries or MCL injuries associated with multi-ligament injury often require surgical repair or reconstruction.

Rehabilitation after medial collateral ligament sprain

The time required to return to function is 4–6 weeks.

Early stage: days 1–7

Key aims
- Maintain ROM—flexion and extension
- Prevent vastus medialis (VM) inhibition, weakening, or atrophy
- Encourage heel–toe gait pattern
- Early mobilization

Strengthening and recruitment
- Static quads (with focus on activating VM)
- Simultaneous ankle dorsiflexion and gluteal recruitment may aid in activating the VM.
- Straight-leg raise
- Inner-range quads: With a ball under the knee, the athletes move their knee into full extension.

Mobility and stretching
- *Heel slides*: The athlete flexes and extends the knee joint through the full pain-free ROM.
- *Static hamstring stretching*: Often the most comfortable position after medial ligament injury is 10–15° flexion. Regular hamstring stretching is important to minimize the degree of secondary hamstring tightness.

Proprioception and gait
Weight transfers
While standing, the athlete slowly transfers weight onto the injured leg.

Heel–toe gait
In the initial stages (days 1–5) crutches may be needed.

Hydrotherapy
- Water at level of sternum
- Walking using heel–toe gait
- Weight transfers (as described above)
- Single-leg standing
- Mini-squats
- Knee flexion and extension in standing

Electrotherapy
- Electrical stimulation: The VM is stimulated using low-frequency electric current
- Electromyographic (EMG) biofeedback is reserved for cases of extreme VM inhibition.
- PRICE regimen should be initiated immediately after injury.

Before moving onto the middle stages of rehabilitation, the athlete must have reached all goals during week 1. The key milestones that MUST be reached by the end of week 1 are as follows:

- Good quad recruitment with minimal inhibition of the VM
- Ability to comfortably transfer weight onto the injured side
- Full knee extension

Middle stage: weeks 2–3

Key aims

- Enhance joint positional sense and proprioception
- Increase strength, ROM, and mobility
- Progress cardiovascular exercises

Mobility, strengthening, proprioceptive exercises

- *Weight transfers*: Standing on both feet, with weight predominantly on the uninjured side. Within the limits of pain, the patient transfers weight onto the injured side. This should progress until it is comfortable to stand solely on the injured side.
- *Single-leg standing/balance*: Standing on the injured side, the athlete balances, minimizing the number of touch-downs. Progress to doing this with eyes closed.

Once the athlete is able to stand comfortably on one leg with eyes closed, more advanced proprioceptive training can begin.

Single-leg standing

- Throw and catch a ball
- Vary type of throw, e.g., underarm, overhead, side pass, chest pass
- Vary the direction of the pass received, e.g., in front, from the side, overhead
- Vary the type of ball used, e.g., tennis ball, medicine ball

Sprinting action (upper body)

- Keeping control through the pelvis, the athlete drives arms forward and back as if he or she were running. To progress, the speed of the arm drives is increased while maintaining balance.
- Upper-body mirroring: The athlete must match the upper-body movements of the therapist.
- Increase complexity and speed of movements.

Dumb bell raises

- Progress from basic movements (bicep curl) to multijoint movement patterns (sword draw)
- Body-blade drills

Single-leg standing on dynamic surface

- Single-leg standing on a dynamic surface, e.g., mini-trampoline (rebounder), wobble board, balance pad/cushion, folded towel; progress as for basic single-leg stands

Progressive strengthening
This requires near full ROM, particularly through dorsiflexion (DF).
- Mini-squats: Ensuring an equal distribution of weight, the athlete should perform a 50% squat (to 45° knee flexion).
- Drop squats: As for a mini-squat, except the speed is increased while maintaining control
- Single-leg squats
- Lunges: Progress to multidirectional lunges.

All of these exercises can be progressed by increasing the demand on the neuromuscular system, e.g., the athlete must perform a single-leg squat on a dynamic surface.

Strength
A measurement of isokinetic knee flexion or extension might be the gold standard at this stage. However, there are a number of simple tests that can act as a good benchmark:
- Number of heel raises/minute (compare to uninjured leg)
- Number of calf raises/minute (compare to uninjured leg)

Balance/proprioception—as for ankle rehabilitation
- Single-leg stand
- Single-leg stand with eyes closed
- Single-leg stand with eyes closed and neck extended
- Wobble board

If the athlete loses balance during the test, they must tap the ground with the uninjured foot. The number of touch-downs/minute is recorded.

Cardiovascular
Biking, cross-training, and an upper-body ergometer are commonly used.

End stage: weeks 3–6
To progress to the end stages of rehabilitation, the athlete must have full pain-free knee flexion, have a good baseline of strength through knee flexion and extension, be able to perform complex proprioceptive exercises in a pain-free state, and have good lumbopelvic and lower-body control and alignment during squatting and advanced proprioceptive exercises.

As for the end stages of ankle rehabilitation, the focus should become less joint specific and more sports specific.

Strength and conditioning
This may be progressed as follows:
- Squat
- Dead lift
- Clean
- Snatch

Ideally, the athlete should begin using the barbell only. Form should be monitored by a trainer or coach. The weight should be increased accordingly, building to the athlete's pre-injury levels.

Running

Prerequisites are as follows:
- Full ankle ROM
- The subject is able to perform march walks and advanced proprioception with good control in a pain-free state.
- Straight-line running:
  - Light jog, building from 30% to 50%; build up to 10–30 minutes
  - Begin progressive running

Running should be on a flat surface, with cones dividing acceleration, maintenance, and deceleration stages.

For the first session, athletes should accelerate from a standing start, up to 60% over the first 30 minutes. They should then aim to maintain this pace over the next 30 minutes, before decelerating slowly to a complete stop. They should build to 90%.

This rehabilitation can be progressed by decreasing the acceleration distance and increasing the maintenance distance, as shown in Table 8.1.

Running exercises
- Curved running
- Figure-eight running
- Shuttles (doggies)
- Run stops: From a 60% run, the athlete must come to a complete stop within 5 steps. To progress, increase the speed of the run and minimize the number of steps.
- Run to lunge: From a 60% run the athlete must come to a complete stop in a lunge position.
- 45° cuts
- 90° cuts
- Spins: Running at 50% the athlete must spin 360° without slowing down.
- T shuffles
- Ladder and cone agility drills

Plyometric exercises

Throughout all plyometric exercises, the athlete is encouraged to keep a "soft" knee, using hips, knees, and ankles to cushion the impact. The athlete's ability to avoid "corkscrewing" by keeping good pelvic, hip, knee, and toe alignment will act as a good guide for their progress.
- 2–1 (two legs to one): Standing in a stationary position the athlete jumps vertically to land on the injured side.
- Hop scotch: This involves multiple 2–1's while moving forward.

Table 8.1 Progression of running program

Acceleration	Maintenance	Deceleration
20 m	40 m	20 m
10 m	30 m	20 m
10 m	40 m	20 m

- 90, 180, 270, 360° rotations: From a stationary position, the athlete jumps vertically and turns 90° clockwise and anti-clockwise before landing.
- Jump–land (from height)
  - Using two foot landing
  - Athlete rotates 45° in the air before landing—add 90 and 180° rotation
  - Single-leg landing
  - Landing on dynamic surface
  - Immediately catching a ball on landing
  - Therapist adds a light perturbation on landing

Field testing

If available, field test results should be compared with preseason or normative data. Useful tests might include the following:

- 10 m, 20 m, 30 m sprint times
- 150 test
- T-shuffle agility drill
- Vertical jump
- Standing broad jump
  - Jumping forward from two feet to land on two feet
  - Jumping forward from the injured foot and landing on two feet
  - Jumping forward from the injured foot and landing on the injured foot
- Lateral broad jump
  - Jumping laterally right or left and progressing as for a standing broad jump

Lateral collateral ligament (LCL)

History and examination

Thinner than the MCL, the LCL is a cord-like structure on the lateral aspect of the knee that resists varus strain.

The LCL is separate from the lateral meniscus and the two are not so often injured in combination as on the medial aspect. The LCL can be injured in combination with cruciate ligaments.

The mechanism of injury is varus loading of the knee and hyperextension.

Posterolateral complex injury can produce significant functional impairment and instability. The posterolateral complex consists of the LCL, arcuate ligament, lateral head of gastrocnemius, biceps femoris tendon, and musculotendinous junction of popliteus muscle.

Treatment

The LCL can be repaired or augmented, usually in association with surgery to the other damaged tissues.

Anterior cruciate ligament (ACL)

History and examination

The ACL is the primary restraint against anterior translation of the tibia. It is also a restraint against internal rotation.

The mechanism of injury is valgus force with a twisting motion (pivoting) or hyperextension of the knee. Most injuries are noncontact injuries. Contact injuries have a higher rate of associated injuries.

Women are thought to be particularly prone to noncontact ACL injuries. Women playing basketball and soccer are 2–6 times more likely than men to sustain ACL rupture. Theories as to why women are more at risk include the following:

- Smaller intercondylar notch
- Increased valgus alignment
- Neuromuscular control
- Hormonal effects on ligament laxity

History that includes a twist and "pop," immediate swelling, and inability to continue sport is 90% predictive for ACL tear.

Physical examination is accurate immediately after injury, but after onset of pain and swelling the accuracy is reduced to 70% accuracy. ACL laxity on clinical examination (see Examination, p. 276) does not mean the knee is necessarily unstable.

Acute ACL injury is associated with lateral meniscal injury. However, because both the ACL and the medial meniscus are restraints against anterior translation, chronic ACL deficiency is associated with a high rate of medial meniscal injury.

Treatment

ACL reconstruction

The ACL is generally not required for normal activities of daily living. Most people after rehabilitation can learn to compensate for the resulting instability. However, because ACL deficiency puts the knee at risk for subsequent medial meniscal injury, individuals who wish to be involved in jumping or twisting activities should consider reconstruction.

A torn ACL does not heal, nor is it amenable to repair. When torn, the ACL is thus reconstructed with tissue obtained from either the patient (autograft) or a cadaveric donor (allograft).

Advantages of autograft include increased graft strength and elimination of disease transmission. Advantages of allograft include avoidance of harvesting morbidity, shorter operative time, and smaller incisions. The most common graft choices are hamstring (semitendinosus and gracilis) and patellar tendon (middle third with attached bony blocks of patella and tibia).

The aim of reconstructive surgery is to restore stability and prevent future injury to the menisci. It has not been proven that ACL reconstruction can prevent long-term osteoarthritis. Reconstruction of an ACL tear is indicated for the following:

- Multi-ligament injuries
- Patients wish to continue activities involving twisting and pivoting
- Persistent instability despite rehabilitation

There is no benefit to early reconstruction; rather, surgery should be deferred until the patient regains full ROM and quadriceps strength. Pre-rehabilitation can be helpful to achieve these criteria prior to surgery.

ACL rehabilitation

Early mobilization with brace protection allows commencement of strengthening and proprioceptive exercises within days, rather than the original periods of weeks or even months.

Open chain exercises should be avoided as this places increased stress on the reconstruction.

With modern rehabilitation, return to sports is now usually possible (90%+) at 6 months postoperatively.

Posterior cruciate ligament (PCL)

History and examination

These injuries are less common than ACL injuries. PCL tears constitute <2% of acute knee injuries.

The PCL is the primary restraint for posterior movement of the tibia on the femur. It also acts as restraint of external rotation.

The mechanism of injury involves falling on a bent knee, hyperextension of the knee, or knee dislocation. The posterolateral corner may be injured in PCL tears.

Usually there is minimal swelling on examination. Posterior sag of the tibia may be seen (see Fig. 8.4).

Treatment

Isolated PCL tears can generally be managed conservatively using a predominantly quadriceps-strengthening program.

Surgical reconstruction is indicated if there is associated posterolateral corner injury.

PCL tears usually lead to long-term osteoarthritis.

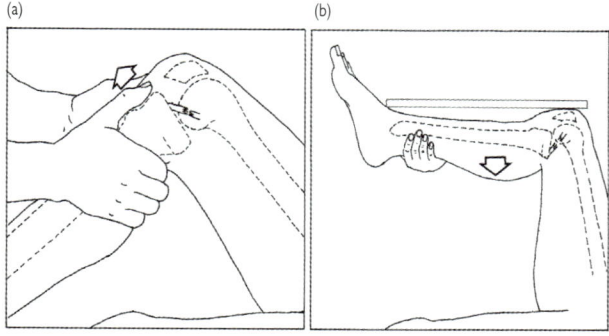

Figure 8.4 (a) Anterior "drawer" test; (b) "sag" test.

Meniscal injuries

History and examination

The menisci are fibrocartilaginous structures interposed between the femur and tibia that act as shock absorbers within the knee. When torn, the meniscus can cause mechanical symptoms of locking and popping as the torn edges flip and become interposed into the joint

There is a bimodal distribution of patients who sustain meniscal injuries. Younger patients with meniscal injury tend to recall a violent twisting motion associated with a "pop." This is because the meniscus is tough and flexible at this age, and requires significant force to tear. Older patients with degenerative, less ductile menisci often do not recall trauma or even pain, but note that mechanical symptoms occurred after activities (such as gardening) that require deep-knee flexion.

Meniscal injuries are not usually associated with effusion. The presence of effusion should prompt the clinician to look for associated chondral or ligament injury.

Articular cartilage injury

History and examination

Articular cartilage is a tissue composed of type II collagen that covers the ends of bones in a joint. It provides a smooth, near-frictionless surface for gliding. Injury to this tissue causes pain and swelling, as well as mechanical symptoms from unstable flaps or loose bodies.

Once injured, articular cartilage does not have the ability to heal. The natural history then is of progressive degeneration and arthritis.

Diagnosis

Injury is diagnosed on MRI scan or at arthroscopy. MRI scans with a 3T (Tesla) strength magnet are preferred for cartilage evaluation. Weight-bearing X-rays can show joint-space narrowing in advanced progression.

Treatment

Articular cartilage is avascular, which is one reason it does not heal when injured. Chondrocytes imbedded within articular cartilage receive nutrition through the synovial fluid in the joint. Gentle activity, which promotes exudation of fluid throughout the extracellular matrix of articular cartilage, is thus important to maintaining the health of the imbedded chondrocytes.

Partial-thickness tears of the cartilage can be treated with arthroscopic debridement, known as chondroplasty. This removes the unstable flaps and thereby aims to limit mechanical symptoms and pain.

Full-thickness tears of the cartilage can be treated with microfracture, autologous chondrocyte implantation, or osteochondral transplantation.

Microfracture is the controlled puncturing of the bone directly under the defect site using picks or awls. This creates a bleeding, which does not heal the cartilage or generate new cartilage. It does, however, create a fibrocartilaginous substitute that can fill the defect site and potentially improve symptoms.

Advantages of microfracture include the ability to perform the procedure arthroscopically on both knees in one operation. Disadvantages include limitation to smaller lesions that have good surrounding cartilage to protect the reparative tissue.

Autologous chondrocyte implantation involves harvesting of cartilage from the patient, isolation and expansion of the chondrocytes in a laboratory, and reimplantation into the cartilage site under a periosteal flap. Advantages include the potential to treat larger defects than those with microfracture, and possible regeneration of tissue with type II collagen, although this is controversial. Disadvantages include increased costs, need for a second procedure, and need for an open procedure.

Osteochondral transplantation involves taking a core of bone and cartilage, from either the patient or a cadaveric donor, and implanting it into the defect site. Advantages include replacement of the defect site with true articular cartilage, more reliable osseous integration, and (in the case of allografts) the ability to replace entire condyles. Disadvantages include technical difficulty, cost, and potential disease transmission with allografts.

Anterior knee pain

Anterior knee pain is a common presenting complaint in sports medicine. Multiple conditions can present as anterior knee pain, including patellar tendonitis, patellar tendinosis, medial plicae syndrome, patellar instability, and patellofemoral pain syndrome.

Tight hamstrings and iliotibial bands, weak hip abductors and external rotators, and flat feet all contribute to malpositioning and excessive strain on the extensor mechanism (see Fig. 8.5). Rehabilitation focusing on core and hip strengthening, hamstring and iliotibial band stretching, and the use of foot orthotics can significantly help most of these conditions.

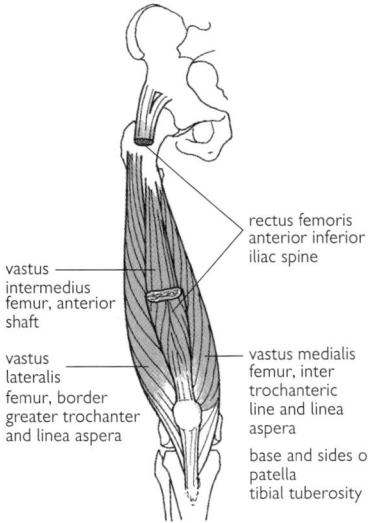

vastus intermedius femur, anterior shaft

vastus lateralis femur, border greater trochanter and linea aspera

rectus femoris anterior inferior iliac spine

vastus medialis femur, inter trochanteric line and linea aspera

base and sides of patella tibial tuberosity

Figure 8.5 Quadriceps femoris. Reproduced with permission from MacKinnon P, Morris J (2005). *Oxford Textbook of Functional Anatomy,* Vol. 1. Oxford, UK: Oxford University Press. ©2005.

Patellar dislocation

History and examination
- Usually a lateral displacement onto the lateral femoral condyle
- Often traumatic and associated with hemarthrosis
- Also in young girls with predisposing factors such as lower limb malalignments and generalized hypermobility

Treatment
The aim of treatment is to reduce the risk of recurrence with vastus medialis strengthening, although recurrent episodes will require surgery.

Hoffa's syndrome

History and examination
The infrapatellar fat pad, known as Hoffa's fat pad, is interposed between the patella and femoral condyle. It acts as a shock absorber against both direct impact and with extension of the knee. Unfortunately, the fat pad is highly innervated and can become quite painful when irritated (typically from a hyperextension injury).

Patients often complain of pain with full extension, which causes impingement of the fat pad between the patella and femur.

On examination, patients will have tenderness to palpation of the fat pad to either side of the patellar tendon. Also, they may have pain at the endpoints of extension.

Treatment
- Rest and anti-inflammatory medications, both NSAIDs and corticosteroids
- Ice therapy to reduce inflammation
- Ultrasound, iontophoresis and transcutaneous electrical nerve stimulation (TENS)
- Taping the superior aspect of the patella will tilt the patella and relieve pressure off the fat pad
- For recalcitrant cases, offer arthroscopic debridement of fat pad

Iliotibial band friction syndrome (ITBFS)

History and examination

ITBFS is also called "runners' knee." It is caused by friction of the iliotibial band (ITB) on the lateral femoral epicondyle (usually at <30° of knee flexion.

This syndrome causes pain over the lateral aspect of the knee during a run, especially on a cambered course. Tightness of the ITB may be present on Ober's test.

Abnormal biomechanics (e.g., leg length discrepancy), excessive training load, and downhill and distance running are other predisposing factors.

ITBFS is usually associated with bursitis at the site of pain.

Diagnosis

Diagnosis is usually made on clinical findings.

Treatment

- NSAIDs
- Myofascial tension massage to ITB
- ITB stretching
- Corticosteroid injection if bursitis is present
- Correction of biomechanical abnormalities and training errors
- For recalcitrant cases, treat with surgical release or lengthening of the ITB

Patellofemoral pain (syndrome)

Patellofemoral pain is a vague, aching pain over the anterior aspect of the knee. It is aggravated by activity, especially distance running, squatting, lunging, going up or down stairs, or sitting for long periods.

The patient may describe a "clicking" or "grating" behind the patella on knee movement. The knee may give way due to pain and quadriceps inhibition.

Clinical features may include tenderness of the medial or lateral facets of the patella, a small effusion, crepitus and stiffness of patellar movement, and wasting of vastus medialis (VM). There may be signs of squinting patellae, hyperrecurvatum, tibial torsion, or hyperpronation in standing.

The usual causes are as follows:
- Overuse (excessive loading of patellofemoral joint [PFJ]).
- Lower limb malalignment—squinting patellae and femoral anteversion, hyperpronation (↑ PFJ forces)
- Patellar maltracking (↓ PFJ contact area)

Patellar tracking

During knee flexion, the patella moves from lateral to medial to travel within the intercondylar notch of the femur at the end of range. The movement of the patella is dependent on passive and active restraints.

Any imbalance of these restraints is most likely to cause the patella to track more laterally. During episodes of loading, patellofemoral symptoms may arise as a result.

Some typical causes of this so-called patellar maltracking are as follows:
- Tightness of passive restraints (iliotibial band, lateral retinaculum)
- Weakness of active restraints (vastus medialis obliquus [VMO])
- Weakness of gluteus medius muscles, leading to increased internal rotation at the hips
- Muscle tightness—hamstrings and quadriceps

If patellofemoral pain occurs on sitting, it is unlikely to be caused by maltracking. Retropatellar pressure is more likely.

The Q angle

This refers to the angle at the junction between two lines drawn from the anterior superior iliac spine to the middle of the patella and a line drawn to the same point from the tibial tubercle (normal is <20° and is increased in femoral anteversion).

A greater than normal angle is associated with patellar maltracking.

Females tend to have a greater Q angle than that of males, which will also predispose them to patellar maltracking and thus patellofemoral pain.

Diagnosis

Diagnosis is made usually on clinical findings.

Treatment

The primary aim is to attempt to correct any abnormal biomechanics:
- Manual treatment and stretching of ITB, hamstrings, gastrocnemius and rectus femoris

- Patellar taping to correct any malposition or tilt can reduce pain by up to 50%
- VM strengthening (± biofeedback)
- Gluteus medius strengthening
- Orthotics to correct hyperpronation
- Proprioception
- Modification of training regime to avoid overuse

Surgery for patellofemoral pain syndrome is not common because of improved rehabilitation techniques.

Patellar tendinopathy

History and examination

Patellar tendinopathy is also known as "jumper's knee." It is an overuse injury.

The underlying pathology is a degenerative tendinosis, not an inflammatory tendonitis. Typically it is seen at the deep origin of the patellar tendon off the distal pole of the patella.

On physical examination, tenderness to palpation is often more pronounced with the knee in extension than in flexion. This is because, in flexion, the superficial layer is pulled taut and shields the affected deeper portion of the patellar tendon (Bassett's sign).

The main complaint is of anterior knee pain aggravated by jumping, bounding, or hopping. Onset is usually insidious, but tears can present acutely.

Eccentric contraction usually reproduces symptoms.

Diagnosis

Ultrasound and MRI scanning are both very effective at confirming the diagnosis.

Treatment

- Often very prolonged
- Physiotherapy—transverse frictions and progressive strengthening to include eccentric exercises
- Correction of biomechanical abnormalities and training errors
- For recalcitrant cases, surgical debridement can remove the degenerative tissue.

Osgood–Schlatter disease

History and examination

This disease involves a traction apophysitis of the tibial tubercle that affects boys more than girls (4:1). It presents between ages 10 and 14 (earlier in girls).

There is insidious onset of anterior knee pain (sometimes bilateral) in a child involved in running and jumping sports.

Pain worsens during and after activity, with difficulty kneeling and jumping.

Clinical findings
- Tenderness and possibly localized swelling over tibial tubercle
- Quadriceps may appear wasted, depending on duration of the symptoms
- May be some restriction in knee flexion
- Pain may be reproduced by resisted knee extension from the flexed position.

Diagnosis

These are not usually required. If performed, an X-ray will show overlying soft tissue swelling (diagnostic) and may demonstrate fragmentation of the tibial tubercle apophysis.

The only indications for X-ray in this group of children are as follows:
- If the diagnosis is in doubt
- If symptoms persist and calcification is suspected
- If an avulsion of the tibial tubercle is suspected

Treatment

- Treatment depends on the stage at presentation.
- A child who has pain with daily living activities will need to avoid running and jumping until the pain subsides.
- Children with minimal symptoms may be able to continue some running and jumping activities at a reduced level.
- Quadriceps and hamstring stretching program will decrease traction force on tibial tubercle.
- Biomechanical abnormalities such as hyperpronation and patella malalignment should be corrected with an exercise program, patellar taping, and orthotics.
- Quadriceps strengthening
- Gradual resumption of activity

Prognosis

Prognosis is usually very good. In about 5% of cases, calcification can develop adjacent to the tibial tubercle, which causes persistence of symptoms and inability to kneel and may require surgical resection.

It is important to reassure the child and parents that this condition does not cause long-term disability but it can be troublesome over one or two seasons during periods of rapid growth.

Sinding–Larsen–Johannson disease ("jumper's knee")

History and examination

- Traction apophysitis affecting inferior pole of the patella
- Less common than Osgood–Schlatter disease but similar presentation
- Pain localized to inferior pole of the patella
- Gradual onset of anterior knee pain exacerbated by activities that load the flexed knee, such as running and jumping
- Focal tenderness inferior pole of the patella
- Swelling rarely present
- Resisted knee extension from flexed position usually reproduces the pain
- Biomechanical factors such as hyperpronation, femoral anteversion, and patellar misalignment may be present

Diagnosis

- Not required

Treatment

- Similar to that in Osgood–Schlatter disease; prognosis is good.

Juvenile osteochondritis dissecans

OCD probably results from a combination of minor repetitive trauma and microvascular compromise affecting the subchondral bone and articular cartilage. The bone becomes sclerotic and fragmented, and loose bodies may form.

History and examination
- More common in boys than girls
- Average age at diagnosis is 13
- Present with knee swelling ± pain
- May or may not have history of injury
- May give history of locking secondary to loose body
- Differential diagnosis is inflammatory arthropathy

Clinical findings
- Effusion
- Tenderness usually localized to medial joint line
- Quadriceps wasting if symptoms prolonged

Diagnosis
- X-ray—look for irregularity; it is important to obtain tunnel views with 45° of flexion
- Medial femoral condyle 75%, lateral femoral condyle 20%, patella and trochlear groove 5%
- May also see loose body
- If the X-ray is normal but clinical history suggests OCD, an MRI should be performed to confirm the diagnosis.

Treatment
Treatment depends on the degree of involvement.

For lesions where the articular cartilage is intact, activity modification and rest are indicated. Cast immobilization may be considered for very large lesions.

For lesions with fluid seen on MRI underneath the lesion that communicates with the joint, retrograde drilling may stimulate blood flow and healing.

For lesions that have completely detached and become loose bodies, arthroscopy removal is indicated to relieve mechanical symptoms. Reattachment may be considered for very large and otherwise intact fragments.

Prognosis
Prognosis depends on the site and size of the defect and age at presentation. Prognosis is favored with younger age and skeletal immaturity.

Bipartite patella and patellofemoral pain syndrome

Bipartite patella results when secondary ossification centers at the superolateral aspect of the patella fail to unite.

History and examination

- Commonly asymptomatic and found incidentally
- Can sometimes be palpated
- May present with patellofemoral pain syndrome, i.e., anterior knee pain exacerbated by climbing stairs, squatting, and prolonged sitting
- May present with localized pain over superolateral aspect of the patella, where fibrous union between ossification centers lies
- Trauma may precipitate the pain, prompting incidental finding upon obtaining radiographs

Diagnosis

An AP radiograph will demonstrate the bipartite fragment.

Treatment

- Strengthening vastus medialis oblique
- Lateral retinacular releases
- Trial of medial patella taping
- If pain persists at the superolateral border of the patella, lateral retinacular release with or without excision of the bipartite fragment may be required.
- Bipartite patella rarely causes long-term disability.

Discoid lateral meniscus

When the lateral meniscus is D-shaped rather than the normal C-shape, it is predisposed to tearing.

History and examination

- May present with a painless clunking in the knee
- May present after a twisting injury, when child complains of lateral joint pain, swelling, clicking, and sometimes locking
- Examination is unremarkable if no tear has occurred
- If associated with a lateral meniscal tear, effusion is often present as well as restricted range of motion
- There may be a positive lateral McMurray's sign

Diagnosis

- X-ray may demonstrate subtle widening of lateral joint space.
- MRI will confirm diagnosis but is not usually necessary.

Treatment

- Treatment is not required if condition is asymptomatic.
- If discoid meniscus is torn, this usually requires excision of the torn lateral meniscal fragment and conversion of the meniscus to a C-shape.
- Discoid lateral menisci may be bilateral.
- After partial lateral meniscectomy, prognosis is favorable.

Ankle and lower leg

Examination of the ankle

Inspection

The ankle contains three joints:
- Talocrural joint
- Inferior tibiofibular joint
- Subtalar joint

With the feet in a symmetrical position, the subtalar joint is in neutral—neither pronated nor supinated. *Pronation* consists of eversion, dorsiflexion, and abduction of the foot. *Supination* consists of inversion, plantarflexion, and adduction of the foot.

Look for evidence of abnormal biomechanics:
- Excessive pronation
- Excessive supination
- Forefoot varus
- Forefoot valgus
- Rearfoot varus
- Rearfoot valgus
- Ankle equines
- Genu varum
- Genu valgum
- Leg length

When:
- Standing
- Walking
- Supine
- Prone

Palpation

Anterior structures
- Ankle joint
- Anteroinferior tibiofibular ligament (AITFL)
- Talus

Lateral structures
- Distal fibula
- Lateral malleolus
- Lateral ligaments—anterior talofibular ligament (ATFL), calcaneofibular ligament (CFL), and posterior talofibular ligament (PTFL)
- Peroneal longus and brevis tendons
- Sinus tarsi
- Base of fifth metatarsal

Medial structures
- Medial ligaments including deltoid ligament
- Tibialis posterior
- Flexor hallucis longus
- Sustentaculum tali

- Navicular tubercle
- Midtarsal joint

Posterior structures (Fig. 9.1)
- Achilles tendon
- Retrocalcaneal bursa
- Posterior talus
- Calcaneum

Active and passive movements
- Ankle dorsiflexion (10–20°)
- Ankle dorsiflexion can be restricted by inflexibility of gastrocnemius and soleus
- Minimum range of ankle dorsiflexion for normal locomotion is 10°
- Ankle plantarflexion (45–50°)
- Dorsiflexion and plantarflexion take place between the talus and tibia and fibula
- Subtalar inversion (10–20°)
- Subtalar eversion (5–10°)
- Inversion and eversion take place at the talocalcaneal, talonavicular, and calcaneocuboid joints
- Inversion is usually double that of eversion

Resisted movements
- Plantarflexion
- Gastrocnemius (knee extended)
- Soleus (knee flexed)
- Flexor digitorum longus, flexor hallucis longus (flex the toes against resistance)
- Dorsiflexion
- Tibialis anterior (dorsiflex the foot against resistance)
- Extensor digitorum longus (dorsiflex the toes against resistance)
- Extensor hallucis longus (dorsiflex the big toe against resistance)
- Inversion
- Tibialis posterior (invert the foot against resistance)
- Eversion
- Peroneus longus and brevis (evert the foot against resistance)

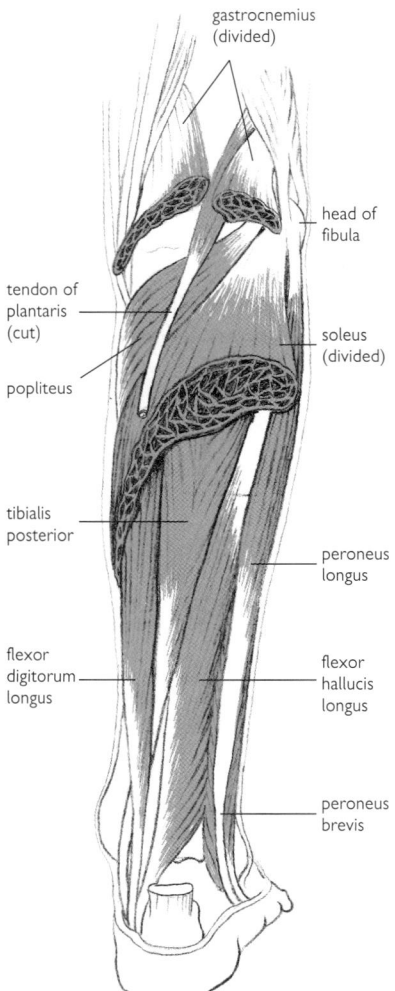

Figure 9.1 Deep muscles of the calf (plantaris may or may not be present). Reproduced with permission from MacKinnon P, Morris J (2005). *Oxford Textbook of Functional Anatomy*, Vol. 1. Oxford, UK: Oxford University Press. ©2005.

Special tests

Anterior drawer test

A positive anterior drawer test in plantarflexion implies injury to the ATFL. It is performed by holding the heel and pulling the foot anteriorly while applying a posterior force to the tibia. A positive anterior drawer test in neutral suggests additional injury to the CFL and possibly the PTFL.

Talar tilt test

The talar tilt test examines for CFL instability. It is performed by holding the calcaneum and inverting the talus on the tibia. A talar tilt of 15° or 5° more than the opposite ankle is positive.

Tinel's test

This test is performed by tapping under the medial malleolus. It is positive when shooting nerve pain or paresthesias occur. It is indicative of tarsal tunnel syndrome.

The squeeze test

This test is positive when compression of the proximal tibia and fibula precipitates distal pain suggesting an injury to the syndesmosis.

Biomechanical examination

Functional tests

- Proprioception
- Lunge
- Hop
- Jump

Ankle sprains are classified as follows:
- *Grade 1*: painful without instability
- *Grade 2*: mild instability
- *Grade 3*: complete rupture

Persistent painful ankle

Pain, swelling, and impaired function may persist for 4–6 weeks after an acute injury. Secondary injuries may be overlooked at the time of the original injury. With persistent symptoms, one should look for occult injury in addition to acute ankle sprain.

Functional instability resulting from inadequate rehabilitation is the most common cause. Other possible causes are listed below.

Osteochondral injuries

Initial radiographs may appear normal. Repeat radiographs or MRI are required for diagnosis.

Osteochondral injuries occur most commonly at the following sites:
- Superomedial talus
- Superolateral talus
- Tibial plafond

Fractures

Initial radiographs may appear normal. Follow-up radiographs or MRI may be required for diagnosis.
- Lateral talar process
- Anterior calcaneal process
- Posterior talar process
- Os trigonum fracture
- Avulsion fracture base of fifth metatarsal

Impingement syndromes
- Anterior impingement syndrome
- Anterolateral impingement syndrome
- Posterior impingement syndrome
- Capsular injury resulting in synovitis can present with anterior impingement on dorsiflexion
- Synovium or ruptured ATFL becomes trapped between the lateral malleolus and talus, provoking anterolateral impingement
- Posterolateral process fracture or os trigonum injury may require CT or MRI to confirm the diagnosis

Tendon dislocation and rupture
- Peroneal tendons
- Radiographs may demonstrate a small bone chip
- Resisted eversion in dorsiflexion precipitates tendon subluxation
- Tibialis posterior tendon
- Occurs with ankle dorsiflexion and inversion
- Subluxation may be demonstrated by resisted plantarflexion

Sinus tarsi syndrome
- Small osseous canal anterior and inferior to the lateral malleolus
- Pain from subtalar ligament injury and fat-pad necrosis
- Diagnosis confirmed by a local anesthetic injection into the sinus tarsi

Other causes

- Anteroinferior tibiofibular ligament (meniscoid lesion)
- Synovitis or ATFL scar tissue produces a meniscal lesion that impinges between the lateral talus and lateral malleolus
- Post-traumatic synovitis
- Calcaneocuboid ligament sprain
- A bony fleck may be seen adjacent to the cuboid
- Peroneal nerve or sural nerve injury

Acute ankle sprain

History and examination

Acute ankle sprains can occur in any sport but are most common in sports that involve a change of direction or jumping, e.g., football, rugby, basketball, netball, and volleyball.

The lateral ligament includes the anterior talofibular ligament (ATFL), calcaneofibular ligament (CFL), and posterior talofibular ligament (PTFL) (see Fig. 9.2). The medial or deltoid ligament is composed of four bands—three superficial and one deep. The interosseous ligaments include the anterior tibiofibular ligament, posterior tibiofibular ligament, and interosseous ligament.

The mechanism of injury is important; an inversion injury suggests lateral ligament sprain, and an eversion injury suggests medial ligament sprain. Compression may suggest an osteochondral injury.

Inversion injuries account for 70%–85% of all ankle injuries. They occur when the foot is plantarflexed and inverted. Inversion injuries lead to sprains of the lateral ligament complex including the ATFL, CFL, and PTFL.

The ATFL is most susceptible to injury. The CFL is injured in 40% of ATFL injuries. Complete tears of the ATFL, CFL, and PTFL result in ankle dislocation and are associated with a fracture.

The location of pain and swelling normally indicates the ligaments injured, most commonly the anterolateral aspect of the ankle involving the ATFL.

Ability to weight bear after the injury in patients <55 years old suggests a sprain and not a fracture.

Clinical examination includes palpation of the ligaments, tendons, and the lateral and medial malleoli, base of the fifth metatarsal, and proximal fibula to consider collateral injuries.

Diagnosis

Radiographs are required if the patient who cannot weight bear or has point tenderness, particularly over the malleoli, tarsal navicular, base of the fifth metatarsal, or proximal fibular.

Repeat radiographs should be considered if there is no improvement or progress is delayed. Radiographs should include the base of the fifth metatarsal to exclude avulsion fracture.

Anteroposterior, lateral, and mortise views are required. Fractures including osteochondral injuries to the medial and lateral talar dome are excluded. Mortise views assess the distal tibial syndesmosis.

If symptoms persist 4–6 weeks after an apparently simple ankle sprain, an MRI is indicated to exclude an osteochondral injury.

Treatment

- Initial treatment consists of rest, ice, compression, and elevation (RICE).
- Provide analgesics or NSAIDs for pain.
- Compression and elevation help reduce swelling.
- Adequate rehabilitation is required to prevent functional instability and injury recurrence.

- Restore range of movement
- Strengthen dynamic ankle stabilizers (ankle evertors and dorsiflexors)
- Proprioception, e.g., wobble board, mini-trampoline
- Functional exercises, e.g., jumping, hopping, twisting
- Athletes can return to sport when they can perform sport-specific actions without pain or instability
- Functional bracing or taping may be required to prevent recurrence

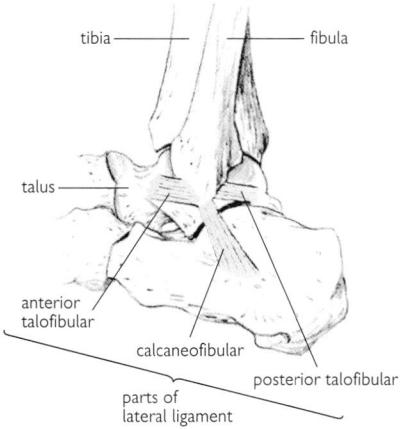

Figure 9.2 Ligaments of the ankle joint, lateral view. Reproduced with permission from MacKinnon P, Morris J (2005). *Oxford Textbook of Functional Anatomy*, Vol 1. Oxford: Oxford University Press, ©2005.

Rehabilitation after ankle sprain (grade 2)

The length of time before returning to sports is based largely on the quality of early management.

Early, intermediate, and late rehabilitation objectives should be highlighted immediately after diagnosis. It is not possible to move on to the later stages of rehabilitation until all early-stage goals are achieved. The athlete should be aware that progressive rehabilitation is necessary to minimize the chances of recurrence.

Anticipated time to return to sports is 3–6 weeks.

Early stage: days 1–7

Key aims
- Minimize swelling.
- Maintain range of movement and general ankle mobility.
- Prevent Achilles tendon stiffness and shortening.
- Begin controlled loading.
- Begin isometric strengthening.
- Enhance joint positional sense and proprioception.
- Maintain upper body strength.

General exercises
The athlete should be encouraged to weight bear or partially weight bear within the limits of pain. The use of crutches may be helpful but should not be to excess. A heel–toe gait pattern should be encouraged at all times. This will prevent the development of a toe-tap gait and minimize shortening of the Achilles tendon.

The RICE regimen should be used as soon as possible after injury:
- The use of horseshoe or focal compression around the malleolus is most effective at preventing swelling accumulating around the healing ligaments.
- Focal compression should be removed before cryotherapy is initiated, to prevent a barrier effect that can reduce the effectiveness of cooling.

Gentle mobility exercises should be encouraged as soon as pain allows. Range of movement through dorsiflexion and plantar flexion (ankle pumps) should be followed by light circling exercises.

The athlete may perform alphabet exercises—this involves using ankle movements to trace each letter of the alphabet in the air. This exercise becomes more challenging with the eyes closed and acts to improve the athletes' awareness of where their ankle is in space.

Cryokinetics is a technique that involves performing mobility exercises immediately after or during cryotherapy. The pain-relieving effect of cooling reduces muscle spasm and inhibition, thereby facilitating the exercises. The athlete should begin static stretching of the Achilles tendon as soon as pain allows. Decreased dorsiflexion is a risk factor for ankle sprain, and in many cases athletes may have already been tight through this range prior to injury.

For upper body strength and conditioning, athletes should be able to perform any upper body exercises that require them to lie (e.g., bench press) or sit (shoulder press).

Middle stage: weeks 2–3

Key aims

- Enhance joint positional sense and proprioception
- Increase strength, ROM, and ankle mobility
- Progress to cardiovascular exercises

Mobility, strengthening, and proprioceptive exercises

- *Weight transfers*: Standing on both feet, with weight predominantly on the uninjured side. Within the limits of pain, the athlete transfers weight onto the injured side. This should progress until it is comfortable to stand solely on the injured foot.
- *Single-leg standing and balance*: Standing on the injured side, the athlete tries to balance, minimizing the number of touch-downs. Progress to eyes closed.

Once the athlete is able to stand comfortably on one leg with eyes closed, more advanced proprioceptive training can begin.

- Single-leg squats
- Lunges: Progress to multidirectional lunges.

All of these exercises can be progressed by increasing the demand on the neuromuscular system. For example, the athlete must perform a single-leg squat on a dynamic surface.

Cardiovascular

Biking, cross-training, and upper body ergometer are used.

End stage: weeks 4–6

To progress to the end stages of rehabilitation, the athlete must have full ankle ROM, a good baseline of strength through all ankle movements, be able to perform complex proprioceptive exercises in a pain-free state, and have good lumbopelvic and lower body control and alignment during squatting and advanced proprioceptive exercises.

In general, as the athlete progress through the later stages of rehabilitation, the focus should become less joint specific and more sport specific.

Medial ligament injuries

The medial or deltoid ligament is injured as a result of an eversion injury, commonly external rotation of the tibia with the foot planted.

The medial ligament is stronger than the lateral ligament and more often accompanied by additional injuries including fractures, e.g., medial malleolus, distal fibula, and talar dome.

Radiographs are mandatory and widening of the ankle mortise (>2 mm between the talus and tibia) represents an unstable ankle and requires surgery.

Treatment of medial ligament injuries is similar to that of lateral ligament injury; however, recovery is much longer—often 6–12 weeks.

Syndesmosis sprain

The anterior tibiofibular ligament is injured as a result of external rotation. Tenderness and swelling are maximal superomedial to the lateral malleolus.

Provocation tests, including the squeeze test and external rotation test (foot externally rotated on a fixed tibia), are positive.

Treatment is similar to that for lateral ligament sprains but recovery can take 6–8 weeks. This injury may lead to diastasis of the ankle joint.

Fractures

A fracture of the lateral, medial, or posterior malleoli is known as a Pott's fracture. Specialist orthopedic opinion is required.

Medial ligament injuries or medial malleolar fractures extending through the interosseous membrane and associated with a fracture of the proximal fibula are called Maisonneuve fractures. Palpate the proximal fibula to avoid missing this potentially unstable ankle injury.

Lateral ankle pain

Peroneal tendinopathy

History and examination

The peroneus longus and brevis muscles dorsiflex and evert the ankle to provide functional lateral ankle stability (see Fig. 9.3). An injury often complicates an acute lateral ankle sprain. The patient may attend with an acute injury or a longer history of chronic subluxation. Rupture of the peroneal retinaculum may lead to subluxation of the peroneal tendons.

Diagnosis is confirmed by demonstrating subluxation of the tendons over the lateral malleolus, by everting the foot against resistance.

Initial treatment is rehabilitation.

Diagnosis

Diagnosis is usually on clinical findings.

Treatment

Surgery is often needed.

Chronic tendinopathy

History and examination

This is the most common cause of lateral ankle pain. Examination confirms tenderness and swelling posterior to the lateral malleolus, and passive inversion and resisted eversion reproduces symptoms.

Precipitating factors include rearfoot varus (supination), a history of ankle ligament sprains, a plantar-flexed first metatarsal, overpronation, and overuse, e.g., jumping sports.

Diagnosis

Diagnosis can be confirmed by musculoskeletal ultrasound or MRI.

Treatment

Treatment is with resisted eversion exercises in plantarflexion to strengthen the peroneals.

Sinus tarsi syndrome

History and examination

A small osseous canal anterior and inferior to the lateral malleolus runs between the talus and calcaneum. It is part of the subtalar joint containing the subtalar ligaments. It may be injured in an acute inversion injury or by repetitive damage from excessive subtalar joint pronation.

Athletes present with diffuse lateral ankle pain after an acute injury or of gradual onset. Symptoms result from subtalar ligament injury, synovial hypertrophy, peroneal nerve entrapment, or degenerative osteoarthritis.

The symptoms include the following:
- Lateral ankle pain
- Pain worse in the morning
- Pain aggravated by eversion
- Local tenderness over the sinus tarsi
- Pain induced by forced passive inversion

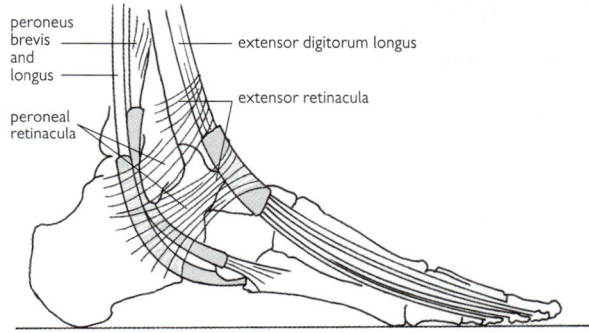

Figure 9.3 Tendons, synovial shealths, and retinacula on the lateral side of the ankle and foot.

The clinical findings may include subtalar instability and a positive Tinel's test. The diagnosis is confirmed by injection of local anesthetic.

Diagnosis
The diagnosis is based on the clinical findings, but the athlete will often have had an ankle X-ray and other diagnosis.

Treatment
- NSAIDs
- Local corticosteroid injections
- Rehabilitation
- Biomechanical assessment

Anterolateral impingement

History and examination
This injury usually results from an acute ankle sprain or recurrent ankle sprains. The patient complains of chronic pain that may persist between sprains or with pain and catching at the anterior aspect of the lateral malleolus. The pain is usually worse on dorsiflexion.

There is synovitis, soft tissue thickening, and scar tissue developing from the injured capsule and anterior talofibular ligament. A meniscoid soft tissue lesion often develops.

Diagnosis
- Clinical assessment is better than MRI.

Treatment
- Injection
- Arthroscopic surgery

Medial ankle pain

Tibialis posterior tendinopathy

History and examination

Medial ankle pain is most often over the retinaculum posteroinferior to the medial malleolus, although the patient may also complain of medial midfoot pain at the site of insertion of the tendon (see Fig. 9.4). The pain is exacerbated by resisted inversion and passive eversion. It may be associated with excessive pronation (rearfoot valgus).

Rupture of tibialis posterior presents with posteromedial tibial pain extending around the medial malleolus to the navicular tubercle. Clinical examination reveals swelling and an inability to raise the heel. Immediate flattening of the medial arch may not be present.

Diagnosis

Ultrasound or MRI confirms the diagnosis.

Treatment

Assess the biomechanics, as physiotherapy and/or orthotics may be required. Rupture of tibialis posterior requires surgical repair.

Flexor hallucis longus tendinopathy

There is usually pain over the posteromedial calcaneum and sustentaculum tali with pain on plantarflexion. This pain is exacerbated by resisted flexion of the first toe with pain on passive extension of the first toe. It is associated with posterior impingement syndrome.

Tarsal tunnel syndrome

History and examination

The posterior tibial nerve becomes trapped in the fibro-osseous tarsal tunnel around the medial malleolus. This compression may be a result of trauma, an inversion injury, overuse, excessive pronation, ill-fitting footwear, or chronic flexor tenosynovitis.

The patient has medial ankle pain radiating into the arch of the foot, heel, and occasionally the toes. The pain is aggravated by prolonged standing, walking, and running. Rarely, there is paraesthesia and numbness over the sole of the foot.

Examination confirms local tenderness and a positive Tinel's sign.

Diagnosis

Radiographs may demonstrate an os trigonum that compresses the tibial nerve. Consider nerve conduction studies.

Treatment

- Appropriate footwear, orthotics
- Injection
- Surgical decompression

Medial plantar nerve entrapment

History and examination

There is pain over the inferomedial calcaneum and this pain may radiate to the arch of the foot. Running aggravates the symptoms and it may be associated with pronation. Recently acquired orthotics can provoke symptoms. A branch of the posterior tibial nerve passes close to the calcaneonavicular ligament.

Examination confirms tenderness, and a positive Tinel's sign is positive.

Diagnosis

Nerve conduction studies confirm the diagnosis.

Treatment

Modification of abnormal biomechanics, injection, or surgical decompression is indicated.

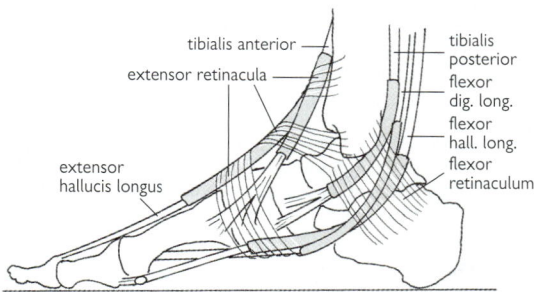

Figure 9.4 Tendons, synovial sheaths, and retinacula on the medial side of the ankle and foot. Reproduced with permission from MacKinnon P, Morris J (2005). *Oxford Textbook of Functional Anatomy*, Vol. 1. Oxford, UK: Oxford University Press. ©2005.

Anterior ankle pain

Extensor tendinitis

History and examination

Tibialis anterior tendinopathy causes pain over the anterior ankle and mid-foot. This pain is exacerbated by dorsiflexion of the foot. It is an overuse injury associated with excessive hill running and may be precipitated by poor footwear. The athlete is tender over the anterior ankle joint and the pain is exacerbated by resisted dorsiflexion.

With tendonitis of the extensor hallucis longus, there is pain on resisted dorsiflexion of the first toes. With tendonitis of the extensor digitorum, there is pain on resisted dorsiflexion of the toes.

Treatment

Management is conservative.

Anterior impingement ("footballer's ankle")

History and examination

Repetitive forced dorsiflexion and plantarflexion of the ankle produces traction osteophytes at the margin of the joint capsule, and exostoses develop on the anterior tibia and talus. It also occurs in basketball, triple jump, long jump, and dance and may follow from ankle instability.

There is pain on running, lunging, or kicking with diffuse anterior ankle joint pain and swelling after activity. The pain is caused by impingement of soft tissues. Examination confirms local tenderness and pain on dorsiflexion. Anterior impingement test is positive (active dorsiflexion with the heel on the ground).

Diagnosis

X-rays can confirm the diagnosis.

Treatment

Physiotherapy, NSAIDs, and corticosteroid injections can improve symptoms. Surgery may be required.

Posterior ankle pain

History and examination

Impingement of the os trigonum or posterior process results from forced plantarflexion of the ankle. This produces posterior ankle joint pain deep to the Achilles tendon. Ballet dancers, jumpers, and fast bowlers are at risk.

Diagnosis

Radiographs demonstrate the ossicle or talar process. Isotope bone scan or MRI can confirm the diagnosis.

Treatment

Management is conservative including rest, physiotherapy, and occasionally corticosteroid injections. If symptoms persist, surgical excision of the ossicle or posterior spur is required.

Shin splints

Although patients may tell you they have shin splints, this is not a diagnosis. It is a general term used to describe shin pain and describes a group of symptoms from a variety of causes. The most common are as follows:
- Stress fractures
- Medial tibial stress syndrome
- Compartment syndromes
- Popliteal artery entrapment

Stress fracture

These are microfractures associated with repetitive stress. The bones are unable to adapt, and breakdown is greater than repair.

The history is of a crescendo-type pain. The pain increases in severity with the duration of exercise. As the condition progresses, the pain begins earlier in exercise. Night pain is a symptom of a severe stress fracture.

Stress fractures occur most commonly in weight-bearing activities such as running or dancing, although they may occur in the ribs of rowers or weight lifters.

Stress fracture of the femoral neck is serious and most often occurs in female runners.

Medial tibial stress syndrome

- Exercise-induced leg pain.
- Pain is felt at the middle to lower third of the medial side of the tibia.
- The medial edge of the tibia may be swollen and tender.
- When symptomatic, there is often a periostitis due to traction with repetitive stress.
- The initial treatment is rest, although surgery with release of the fascia may be required.

Compartment syndromes

- Exertional pain
- Swelling in the anterior compartment
- Pain on active dorsiflexion of the ankle
- There may be tenderness in the muscle on palpation with hypertrophy.
- There may be increased anterior compartment pressure.
- Treatment is altering the type and/or intensity of activity. Alternately, fasciotomy (or fasciectomy if severe) of the involved compartment is perfomed.

Other compartment syndromes include posterior compartment syndrome, where there is pain during and after running in the posterior compartment. Peroneal compartment syndromes have also been described.

Diagnosis

X-rays may show some changes with increased callus formation or simply resorption at the edges of the fracture. A bone scan may show a hot spot. CT scanning and MRI may also be helpful in identifying the lesion.

Resting and post-exercise compartment pressure measurements are useful.

Prevention

Lower limb stress fractures associated with running may be prevented by looking at the impact and biomechanics.

Impact may be reduced by running on a forgiving surface; grass is best. Footwear needs to give adequate shock absorption.

Biomechanical anomalies such as hyperpronation of the foot or increased Q angle may increase the impact of stress.

Treatment

- Alter training to reduce impact
- Run on a forgiving surface
- Lose weight
- Wear good, supportive running footwear
- Orthotics may improve biomechanics

Achilles tendinopathy

History and examination

The Achilles tendon is formed by the insertion of the soleus and gastrocnemius. Plantaris inserts into the Achilles tendon. The tendon is surrounded by a paratendon.

At first, there is gradual development of pain and stiffness after rest, which may occur, for example, in the morning. In the early stages the symptoms usually improve with exercise. As the condition progresses, there may be pain after exercise and, finally, pain during exercise.

On examination, there is local tenderness and swelling. Predisposing factors are overpronation, lack of calf flexibility, and restricted dorsiflexion. Footwear may also contribute. Other contributory factors include a change in training pattern with increased exercise and reduced recovery.

Diagnosis

The diagnosis may be confirmed by ultrasound or MRI.

Treatment

Relative rest, ice, and elevation. An eccentric exercise program is most effective. The next stage is of functional and sport-specific rehabilitation. It is important to correct predisposing factors.

With delayed recovery some clinicians suggest ultrasound-guided Aprotinin injection. Steroid injections are controversial because of reported incidence of increased risk of tendon rupture.

Finally, surgery remains an option.

Achilles tendon rupture

History and examination

The Achilles tendon is the most frequently ruptured tendon. The patient has a sudden, acute pain in the Achilles tendon with an audible snap or tear that is often described as "like being hit or kicked in the back of the leg."

On examination there is swelling and a palpable defect. There is reduced function with an inability to plantarflex the ankle. Simmond's calf squeeze test is positive.

With a partial tear there is acute onset of pain, tenderness, and swelling, but examination confirms no defect and normal function.

Diagnosis

Ultrasound or MRI confirms the diagnosis.

Treatment

- *Surgery*: Either open or percutaneous repair. Surgery is probably the treatment of choice for physically active young adults.
- *Nonoperative*: Rehabilitation is prolonged.

Retrocalcaneal bursitis

History and examination

Inflammation of the bursa between the Achilles tendon and the calcaneum causes symptoms similar to Achilles tendinopathy. The patient is tender over the Achilles tendon insertion. Retrocalcaneal bursitis can coexist with Achilles tendinopathy.

Haglund's deformity consists of Achilles tendinopathy, and retrocalcaneal bursitis associated with retrocalcaneal exostosis, or prominent calcaneum.

Treatment

* Physiotherapy, NSAIDs, heel lifts, and injection of corticosteroid
* Surgical intervention is indicated after 6 months of failed nonoperative treatment

Chronic exertional leg pain

* Chronic exertional compartment syndrome
* Medial tibial stress syndrome
* Stress fracture
* Popliteal artery entrapment

Anterior compartment syndrome

History and examination

This syndrome affects the anterior compartment, which includes tibialis anterior, extensor digitorum longus, extensor hallucis longus, and peroneus tertius. The patient may describe exercise-induced discomfort or dull, aching, cramp-like pain lateral to the anterior border of the tibia.

The symptoms develop within 10–30 minutes of exercise and are often associated with an increase in the intensity. The athlete may describe a feeling of tightness. The symptoms are often reproducible and bilateral (50%–60%) and resolve slowly on stopping exercise.

As the syndrome becomes more severe, symptoms take longer to resolve but are usually gone by the next day. There may be numbness on the top of the foot and weakness of ankle dorsiflexion suggesting nerve compression. It occurs most often in repetitive loading sports such as running, football, and cycling.

Clinical examination is often normal. There may be tightness of the anterior compartment. Muscle herniation is sometimes seen in the distal third of the anterior compartment where the superficial peroneal nerve exits the compartment.

Examination after exercise may demonstrate fullness of the compartment with discomfort on passive stretching.

Posterior compartment syndrome

History and examination

The lateral compartment, consisting of peroneus longus and brevis, and the superficial compartment of gastrocnemius and soleus, is less frequently affected.

The patient may describe a cramp-like discomfort of the calf and medial border of the tibia and a tightness that increases with exercise. There may be associated weakness and paraesthesia.

Examination is often normal, or there may be tenderness over the medial border of the tibia. Occasionally, small muscle hernias are present.

Diagnosis

Compartment syndrome consists of increasing pressure in the limited myofascial compartment that causes reduced tissue perfusion and abnormal neuromuscular function.

Intracompartmental pressure studies should be conducted. A catheter is inserted into the relevant compartment and the muscles exercised to reproduce the pain. Normal compartment resting pressures are between 0 and 15 mmHg. The diagnosis of chronic compartment syndrome is supported by a pre-exercise pressure >15 mmHg, maximum pressure 1 minute after exercise >30 mmHg, and a resting 5-minute post-exercise pressure >20 mmHg.

Plain radiographs may demonstrate a stress fracture.

An isotope bone scan may reveal increased linear uptake consistent with medial tibial stress syndrome or focal uptake indicative of a stress fracture.

Treatment

Conservative treatment consists of activity modification to avoid symptoms. Physiotherapy often includes stretching and deep massage. Assessment includes the correction of biomechanical abnormalities.

If conservative treatment fails then surgery is indicated. Surgical fasciotomy relieves symptoms and allows the athlete to return to previous levels of activity.

Popliteal artery entrapment

Popliteal artery entrapment often mimics the symptoms of chronic exertional compartment syndromes. Symptoms may be unilateral or bilateral. There are many anatomical variants that cause popliteal artery entrapment.

Diagnosis is made by lower extremity arteriography while the ankle is dorsiflexed and plantarflexed.

Surgical decompression relieves the symptoms and the athlete usually may return to previous levels of activity.

Foot

Fracture of the calcaneus

History and examination

Acute fractures generally occur as the result of a high-energy compressive force such as a fall from height or motor vehicle accident. Extra-articular calcaneal fractures can occur with torsional forces and are those more likely to be seen in sports.

Diagnosis

- X-ray aids the initial diagnosis.
- CT is best for defining the exact fracture configuration.

Classification

Extra-articular

- *Anterior process*: Following adduction of the transverse tarsal joint (midfoot) on the hindfoot there is an avulsion of the anterior process of the calcaneus via the bifurcate ligament.
- *Calcaneal tuberosity*: Avulsion occurs via the tendo-achilles; this is seen in the older population.

Intra-articular

- The typical high-energy group
- Varying degrees of comminution and articular involvement

Treatment

The type of treatment depends on the severity of the fracture, the degree of articular displacement, and the general medical condition of the patient.

Conservative treatment involves initial management of swelling in the acute stage, followed by non–weight bearing on crutches, progressing to increasing weight bearing as union occurs (complete union takes approximately 3 months).

Open reduction is considered when there is significant loss of normal calcaneal morphology or articular displacement, in those patients whose local soft tissue and general health are amenable to surgery.

Fracture of the metatarsal bones

For anatomy of the tarsal bones, see Figure 10.1.

History and examination

These fractures occur commonly in many sports. They may be caused by direct trauma (e.g., a kick in football), a twisting injury (usually resulting in a spiral fracture or avulsion), or by repetitive forces (stress fracture).

The base of the fifth metatarsal is worth separate attention. Avulsion fractures may complicate acute ankle sprains. Its particular blood supply can result in delayed union or nonunion. See also Jones fracture of the fifth metatarsal (p. 351).

Diagnosis

X-ray can confirm the diagnosis.

Treatment

Patients generally respond well to conservative measures—strapping or use of a walking cast or functional brace for a period of 2 or 3 weeks, followed by return to sports in approximately 6–8 weeks.

Complications are rare—see Jones fracture of base of fifth metatarsal (p. 351).

Fitness should be maintained through non–weight bearing activities such as cycling, aqua jogging, or swimming.

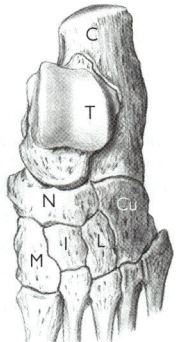

C = calcaneus
T = talus
N = navicular
Cu = cuboid
M = medial cuneiform
I   = intermediate cuneiform
L = lateral cuneiform

Figure 10.1 Tarsal bones, dorsal view. Reproduced with permission from MacKinnon P, Morris J (2005). *Oxford Textbook of Functional Anatomy*, Vol. 1. Oxford, UK: Oxford University Press. ©2005.

Lisfranc fracture: dislocations

History and examination
- Fracture or dislocation occurring at the tarsometatarsal joints
- Relatively uncommon in sports
- Usually occurs in sports as the result of a combined axial load and twist on a plantarflexed foot

Diagnosis
Plain X-ray appearances are subtle and may be missed. Careful assessment of the relationship between the base of the metatarsals and their corresponding cuneiforms is needed to detect any diastasis or bone fragment occurring at this articulation.

Occasionally, plain X-rays can be normal and a high clinical suspicion is required to avoid missing the diagnosis.

CT or MRI scan is very helpful in confirming the diagnosis and planning treatment.

Treatment
Treatment is aimed at restoring the exact anatomical alignment and may be conservative for minor (grade 1 and 2 sprains) injuries or internal fixation of any unstable injuries.

It is crucial that normal anatomical alignment is obtained and then maintained while the injury heals.

Fat pad contusion

History and examination
The contusion occurs either as a result of landing from a jump directly onto the heel or from repetitive heel strike on hard surfaces (especially in heavy individuals or those wearing inadequate footwear).

Fat pad atrophy may be precipitated by steroid injection (e.g., for plantar fasciitis) and is irreversible.

Tenderness is felt more proximally than with plantar fasciitis.

Diagnosis
Imaging is not necessary. The diagnosis is based on clinical findings.

Treatment
Treatment includes the use of shock-absorbing heel cushions, taping, and modification of training surfaces.

Footwear with a firm heel counter should be worn to prevent splaying of the heel pad.

Midtarsal joint sprains

History and examination

Sprains may occur as a result of an acute injury or from repetitive stress in an individual with an overpronated gait. They generally involve the calcaneonavicular ligament.

Diagnosis

Diagnosis is based on clinical findings, although X-rays may be undertaken to exclude other causes of mid-foot pain.

Treatment

Conservative treatment involves electrotherapeutic modalities and taping and orthotic supports.

Occasionally, corticosteroid injection is required if there is a persistent synovitis of one of the midtarsal joints.

Turf toe

History and examination

- An acute dorsiflexion sprain injury of the first metatarsophalangeal joint
- Common on artificial surfaces where the traction between the surface and the shoe is great
- Involves injury to both the metatarsophalangeal joint and the associated plantar plate complex
- While most cases are typically stable sprains, more severe injuries may result in instability of the first metatarsophalangeal joint (MTPJ) (Lachman test of the joint)

Diagnosis

An X-ray is needed to exclude a fracture. MRI is used to assess the plantar plate soft-tissue complex.

Treatment

Turf toe is managed conservatively with ice, analgesics, rest, and taping to limit joint movement on return to sports (generally after 2–4 weeks). These injuries can result in persistent discomfort on return to running.

Choice of footwear is important in preventing these injuries, with a rigid insole limiting excessive movement at the first MTPJ (especially in those with hallux limitus).

Hallux rigidus ("footballer's toe")

History and examination

Hallux rigidus occurs after repeated minor injuries to the first MTPJ, resulting in early degenerative changes and restricted movement, especially dorsiflexion. It is very common in sports such as soccer, where repetitive stress occurs during kicking and sprinting.

This condition may cause the athlete to change their normal gait pattern to push off on the lateral border of the forefoot rather than at the hallux.

Diagnosis

X-rays will demonstrate osteophyte formation and joint-space narrowing.

Treatment

Treatment is very difficult—NSAIDs and corticosteroid injection can give temporary relief. Referral to a podiatrist is indicated as orthotics can be used to unload the joint.

In more severe cases, surgical options include removal of the osteophytes, osteotomy of the first metatarsal, or MTP fusion (although this has implications for push-off power).

The term *hallux limitus* is used to describe less severe cases of this condition.

Normal walking

The normal gait cycle consists of a stance phase initiated by heel strike (usually toward the lateral border of the heel with the foot slightly supinated), followed by flat foot, heel-off, and finally toe off, before the gait cycle is completed by the swing phase, which leads to another heel strike.

There is a period of double-legged support, followed by an intermediate single-leg phase, before another double-leg phase.

During distance running this gait cycle is maintained (except for elimination of the double-leg phase). In sprinting the stance phase tends to consist of a midfoot or forefoot rather than a heel strike (i.e., sprinters tend to run more on their toes).

Following heel strike, the foot pronates (see Fig. 10.2) to allow full contact with the ground, before supinating to form a rigid lever, allowing toe-off to occur.

This complex series of movements enables the foot to change from a flexible, shock-absorbing platform at heel-strike through to a rigid lever allowing maximal propulsion at push-off.

The subtalar joint is important in dissipating shock following foot strike. Stiffness of the subtalar joint will reduce the ability to absorb shock. It plays an important role in using the rotary forces of the lower limb to realign the joint planes throughout the hind- and midfoot during the gait cycle to allow for these alterations in foot compliance.

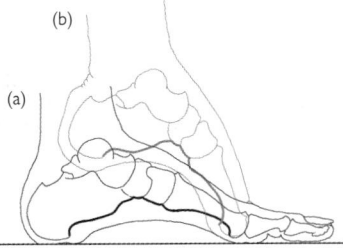

Figure 10.2 (a) Medial longitudinal arch of the foot when standing. (b) Change in medial arch and dorsiflexion of metatarsophalangeal joint when standing on tiptoe and at the start of locomotion. Reproduced with permission from MacKinnon P, Morris J (2005). *Oxford Textbook of Functional Anatomy,* Vol. 1. Oxford, UK: Oxford University Press. ©2005.

Pronation

Pronation is a triplanar movement occurring at the subtalar joint. Pronation is a normal component of the gait cycle. Pronation consists of eversion, dorsiflexion, and abduction of the foot. Pronation should not occur past the latter stages of midstance, as the normal foot should then supinate in preparation for toe-off.

Excessive (over) pronation may contribute to, or be a consequence of, biomechanical anomalies elsewhere in the kinetic chain, placing abnormal stresses on other structures (e.g., causing internal rotation of the lower limb and placing abnormal stress on the medial structures of the foot and ankle).

Overpronation or hyperpronation has been implicated as a causative factor in the development of many lower limb problems, including achilles tendinopathy, plantar fasciitis, metatarsalgia, sesamoiditis, tibialis posterior tendinopathy, medial tibial periostitis and stress fractures, patellofemoral pain, and iliotibial band friction syndrome.

Overpronation can be corrected by the use of orthoses placed in the individual's shoe. Orthoses can be either preformed or (preferably) custom-cast to suit the individual athlete.

Many asymptomatic athletes overpronate—there is little or no evidence for the use of orthoses to correct this as a preventative measure.

Supination

Supination also occurs at the subtalar joint and normally occurs toward the end of the midstance phase of the gait to allow the foot to form a rigid lever in preparation for toe-off. The supinated foot is plantarflexed, inverted, and adducted.

Typically these individuals have a cavoid (high-arched), rigid foot with poor shock absorption that predisposes to metatarsal stress fractures. Excessive supination may also contribute to the development of iliotibial band friction syndrome.

Supination is much more difficult to correct with orthoses— individuals should buy shoes with maximum shock absorption.

Footwear

Different sports require different footwear. Shoes should be further tailored to the requirements of the individuals.

Shoes consist of an upper (the part covering the foot) and a sole (consisting of inner sole, mid-sole, wedge, and out-sole). The mid-sole is the main shock absorber and can be made of various materials with different inserts. The out-sole is designed for both traction and shock absorption, whereas the wedge increases heel height and aids shock absorption. The upper should have a toe box providing adequate room and a firm heel counter to stabilize the subtalar joint and help prevent excessive pronation.

The shape of the shoe can be straight or curved—a straight-last shoe provides more stability. *Board lasting* and *slip lasting* describe the way the upper of the shoe is attached to the sole. In board lasting the upper is attached to a hard inner sole board and is heavier and more stable.

Those with a tendency to overpronate require a running shoe providing more control—i.e., a straight (rather than curved) last construction, a combined-last inner sole (i.e., board last to metatarsals, allowing more flexibility at the forefoot) with added medial support and a firm heel counter.

Tennis and other court shoes are generally constructed to provide more control and will be of a full board last construction. Running shoes do not contain these stabilizing constructions and are not designed to allow sudden changes of direction, making them unsuitable for sports involving a lot of twisting.

A high heel tab should generally be avoided, as this may cause impingement on the Achilles tendon when the ankle is fully plantarflexed.

Shoes should be individual and sport specific—those designed for distance running should provide stability and shock absorption, whereas those aimed at sports involving sudden changes in direction should provide good traction between the foot and the playing surface to avoid slipping.

Running shoes lose their shock-absorbing qualities after about 500 kilometers and should be changed frequently. Using worn-out footwear may lead to injury.

Boots with "blade"-type cleats may increase the likelihood of some lower limb injuries, in addition to causing tibial lacerations.

Shoes designed for aerobic classes become worn after approximately 100 hours of activity.

Gait analysis

A detailed description of the techniques used in formal gait analysis is beyond the scope of this book. However, from the discussion under Normal walking (p. 341) and Footwear (p. 343), it is clear that the physician should have some understanding of the normal biomechanics of walking and running and should be able to recognize abnormal gait patterns and refer appropriately for more detailed podiatric assessment.

Pronation is a normal component of the gait cycle, and there is no evidence supporting the prescription of foot orthoses as a preventative measure in asymptomatic athletes who "overpronate." These are generally individuals who have adapted and learned to cope with their "abnormal" gait, and the introduction of orthoses into their shoes may cause considerable secondary problems.

Athletes should first be assessed standing from the front and then the posterior aspect.

Alignments such as persistent femoral anteversion will be obvious, producing a "squinting patellae" appearance.

A pelvic tilt may be due to a leg-length discrepancy. This can be formally measured from the anterior superior iliac crest to the medial malleolus with the athlete supine.

From the posterior aspect, the shape of the longitudinal arch and the angle between the Achilles and the calcaneus can be assessed. Athletes who overpronate will tend to have a flat-footed appearance with valgus heel position, producing the "too many toes" sign.

The athlete should be asked to perform a half squat with the heels flat. This will reproduce the position of the foot in the mid-stance phase of running and will demonstrate any tendency to overpronate.

The athlete should be observed walking in bare feet and, if possible, while treadmill running in normal training shoes.

The athlete who supinates excessively will typically have a rigid high-arched foot with rearfoot varus alignment.

Core stability should be assessed, for example, by asking the athlete to perform a one-leg squat and observing the degree of pelvic tilt and twisting that occurs during this maneuver.

Any abnormal gait patterns identified in a symptomatic athlete should prompt referral to a podiatrist for more formal gait analysis.

Several different types of orthoses are available, with the most appropriate usually being made from a cast of the athlete's foot taken in the subtalar neutral position.

Plantar fasciitis

History and examination

Plantar fasciitis is a chronic overuse injury resulting from repetitive traction on the plantar fascia attachment to the calcaneus. It is often found in individuals with pes planus or a tendency to overpronate, and may be initiated by wearing sandals or soft shoes.

Older or middle-aged athletes are more commonly affected.

The classical symptom is heel pain and stiffness that is worse in the mornings. Individuals report that they have to walk on their toes for the first few strides, with their symptoms improving as they "warm up."

Pain may be present during the day if walking long distances or after a period of sitting.

Patients with plantar fasciitis have point tenderness at the plantar fascia attachment to the calcaneus anteromedially. They may also experience tenderness at the plantar fascia origin when the great toe is dorsiflexed.

The differential diagnosis includes calcaneal stress fracture, tarsal tunnel syndrome, medial or lateral plantar nerve entrapment, Reiter's disease, and lumbar radiculopathy.

Diagnosis

X-ray often reveals a calcaneal spur in asymptomatic individuals (approximately 15% of the general population will have a heel spur) and the presence of a spur is NOT related to the development of pain.

There is an association with inflammatory conditions and enthesopathies such as gout, rheumatoid arthritis (RA), ankylosing spondylitis, and Reiter's syndrome (especially if heel pain is bilateral), so further diagnosis may be appropriate.

Treatment

Treatment is nonsurgical in virtually every case. A tension night splint (holding the foot in dorsiflexion) is very useful in relieving morning pain and stiffness.

Stretches for the calf and Achilles tendon and plantar fascia should be advised, and heel cups or orthoses to correct abnormal foot biomechanics are indicated.

Strapping techniques to support the plantar fascia are very useful in providing short-term symptomatic relief. Taping begins at the level of the metatarsal heads and continues to the heel, forming a fan to support the plantar fascia. It is quick and easily applied by the patient and may also be used on return to impact activities.

Intrinsic foot exercises should be advised—easily performed using a towel on the floor and instructing the athlete to pull this towards him using his toes.

Extracorporeal shock wave therapy has recently been reported as being a promising treatment option. Electrotherapeutic modalities are usually ineffective.

Cortisone injections may be useful but can cause rupture of the plantar fascia or fat pad atrophy, which may lead to permanent heel pain. The preferred technique is to use a medial approach rather than inject directly through the heel pad, which has a plentiful nerve supply. Injection is usually reserved for patients who have failed to respond to other conservative measures.

Surgery is very occasionally required for refractory cases (i.e., at least 12 months' duration). Results are generally good, although long-term problems following surgery have been reported.

Extensor tendinopathy

History and examination

Overuse of the extensor tendons can be caused by uphill running, and, in some cases, an acute peritenonitis can occur, causing crepitus and swelling.

Pain can also arise from ill-fitting shoes or laces tied too tightly.

Treatment

Attention to footwear is important; soft padding may prevent excessive pressure.

Steroid injection along the tendon sheath is often helpful in cases of peritenonitis. Referral for physiotherapy including eccentric strengthening exercises is indicated.

Surgery is very rarely necessary.

Stress fractures of the calcaneus

History and examination

Stress fractures of the calcaneus are relatively uncommon, having been described mostly in military populations. The history is of an insidious onset of heel pain on impact activities.

On clinical examination there will be pain compressing the calcaneus from the sides, slightly proximal and posterior to where tenderness from plantar fasciitis would be maximal.

Diagnosis

X-rays usually show a sclerotic line parallel to the posterior margin of the calcaneus on the lateral view.

Isotope and/or MRI scanning may be necessary to make the diagnosis.

Treatment

Treatment is conservative, with return to impact activities as the symptoms and signs permit (usually 6–8 weeks). There is no need to advise a period of non–weight bearing, though severe cases may benefit from a period in a Cam-type boot.

Fitness can be maintained through nonimpact training—aqua jogging and cycling.

On return to impact activities, footwear that provides adequate shock attenuation should be worn.

Stress fractures of the navicular

History and examination

The exact cause of navicular stress fractures is unclear. They occur through the sagittal plane of the central third of the bone, an area that is felt to be relatively avascular.

Impingement and shearing of the navicular between the talus and first, second, and third rays is thought to occur in sprinting and jumping activities. The fractures occur most commonly in sprinters and jumping athletes, but also in soccer players.

Fractures usually present insidiously with midfoot pain and localized tenderness over the proximal, dorsal surface of the navicular (the so-called N spot).

Diagnosis

Plain X-rays are often negative and the diagnosis should be confirmed with isotope scanning, CT, or MRI.

Treatment

These fractures are prone to nonunion and require aggressive treatment—initially strictly non–weight bearing in a cast for 6–8 weeks. Fitness can be maintained through cycling during this phase.

Once the cast is removed the N spot is again palpated. If there is residual tenderness, a further 2-week period of immobilization is needed.

If there is no localized tenderness, gradual weight-bearing activities can be resumed, with return to full training over the next 6–8 weeks.

Nonunion or delayed union is a major problem and surgery may be required for those fractures that fail to unite with conservative treatment.

Recovery from these injuries is often prolonged. A gradual return to impact activities is required and footwear should be carefully checked to ensure that it is appropriate to the individual.

Orthoses are indicated for those athletes who have an excessively overpronated gait.

Stress fractures of the metatarsals

History and examination

These are very common in athletes, most often involving the second ("March fracture") and third metatarsal shafts.

Stress fractures of the second metatarsal are especially common in ballet dancers.

These fractures present with increasing pain on impact activities and localized tenderness over the affected bone.

Diagnosis

Plain X-rays may not be positive for 3 or 4 weeks and isotope scans are used to make an earlier diagnosis. MRI can also be used with high sensitivity.

Treatment

Conservative treatment consists of strapping or use of a cast brace or walker with return to impact activities over a period of 6–8 weeks.

Fitness can be maintained with low- or nonimpact exercise, such as aqua jogging. Return to full activity can be expected over 8–10 weeks.

Jones fracture

History and examination

This is a fracture at the junction of the metaphysis and diaphysis of the proximal fifth metatarsal. It can result from either a stress fracture at this point or present acutely as the result of an inversion/plantarflexion injury.

These fractures represent a special group, as they are prone to nonunion (reported rate of 7%–28%) because of the vascular arrangement at this area (it is supplied by the terminal branches of the nutrient artery to the fifth metatarsal and a fracture at this zone can disrupt this terminal supply resulting in an avascular area).

Diagnosis

With stress fracture, plain X-rays may not be positive for 3 or 4 weeks. Isotope scans or MRI is used to make an earlier diagnosis in this situation.

Treatment

These fractures should be immobilized in a short leg cast, with non–weight bearing for 8 weeks. Subsequent nonunion is treated with intramedullary screw fixation or bone grafting.

Early surgical intervention should be considered in the professional or elite athlete.

Metatarsalgia

History and examination

Forces while walking are normally transmitted predominantly through the first metatarsal head (one-third of total) with remainder two-thirds being evenly distributed among the metatarsal heads of the lesser four toes.

Alterations in normal foot anatomy or kinematics (such a short first metatarsal or loss of the normal transverse arch of the forefoot) can result in excessive stress being placed on the MTPJs of the lesser toes, causing synovitis and pain.

The second and third MTPJs are commonly affected, and there may be callous formation on the plantar surface of these joints, reflecting the excessive stress.

Diagnosis

Diagnosis is based on clinical examination. There is pain compressing the metatarsal heads and manipulation of the affected joints.

Treatment

Treatment includes use of a metatarsal pad, bar, or dome (placed on the plantar surface of the foot, proximal to the MTPJs to restore the normal transverse arch and/or unload the metatarsal heads) and orthoses to correct any overpronation.

Occasionally, a cortisone injection into the affected MTPJ may give good relief by settling the secondary synovitis.

Morton's (interdigital) neuroma

History and examination

Symptoms occur from irritation of the digital nerve, resulting in an inter-digital neuroma. This results from repetitive trauma to the digital nerve against the deep transverse metatarsal ligament.

Typically the neuroma occurs between the third and fourth metatarsal heads (although it can occasionally affect the second interspace) and causes pain and interdigital paraesthesia.

Clinical examination most commonly reveals tenderness in the third web space, altered sensation in the digital cleft (in 40%), and the classic sign of a Mulder's click occurring with ballottement of the nerve between compressed third and fourth metatarsal heads (frequently, though not always, present)

Diagnosis

Diagnosis is clinical but can be confirmed by MRI scan.

Treatment

Initial treatment is nonoperative. Metatarsal pads and orthotic correction of any abnormal gait pattern should be advised, along with a wide toe box in footwear. Cortisone injection frequently gives good initial relief, although the reported cure rate at 2 years is around 30%.

Surgical excision is the definitive treatment and involves excision of the neuroma.

Sesamoid injury

History and examination

The medial and lateral sesamoid bones lie within the tendon of flexor hallucis brevis, and injuries are frequent in sports. They act to increase the efficiency of the tendon and to stabilize the first MTP joint.

The medial sesamoid is most commonly affected by repetitive loading leading to the development of sesamoiditis/osteonecrosis or stress fracture (the medial sesamoid transmits more force with weight bearing than the lateral sesamoid). Athletes who overpronate are particularly vulnerable to these problems.

On clinical examination there will be tenderness to direct palpation over the medial sesamoid, decreased strength of plantarflexion, and pain on passive dorsiflexion of the MTP. The patient may tend to walk on the lateral border of the foot in an attempt to unload the painful area.

Diagnosis

Specific "sesamoid views" on plain X-ray may show fragmentation or fracture of the involved bone. However, a bipartite sesamoid is a common finding and differentiation from a stress fracture may be difficult (the fibrous joint of a bipartite sesamoid is also prone to injury).

Isotope or MRI scanning can be used to make the diagnosis.

Treatment

These stress fractures are prone to nonunion and initial treatment should be in a non–weight-bearing cast for 6 weeks followed by gradual resumption of impact activities if bony tenderness is no longer present.

Overpronation should be corrected with orthoses and padding may be used to unload the area on return to training. A stiff sole or rocker-bottom shoe can also be used to protect the sesamoid during healing and graduated return to activity.

Sesamoiditis may occasionally respond to a cortisone injection.

Generally, excision of the sesamoid bones should be avoided, as there can be significant problems following such procedures (although excision of a partial fragment can produce good results).

Cuboid syndrome

Occasionally the lateral aspect of the cuboid may be subluxed dorsally from excessive pull of the peroneus longus tendon. This results in lateral foot pain when weight bearing.

Treatment is by manipulation of the subluxed cuboid and taping may be used post-reduction to hold the cuboid in place.

Any biomechanical problems, such as overpronation, should be addressed.

Os naviculare syndrome

An accessory ossicle at the tuberosity of the navicular occurs in approximately 10% of the population and is generally asymptomatic. It may be either a sesamoid within the tibialis posterior tendon or a developmental variation of the navicular, with the accessory bone being connected to the navicular by cartilage (synchondrosis) or bone (bicornuate navicular).

Pain may occasionally occur as a result of traction from the tibialis posterior tendon, especially in an individual with an overpronated gait.

Treatment is aimed at reducing the traction with activity modification and orthoses to correct the abnormal gait pattern.

A traction apophysis may occur at this site in the adolescent athlete. Treatment is along similar lines.

Surgical excision may occasionally be necessary, with care being taken to preserve the insertion of tibialis posterior.

Sever's disease (traction apophysitis calcaneum)

History and examination

This is the second most common traction apophysitis after Osgood–Schlatter disease. It usually presents in children who are between 10 and 13 years of age.

Unilateral or bilateral heel pain related to running and jumping activity occurs. Pain may be associated with limping. Heel pain is often worst on rising from bed. In severe cases, swelling develops over the posterior calcaneum.

Hyperpronation and pes planus may be associated. Calf and hamstring flexibility are usually poor. There is focal tenderness at the posterior border of the calcaneum at insertion of the Achilles tendon. Ankle dorsiflexion may be reduced.

The differential diagnosis includes a calcaneal stress fracture.

Diagnosis

Imaging is rarely required. X-rays will demonstrate fragmentation of the calcaneal apophysis.

Treatment

- Limit running and jumping activities
- A heel raise in the shoe will decrease pain
- Ice heels after activity
- A calf and hamstring stretching program should be implemented
- Calf strength program

Prognosis

There are no long-term complications. Activity may need to be modified during vulnerable periods.

Iselin's disease (traction apophysitis affecting base of fifth metatarsal)

History and examination
- Presents with pain over lateral aspect of foot at site of insertion of peroneus brevis tendon into base of fifth metatarsal
- Pain reproduced by passive foot inversion and resisted eversion

Diagnosis
- Not required

Treatment
- Unloading tendon with standard ankle taping in eversion (as is done for the prevention of lateral ligament injuries)
- Exercise program to stretch and strengthen the peroneal muscles
- Prognosis is good

Traction apophysitis navicular (insertion tibialis posterior tendon)

History and examination
- Presents with medial midfoot pain
- Pain reproduced by passive foot eversion and resisted inversion
- Flat feet and hyperpronation commonly associated
- No diagnosis is required

Treatment
- Unload tibialis posterior tendon with orthotic device
- Program to stretch and strengthen tibialis posterior
- Prognosis is good

Tarsal coalition

This congenital abnormality results in bony, cartilaginous, or fibrous fusion of two tarsal bones. It causes abnormal mechanics around affected bones due to limitations of movement at the site of the coalition.

The most common coalitions are calcaneonavicular (CN) (2/3) followed by talocalcaneal (TC) (1/3) and calcaneocuboid (rare).

The abnormality is bilateral in 40%–50% of patients and a family history is common.

History and examination

Presentation is of ankle and hindfoot pain. The exact site depends on the site of the coalition (calcaneonavicular coalitions cause lateral pain, whereas talocalcaneal coalitions result in pain posterior to the medial malleolus).

Symptoms develop when the coalition begins to ossify (CN ages 8–12, TC ages 12–16, and talonavicular [TN] ages 3–5). It may also present with recurrent ankle sprains or a painless, rigid flat foot.

Tarsal coalition may be asymptomatic in childhood and only present in adult life as a result of degenerative changes caused by altered foot mechanics.

Diagnosis

X-rays are useful when appropriate views are requested. Series should include the following:
- AP
- Lateral—look for talar beaking, elongation of the anterior process of the calcaneus, and the C-sign of talocalcaneal coalitions
- Oblique—visualizes the CN coalition
- Harris-Beath view—visualizes the middle and posterior facets of the subtalar joint

CT scanning is the gold standard. MRI will show cartilaginous and fibrous coalitions not seen with other modalities.

Treatment

Initial treatment is nonoperative. The aim is to reduce stresses on the coalition. Arch supports, orthotics, and short-leg walking casts or boots can all be used.

Surgery is indicated when there is failure of nonoperative measures and interference with activity. Options include resection of the coalition (in younger patients with no evidence of secondary degenerative changes) or fusion of the affected joint.

Prognosis

Tarsal coalition is commonly missed in childhood and presents as severe arthritic change in the tarsal joints of adults.

Freiberg's disease

Freiberg's disease is also called Freiberg's infraction or Freiberg's osteochondritis.

History and examination

Freiberg's disease is an avascular necrosis of the metatarsal head, most commonly presenting between the ages of 12 and 18 years, and is more common in women (the only osteochondritis that is more common in females). Initial synovitis is followed by sclerosis, resorption, and collapse of the metatarsal head, leading to secondary degenerative changes.

The second metatarsal head is most commonly affected, although the third can also be involved.

Freiberg's disease is usually seen in running athletes and dancers, probably secondary to compressive forces at the metatarsal heads, and the fact that the second metatarsal is the least mobile.

There is gradual-onset forefoot pain, which worsens with push-off and dancing en-pointe. Focal tenderness and decreased ROM occur over the involved metatarsal head.

Morton's foot (in which the second metatarsal is longer than first) is commonly associated and increases the load on the second metatarsal head.

Diagnosis

The X-ray is often normal initially. It later shows fragmentation of the epiphysis, followed by flattening of the metatarsal head and widening of the shaft.

If the X-ray is normal early in the course of symptoms, a bone scan or MRI will confirm the diagnosis.

Treatment

In the acute phase, rest from all impact activity is necessary. Limit activity and modify footwear (use a metatarsal bar to unload the metatarsal head and avoid high-heeled shoes). In severe cases, immobilization may be required.

Persistent pain may necessitate surgical intervention, but this should be delayed until after reossification has occurred.

Surgical options include synovectomy, joint debridement, metatarsal osteotomy, head reshaping, or head excision.

Long-term prognosis is variable, from healing with little deformity to progressive destruction of the metatarsal head and chronic symptoms.

Kohler's disease

- Avascular necrosis of navicular
- More common in boys than girls
- Ischemia and stress have been implicated as causative factors

History and examination

- Presents earlier than other osteochondroses (around age 3–5)
- Presents with a painful limp and focal tenderness over the navicular
- Passive eversion and resisted inversion often reproduce the pain

Diagnosis

X-ray shows patchy sclerosis of the navicular, followed by compression and collapse.

Treatment

- Symptomatic
- Analgesia
- Rest from running activities
- Medial arch-support orthotic improves pain by unloading the navicular

Prognosis

- Excellent prognosis
- Despite marked abnormalities on initial imaging, navicular returns to its normal shape before growth is complete

Subungual hematoma

- This is a painful condition. The hematoma should be drained by piercing the nail with a needle or heated paper clip to prevent loss of the nail, which would otherwise occur in 2 or 3 weeks.
- Dress the nail to avoid infection.
- Black nails can also occur as the result of wearing poorly fitting shoes.

Ingrown toenails (onychocryptosis)

- This usually affects the great toe and is caused by ill-fitting shoes or injudicious nail clipping.
- The toenail can readily become infected and require antibiotic treatment.
- It may require wedge resection of part of the nail and ablation of the nail bed with phenol to prevent regrowth.
- Prevention through proper and regular nail care is the best solution.

Medical issues in athletes

What happens when we exercise?

The individual response to exercise depends on a number of factors:
- Type of exercise stress encountered
- Level of training and conditioning, and nutritional and hydration status
- Age, gender, body type, muscle fiber–type ratios
- Genetic factors and environmental conditions
- Psychological factors

Physiological responses to exercise stress will vary according to these factors. The complex interactions of the body's homeostatic mechanisms and responses can be briefly summarized in the time line below.

Short-term—seconds to minutes (stress reaction)

- *Autonomic nervous system response:* sympathetic increase with parasympathetic decrease resulting in the fight-or-flight response and reduced vegetative functions
- *Cardiovascular responses:* increased cardiac output to exercising muscles and reduced blood flow to other organ systems. As core temperature increases, there is increased blood flow to the skin for thermoregulation.
- *Respiratory responses:* increased rate and depth of respiration to meet demands for gas exchange
- *Metabolic and respiratory responses:* buffering of lactic acid produced by the active muscles

Medium-term—minutes to hours (resistance reaction)

Hormonal responses

These responses accentuate and prolong the autonomic neural responses (above). Catecholamines are released from the adrenal medulla, and adrenocorticotrophic hormone (ACTH) and growth hormone (GH) from the pituitary with increased substrate availability for energy metabolism to provide fuel for longer-duration exercise.

Activation of the renin angiotensin and antidiuretic hormone (ADH) mechanisms help preserve fluid and electrolyte balance and maintain blood pressure.

Long-term—days to weeks (adaptation)

Through repeated acute bouts of exercise (training) the body adapts to the exercise stimulus. Adaptation results from gene activation in various tissues under stress. Cellular structural changes in muscle and other tissues bring about strength and endurance changes; changes in neural regulation optimize muscle activation patterns; and renal mechanisms are probably responsible for cardiovascular responses to training through changes in plasma volume and venous return.

Basic principles of training

Training is the use of progressive overload to stress the major energy systems used in an activity. Training usually results in adaptation of the energy system and improvement in performance.

Overload

A greater-than-normal load with appropriate rest leads to adaptation. Exercise intensity should be near maximal and increased as fitness increases.

Progression

Frequency, intensity, time (duration), and type of training are manipulated to create a progression in load. The athlete should build up duration or volume of training and, with a basic foundation, then reduce volume but increase intensity and speed.

Specificity

The metabolic and neuromuscular demands of exercise are usually specific to the sport or activity. Training must reflect the elements found within the sport.

Individuality

Training load should be prescribed according to age, gender, level of skills, experience, and conditioning and then adjusted according to individual response. Elite-level training programs should not be imposed on juniors, beginners, or intermediate-level athletes.

Rest

Regeneration and adaptation occurs when resting. Rest should be an actively programmed part of training.

Periodization

Plan the season and build the necessary skills, strength, and endurance (distance) or speed systematically in a series of well-planned phases.

Fitness deterioration with aging

In most humans there is a physiological decline in performance from the mid- to late 30s onward. However, exceptional performance is still possible in later years, e.g., men and women over 80 have run marathons in under 5 hours.

Stature

Stature declines by approximately 1 cm per decade after 40 years. This is partly due to degenerative changes in intervertebral discs and partly from loss of vertebral bone height.

Body fat

The body fat percentage rises steadily to 23%–25% in males and 32%–40% in females by age 60–70 years, while lean body mass steadily declines.

Skin

The rete pegs anchoring the epidermis to the dermis become shorter with age, leading to a greater propensity to blister formation and skin tearing. Melanocytes disappear at the rate of 2% per year and the cutaneous inflammatory response diminishes. Therefore, the elderly are more susceptible to sunburn and yet show less of the acute effects of sunburn than the young.

Muscle

In comparison to performance-matched younger athletes, the muscle of elderly athletes tends toward a predominance of slow-twitch type fibers, with greater muscle capillarization. This is thought to be due to reinnervation of muscle by type 1 nerve following type 2 nerve degeneration.

Aging also causes a decrease in myosin ATPase levels and size and number of mitochondria. Between the ages of 60 and 90 years there is greater loss in muscle power than muscle strength, 3.5% vs. 1.8% per year, respectively.

In both sexes, decreased strength is not usually apparent until 40 years of age, with concentric force production lost more rapidly than that of eccentric force.

Over age 40, decrement is approximately 25% by age 65, with a further proportionate drop after age 65. In women, strength loss is further accentuated by menopause.

These changes are reversible, however, and an increase in local muscular endurance and doubling of force development with 6–8 weeks of initiation of strength training programs is well documented in those 56–70 years old. This ability to increase strength with training in the elderly is extremely important for mobility, balance, and independence.

Respiratory

In the lung, connective tissue elasticity decreases, alveolar size increases, and the number of pulmonary capillaries decreases, leading to an increase in the work of ventilation and decreased perfusion quality.

Cardiovascular

Heart rate max declines with age because of decreased sympathetic tone, marked reduction in sinoatrial (SA) nodal cells, and decreased sarcoplasmic uptake of calcium. Age-related cardiac hypertrophy can paradoxically reduce stroke volume through decreased chamber size.

Aerobic performance

Oxygen uptake decreases because of the cardiorespiratory factors mentioned previously. From age 20 years the average maximal consumption of oxygen (VO_2max) of 750 mL·kg^{-1}·min^{-1} of an untrained male decreases by approximately 5 mL·kg^{-1}·min^{-1} per decade. The same decrements apply to the trained male, but because of higher starting aerobic capacity, their VO_2max values remain consistently higher than in the untrained, and are 20 mL·kg^{-1}·min^{-1} higher at age 40 years and 10 mL·kg^{-1}·min^{-1} higher at age 70 years.

Response to training

Training effects are still apparent in the elderly. Despite the aerobic decrements, elderly people can improve their VO_2max by 15% and training load by 80% after 3 months of aerobic training. There are also similar changes seen in lactate threshold and anaerobic performance indices with appropriate training.

Overtraining syndrome

History and examination

This syndrome is a condition of fatigue and underperformance that occurs following a period of hard training and competition. It affects mainly endurance athletes. The symptoms do not resolve after 2 weeks adequate rest and may be associated with frequent infections and depression. No causative medical condition can be identified.

Normal training is usually cyclical (periodization), allowing adequate time for recovery, and with progressive overload to improve performance. During these cycles, there may be transient symptoms and signs of overtraining known as "overreaching."

With overtraining syndrome, there may have been a sudden increase in training, prolonged heavy training, and other physical and psychological stresses. Most athletes recover fully after 2 weeks of adequate rest. The diagnosis of overtraining syndrome is made when the symptoms and signs persist after 2 weeks of relative rest. While the main complaint is of underperformance, there are other associated features:

- Sleep disturbance is common.
- There may be loss of competitive drive, loss of appetite, and increased emotional lability, anxiety, and irritability.
- The athlete may complain of frequent upper respiratory tract infections or other minor infections, sore throats and lymphadenopathy, myalgia, arthralgia and heavy legs. The athlete may also report a raised resting heart rate.
- There may be symptoms of depression and reduced concentration, as well as loss of libido.

Clinical examination is frequently normal.
- Cervical lymphadenopathy is common but nonspecific.
- Increased resting heart rate
- Increased postural fall in blood pressure and postural rise in heart rate
- Slow recovery of pulse rate to normal after exercise
- Reduced sub-maximum oxygen consumption
- Reduced maximum power output

Diagnosis

There is no specific diagnostic test. Clinical diagnosis excludes other causes of fatigue and reassures the athlete.
- Routine hematological screen. Many athletes have a relatively low hemoglobin count and packed cell volume. This athletic anemia is physiological from hemodilution and does not affect performance.
- Creatine kinase levels are often high, reflecting the intensity, volume, and type of exercise.
- Post-viral illness is confirmed by appropriate viral titers.
- Stress hormones, e.g., adrenaline and cortisol, are generally higher in overtrained athletes than in controls. A low testosterone–cortisol ratio has also been noted in underperforming athletes.
- Low levels of glutamine have been found in overtrained athletes compared to levels in controls.

Treatment

Reassure the athlete that there is no serious pathology and that the prognosis is excellent. The symptoms normally resolve within 6–12 weeks but can persist if athletes return to intensive training too quickly.

- Relative rest for a minimum period of 6 weeks
- Exercise aerobically at a pulse rate of 120–140 for a short period each day, depending on the clinical picture and rate of improvement with the emphasis on volume, not intensity of exercise
- Avoidance of athlete's own sport and use of cross-training to prevent too rapid an increase in exercise intensity
- Vitamins and supplements are recommended, but there is no evidence that they are effective.

Prevention and monitoring

Athletes tolerate different levels of training, competition, and stress throughout the season. While there is no single test to detect overtraining, athletes can monitor fatigue, muscle soreness, sleep, perceived exertion during training, and performance.

Because it is difficult to predict those athletes who will progress from overreaching to becoming overtrained, adequate rest is essential. Training intensity and periodization are the most important factors in minimizing the risk of overtraining. Awareness of the condition and monitoring the response to training may help to prevent overtraining syndrome.

- The profile of mood states (POMS) may be helpful but is not a reliable diagnostic tool.
- Laboratory investigations are not reliable enough for routine monitoring of athletes.
- Athletes can monitor their heart rate but this is nonspecific.

Exercise-induced bronchospasm

Definition

Exercise-induced bronchospasm (EIB) or *exercise-induced asthma (EIA)*: a transient increase in airway resistance following vigorous exercise.

Intrinsic asthma (IA) or *allergic asthma*: chronic airway restriction assumed to be due to some endogenous cause such as allergies.

Epidemiology

Exercise-induced bronchospasm occurs in 80%–90% of asthmatic persons and 40%–50% of those with allergic rhinitis. EIB has an incidence of 5%–19% in elite athletes.

Etiology

The exact cause is not well understood and may have multiple etiologies specific to the individual. The airways are much more sensitive in EIB than in normal individuals, although normal people can have an EIB under the right conditions (i.e., respiratory infections, cold air). Following are factors that may contribute to EIB.

Hyperventilation as the cause of airway drying:
• EIB is worsened in some when exercising in cold dry air.
• The increased osmolarity of the mucous somehow causes a release of bronchoconstrictors.
• Hyperventilation alone can cause bronchospasm.
• Hyperventilation with moist warm air inhibits the bronchoconstriction (which explains why indoor swimming is relatively nonasthmagenic).

The osmolarity of airways does not recover immediately after exercise:
• Prostaglandin E2 may be protective.
• Leukotriene B4 is increased following exercise.
• Leukotriene inhibitors have been shown to decrease bronchoconstriction during exercise.

Post-exercise rewarming as a source of bronchoconstriction:
• Rapid rewarming may cause reactive hyperemia and edema in airway mucosa and submucosa.
• This may result in luminal narrowing and reactive asthma.
• Hyperventilation also increases the amount of allergens and pollutants that may reach the pulmonary tree.

Exercise-induced mediator release from mast cells and basophils can also occur. Parasympathetic mediation can occur through vagus nerve innervation.

Clinical presentation (see Table 11.1)

In normal people and those with EIB with no baseline pulmonary function test (PFT) changes, exercise increases pulmonary functions (peak expiratory flow rate [PEFR] and forced expiratory volume in 1 second [FEV_1] by <5%. In those with baseline obstruction it may increase by >25%.

From 28% to 52% of those with EIB experience a decline in PFT values by the end of exercise. This pattern may intensify over the next 3–20 minutes and may last 20–30 minutes.

Table 11.1 Clinical clues to exercise-induced bronchospasm (may be present during or after exercise)

Obvious clinical clues	Subtle clinical clues
• Wheezing	• Abdominal pain
• Cough	• Athlete feels "out of shape"
• Dyspnea on exertion	• Cannot run 5 minutes without stopping
• Chest tightness	• Chest congestion
	• Chest discomfort or pain
	• Increased difficulty in cold air
	• Problems with running but not swimming
	• Lack of energy
	• Frequent colds

After exercise there may be a decrease in pulmonary function by up to 10% in normal subjects (this decrease is higher in EIB).

Refractory period
After exercise, approximately 50% of those with EIB are resistant to further bronchospasm. This usually lasts <3 hours.

Late-phase reaction
A second increase in airway reactivity may be seen in up to 50% of children 4–12 hours after the acute episode.

The release of inflammatory mediators by bronchial smooth muscle such as eosinophilic chemotactic factor of anaphylaxis, platelet-activating factor, and some leukotrienes has been theorized as a cause.

Diagnosis

History
The athlete may be unaware of any bronchospasm. More significant symptoms include shortness of breath, cough, lack of endurance, or wheeze, during or immediately following sustained exercise.

They may feel vague chest tightness or feel out of shape when exercising. Children may simply avoid strenuous play, have chest pain, or experience abdominal pain.

Multiple stimulants have been identified (see Table 11.2).

Pulmonary function tests
- Medications are withheld for 8–24 hours before testing.
- Baseline PFTs are done first and results should be within 80% of predicted values (or intrinsic asthma may be present).
- Use a bicycle or ergometer for testing exercise stress (or whatever activity is most asthmagenic).
- The athlete exercises until 80%–90% of maximum heart rate is achieved.

Table 11.2 Stimulants that can contribute to exercise-induced bronchospasm

• Exercise	• Primary pollutants
• Cold air	• Secondary pollutants
• Low humidity	• Other pollutants
• Respiratory infections	• Strong odors and other airborne irritants
• Fatigue	
• Emotional stress	• Allergens
• Athletic overtraining	

- Heart rate is maintained for 6–8 minutes.
- PFTs are measured immediately after exercise and then every 5 minutes for 20–30 minutes.

EIB is present if there is a 15% or more decrease in peak expiratory flow rate (PEFR) or forced expiratory volume after 1 second (FEV_1).
- 15%–20% decrease is mild EIB.
- 20%–40% decrease is moderate EIB.
- >40% decrease is severe EIB.

Methacholine challenge test
- If the suspicion is high for EIB and exercise testing is negative, a methacholine challenge test may be performed.
- This is a more sensitive test, but less specific.
- Intubation equipment must be available.

Treatment
For an EIB treatment algorithm see Table 11.3.
Nonpharmacological
Regular exercise programs
- Regular exercise programs produce a significant reduction in bronchoconstrictions.
- They increase tolerance and threshold levels for exercise.
- Decreased medication needs
- Improvement in aerobic capacity

Considerations
- Wearing a facemask for outdoor exercise may increase temperature and humidity of air and filter out allergens and pollutants.
- A warm shower immediately after exercise may reduce bronchospasm.
- Don't exercise in early morning or late evening if conditions are cold.
- Encourage indoor sports in winter.
- Avoid areas where pollutants and allergens are high.
- Encourage water sports or sports that allow intermittent rest periods (most team sports, tennis, weight lifting, racquetball, etc.).
- Short bursts of activity can produce refractory periods lasting up to 3 hours.

Table 11.3 Treatment algorithm for exercise-induced bronchospasm

Nonpharmacologic corrections (see text)
EIA continues
⇩
β_2 agonist (B2A)
EIA continues
⇩
Add cromolyn or nedocromil for a child or late responder, or when there is history of response to cromolyn (may double B2A and cromolyn if needed)
EIA continues
⇩
Add inhaled glucocorticoid (also good for late-phase symptoms)
EIA continues
⇩
Add leukotriene inhibitor
EIA continues
⇩
Add long-acting β_2 agonist
EIA continues
⇩
Add ipratropium bromide. By now, most asthmatics' symptoms should be controlled. If not, consider oral steroid burst, alternative cause, or referral
⇩
Effective control of EIA
(check inhaler technique and lung function regularly)

- Warm up before any exercise for 10–15 minutes and cool down for 8–10 minutes.
- Nose breathing may increase temperature and humidity of inspired air.
- Encourage the athlete to try to "run through" their asthma to take advantage of the refractory period.

Pharmacological

Short-acting B_2 agonists, metered-dose inhaler (MDI; albuterol, terbutaline, metaproterenol, bitolterol, etc.):
- Drug of choice for prophylactic and acute treatment
- Initial treatment is with β_2 agonist MDI 15–60 minutes before exercise
- Effective in about 95% of patients
- May provide protection for 3–6 hours
- May cause tachycardia or slight tremor

Mast cell stabilizers, MDI (cromolyn sodium and nedocromyl sodium):
- If the patient is a child or a late responder or has responded to cromolyn in the past, add cromolyn 15–30 minutes before exercise.
- 70%–80% are protected
- May prevent late-phase reaction and thus may be more effective in children

- Decreased duration compared to β_2 agonist.
- Not effective for acute attacks
- May be most effective in combination with β_2 agonists

Long-acting β_2 agonists, MDI (salmeterol):
- Taken 45–60 minutes before exercise
- May give protection for up to 6 hours
- Cannot be used for acute episodes
- Expensive

Leukotriene inhibitors, oral (montelukast, zafirlukast, zileuton):
- Leukotriene receptor antagonists
- Shown to improve airway edema and smooth muscle constriction and reduce inflammation
- Blocks leukotrienes D4 and E4 as well as slow-reacting substance of anaphylaxis
- Recently advocated as treatment for EIB
- May have some drug interactions and liver toxicity

Glucocorticoids, oral and inhaled (beclomethasone, flunisolide, fluticasone, triamcinolone):
- Those athletes with a baseline obstruction on PFT (and maybe late-phase reactors) should be on an inhaled bronchodilator and an inhaled glucocorticoid.
- Oral glucocorticoids are used acutely for gaining control in inflammatory asthma.
- Inhaled glucocorticoids are used for maintenance of control.
- Both will decrease the reactivity of the airways.

Theophylline, oral:
- May be of some benefit in some patients
- Serum levels must be monitored
- Toxic in high doses
- Not presently used often for EIB

Anticholinergic agents, MDI (ipratropium bromide):
- Add ipratropium bromide 1–2 hours before exercise
- Not effective in all patients
- Especially effective for chronic obstructive pulmonary disease (COPD), bronchitis, and emphysema
- May be used for acute attacks

Iron deficiency anemia

Background

The capacity of the body to transport oxygen is one of the factors that limits physical performance. Oxygen is transported in the blood by the pigment of the red blood cells (hemoglobin). If the concentration of hemoglobin is reduced, the oxygen-transporting capacity of the body is impaired, and the capacity to perform drops.

Anemia is said to occur when the concentration of hemoglobin falls below that specified as normal for the individual's age and gender. Iron deficiency is the most common form of true anemia among athletes. Stores of iron are often depleted before clinical signs are apparent.

Iron occurs in small quantities in the body, totaling about 1.5–1.75 oz (4–5 g) in the adult. It is required for the manufacture of not only hemoglobin but also the related compound myoglobin, found in muscle tissue. Both of these substances bind oxygen and play an important role in its transport. Iron is stored mainly in hemoglobin and bone marrow.

Iron deficiency anemia is most prevalent among menstruating women and males between the age of 11 and 14.

Three conditions occur during anemia: erythrocytes (red blood cells) are too small, hemoglobin is decreased, and ferritin concentration is low. Ferritin is an iron–phosphorous–protein complex that normally contains 23% iron.

There are many ways that athletes can be iron deficient. Gastrointestinal (GI) losses are common in runners because of bowel ischemia. Aspirin or nonsteroidal anti-inflammatory drugs (NSAIDs) may cause GI blood loss. Inadequate dietary intake of iron is the primary cause of iron deficiency.

The recommended daily allowance (RDA) is 15 mg/day for females and 10 mg/day for males. The average diet contains 5–7 mg or iron per 100 kcal. Because female athletes often eat less than they need, they also fail to consume enough iron. If the athlete is a vegetarian they may run the risk of lacking in iron.

The diagnosis of anemia can be confirmed by measuring the hemoglobin levels of the body. An iron deficiency can be identified by blood cell analysis and by determining the serum ferritin level. Young people store only small amounts of iron, and low serum ferritin levels are therefore normal in individuals under the age 20.

Signs and symptoms

Early on, the athlete's performance begins to decline. Athletes with mild iron-deficiency anemia may have a slight drop-off in maximum performance. Determining serum ferritin is the most accurate test of one's iron levels. The athlete's mean corpuscular volume (MCV), which is the average volume of individual cells in cubic micron, and the relative sizes of the erythrocytes are measured.

Treatment

The following are some ways to manage iron deficiency: ensure a proper balanced diet, include more red meat or dark poultry in the diet; avoid coffee and tea, as they effect iron absorption from grains; ingest vitamin C sources, which enhance iron absorption; and take an iron supplement, consisting of ferrous sulfate 325 mg.

Footstrike anemia

The cause of footstrike anemia, as its name implies, is the impact of the foot as it strikes the floor surface. Impact forces serve to destroy normal erythrocytes within the vascular system.

The hemolysis is characterized by mildly enlarged red cells, an increase in circulatory reticulocytes, and a decrease in the concentration of haptoglobin, which is a glycoprotein bound to hemoglobin and released into the plasma. Even if the athlete wears a well-designed and well-constructed shoe, this condition can occur.

Footstrike anemia can be managed by running on soft surfaces, wearing well-cushioned shoes and insoles, and running as lightly as possible on the feet.

Sickle cell anemia

Background

The top causes of nontraumatic sports deaths in high school and college athletes are cardiovascular conditions, hyperthermia (heatstroke), acute rhabdomyolysis tied to sickle cell trait, and asthma. Sickle cell trait is the inheritance of one gene for sickle hemoglobin and one for normal hemoglobin.

During intense exercise, the sickle hemoglobin can change the shape of red cells to a "sickle" shape. Sickle cells can block blood vessels and lead to collapse and the rapid breakdown of muscles starved of blood. Heat, dehydration, altitude, and asthma can increase the risk for and worsen sickling.

The sickle gene is common in people whose origin is from areas where malaria is widespread. Over the millennia, carrying one sickle gene fended off death from malaria, leaving 1 in 12 African-Americans (vs. 1 in 2000 to 1 in 10,000 white Americans) with sickle cell trait. The sickle gene is also present in those of Mediterranean, Middle Eastern, Indian, Caribbean, and South and Central American ancestry. Of 136 sudden, nontraumatic sports deaths in high school and college athletes over a decade, seven (5%) were from exertional sickling.

With sickle cell trait, strenuous exercise causes stress on the red blood cells that lead to sickling. These stresses include severe hypoxemia, metabolic acidosis, hyperthermia in muscles, and red-cell dehydration.

A sickle cell crisis may occur at the following times:

- Early in the season
- During intense sustained strength training
- When a sporting event takes place at a higher altitude than what a player is accustomed to

Symptoms

A sickle cell crisis has been mistaken for a cardiac event or heat illness. But unlike a sickle cell crisis, a cardiac event is usually a sudden event. Unlike heat illness, sickling is not associated with a rise in core temperature. Sickling is often confused with heat cramping, but there are ways to distinguish the two conditions:

- Heat cramping often has a prodrome of muscle twinges and sickling does not.
- Heat cramping pain is more severe.
- Heat crampers hobble to a halt with tight muscles, and sickling players slump to the ground with weak muscles.
- Heat crampers have muscles that are visibly contracted and firm, whereas sicklers have muscles that appear and feel normal.

Prevention

An athlete with a sickle trait should not be disqualified, but precautions must be taken. For the athlete with sickle cell trait, it is recommended that each athlete do the following:

- Start the preseason training sessions slowly and allow longer periods of rest and recovery between repetitions.

- Athletes need to stop the workout if symptoms of muscle cramping, pain, swelling, weakness, tenderness, shortness of breath, or fatigue occur.
- Heat stress, dehydration, asthma, illness, and altitude predispose the athlete with sickle trait to an onset of crisis in physical exertion.
  - Adjust work–rest cycles for environmental heat stress
  - Emphasize hydration
  - Control asthma
  - No workout if an athlete with sickle trait is ill
  - Watch closely the athlete with sickle cell trait who is new to the altitude. Modify training and have supplemental oxygen available for competitions.

Educate to create an environment that encourages athletes with sickle cell trait to report any signs or symptoms such as fatigue, difficulty breathing, leg or low back pain, or leg or low-back cramping.

Treatment for a sickle cell crisis

A sickle cell crisis needs to be treated as a medical emergency:
- Check vital signs.
- Administer high-flow oxygen, 15 lpm (if available), with a non-rebreather face mask.
- Cool the athlete.
- If the athlete is obtunded or as vital signs decline, call 911, attach an automated external defibrillator (AED)
- Start an intravenous (IV) line.

Summary

There is no contraindication to participation in sports for the athlete with sickle cell trait. Red blood cells can sickle during intense exertion, blocking blood vessels and posing a grave risk for athletes with sickle cell trait. Screening and simple precautions may prevent deaths and help athletes with sickle cell trait participate in their sport safely.

Diabetes mellitus

Background

Diabetes mellitus (DM) is a chronic endocrine disorder characterized by hyperglycemia. Persons with diabetes are at risk for macrovascular, microvascular, and neuropathic complications.

Chronic hyperglycemia leads to long-term damage and failure of various organs, especially the eyes, kidneys, nerves, and heart. Type 2 diabetes typically occurs in adults 40 years of age and older. Type 1 diabetes typically occurs in children and young adults and is the rarer form of the disease, but the sports medicine team is more likely to encounter athletes with type 1 than with type 2 diabetes.

The main goal in managing diabetes is to keep blood glucose levels at or as close to normal levels as possible without causing hypoglycemia. This is often challenging because of the physical demands during exercise affecting the glucose levels. The sports medicine team should know each athlete that is a diabetic and a plan should be in place for each athlete.

Diabetes care plan

Each athlete with diabetes should have a diabetes care plan for practices and games. The plan should include the following:

- Blood glucose monitoring guidelines. Address frequency of monitoring and pre-exercise exclusion values.
- Insulin therapy guidelines. These should include the type of insulin used, dosages and adjustment strategies for planned activities types, and insulin correction dosages for high blood glucose levels.
- List of other medications. Include those used to treat other diabetes-related conditions.
- Guidelines for hypoglycemia recognition and treatment
- Include prevention, signs, symptoms, and treatment of hypoglycemia, with instructions on the use of glucagon.
- Emergency contact information. Include parents' and/or other family and physician telephone numbers.

Supplies for medical bags/kits

Supplies to treat diabetes-related emergencies should be available at all practices and games. The athlete (or athlete's parents or guardians, in the case of minors) provides the following items:

- A copy of the diabetes care plan
- Blood glucose monitoring equipment and supplies. Check the expiration dates of supplies, such as blood glucose testing strips and insulin, on a regular basis.
- Supplies to treat hypoglycemia, including sugary foods (e.g., glucose tablets, sugar packets) or sugary fluids (e.g., orange juice, non-diet soda) and a glucagon injection kit
- Supplies for urine or blood ketone testing
- A sharps container to ensure proper disposal of syringes and lancets.

Hypoglycemia

Hypoglycemia is the most severe acute complication of intensive insulin therapy in diabetes, and exercise is its most frequent cause. Under most circumstances, hypoglycemia is the result of too much insulin, both during and after exercise. Several factors contribute to too much insulin.

First, the rate at which subcutaneously injected insulin is absorbed increases with exercise due to increases in body temperature and in subcutaneous and skeletal muscle blood flow.

Second, exogenously administered insulin levels do not decrease during exercise in persons with type 1 diabetes. This is in contrast to exercise in persons without diabetes, in whom insulin levels decrease during exercise to prevent hypoglycemia. The inability to decrease plasma insulin levels during exercise in type 1 diabetes causes relative hyper-insulinemia.

Finally, exercise improves insulin sensitivity in skeletal muscle.

Exercise-associated improvements in insulin sensitivity may last for several hours to days after exercise. Some athletes experience a phenomenon known as post-exercise late-onset hypoglycemia, which may occur while the athlete is sleeping. Athletes who experience nighttime hypoglycemia require additional blood glucose monitoring in addition to a snack.

Managing blood glucose levels during practices and games and preventing hypoglycemia are challenges. Typically, hypoglycemia prevention requires a three-part approach of blood glucose monitoring, carbohydrate supplementation, and insulin adjustments.

Hypoglycemia normally produces noticeable autonomic or neurogenic symptoms. Autonomic symptoms include tachycardia, sweating, palpitations, hunger, nervousness, headache, trembling, and dizziness. These symptoms typically occur at blood glucose levels <70 mg/dL (<3.9 mmol/L) in persons with diabetes.

As glucose continues to fall, symptoms of brain neuronal glucose deprivation (neurogenic symptoms) occur and may cause blurred vision, fatigue, difficulty thinking, loss of motor control, aggressive behavior seizures, convulsions, and loss of consciousness. If hypoglycemia is prolonged and severe, brain damage and even death can result.

Athletes should measure blood glucose levels before, during, and after exercise. Athletes who exercise in extreme heat or cold or at high altitude or experience post-exercise late-onset hypoglycemia, which may lead to nighttime hypoglycemia, require additional monitoring.

- Measure blood glucose levels 2 to 3 times before exercise at 30-minute intervals to determine directional glucose movement.
- Measure glucose levels every 30 minutes during exercise, if possible.
- Athletes who experience post-exercise late-onset hypoglycemia should measure glucose levels every 2 hours up to 4 hours post-exercise. Athletes who experience nighttime hypoglycemia should measure blood glucose values before going to sleep, once during the night, and immediately upon waking.

When using an insulin pump, the following insulin-reduction strategy may be used.

- Reduce basal rate by 20%–50% 1–2 hours before exercise.
- Reduce bolus dose up to 50% at the meal preceding exercise.
- Suspend or disconnect the insulin pump at the start of exercise.
  Athletes should not suspend or disconnect from the pump longer than 60 minutes without supplemental insulin.

Also, athletes using a multiple daily injection may reduce the bolus dose up to 50% at the meal preceding exercise.

Hyperglycemia and ketosis

Hyperglycemia with or without ketosis can occur during exercise in athletes with type 1 diabetes. Hyperglycemia during exercise is related to several factors.

First, exercise can cause additional increases in blood glucose concentrations and possible ketoacidosis in athletes with poor glycemic control and in those who have not taken enough insulin. Without adequate insulin levels, blood glucose levels continue to rise because of exaggerated hepatic glucose production and impairments in exercise-induced glucose utilization.

Second, even in well-controlled athletes with type 1 diabetes, high-intensity exercise may result in hyperglycemia. High-intensity exercise may lead to significant increases in catecholamines, free fatty acids, and ketone bodies, all of which impair muscle glucose utilization and increase blood glucose levels. This exercise-associated rise in glucose levels is usually transient in the well-controlled diabetic athlete, declining as counterregulatory hormone levels decrease, typically within 30–60 minutes.

Third, the psychological stress of competition is frequently associated with increases in blood glucose levels before competition.

While effects of hyperglycemia vary from one athlete to another, hyperglycemic signs and symptoms include nausea, dehydration, reduced cognitive performance, slowing of visual reaction time, and feelings of sluggishness and fatigue. Symptoms of hyperglycemia with ketoacidosis may include those listed above as well as rapid breathing (known as Kussmaul breathing), fruity odor of the breath, unusual fatigue, sleepiness, inattentiveness, loss of appetite, increased thirst, and frequent urination.

Treatment for mild hypoglycemia

In mild hypoglycemia the athlete is conscious and able to follow directions and swallow.

- Administer 10–15 g of fast-acting carbohydrate—e.g., 4–8 glucose tablets, 2 T honey.
- Measure blood glucose level.
- Wait approximately 15 minutes and re-measure blood glucose.
- If blood glucose level remains low, administer another 10–15 g of fast-acting carbohydrate.
- Recheck blood glucose level in approximately 15 minutes.

- If blood glucose level does not return to the normal range after the second dosage of carbohydrate, activate emergency medical system.
- Once the blood glucose level is in the normal range, the athlete may wish to consume a snack (e.g., sandwich, bagel).

Treatment for severe hypoglycemia

Severe hypoglycemia is when the athlete is unconscious or unable to follow directions or swallow.

- Activate emergency medical system.
- Prepare glucagon for injection following directions in the glucagon kit. The glucagons kit has either (1) a fluid-filled syringe and a vial of glucagon powder, or (2) a syringe, 1 vial of glucagon powder, and 1 vial of fluid.
  - Inject the fluid into the vial of glucagon. If the vial of fluid is separate, draw fluid into the syringe and inject it into the vial of glucagon powder.
  - Gently shake the vial until the glucagon powder dissolves and the solution is clear.
  - Draw fluid back into the syringe and then inject glucagon into the arm, thigh, or buttock.

Glucagon administration may cause nausea and/or vomiting when the athlete awakens. Place the athlete on their side to prevent aspiration.

Hyperglycemia and exercise

Blood glucose levels

Fasting blood glucose level is >250 mg/dL (13.9 mmol/L):

- Test urine and/or blood for ketones.
- If ketones are present, exercise is contraindicated.
- If ketones are not present, exercise is not contraindicated.

Blood glucose value is >300 mg/dL (16.7 mmol/L) and without ketones:

- Exercise with caution and continue to monitor blood glucose levels.

Summary

Physical activity is beneficial for individuals with diabetes, but such exercise can make blood glucose management difficult. Maintaining the delicate balance between hypoglycemia, euglycemia, and hyperglycemia is best achieved through a team approach. Athletes with diabetes can benefit from a well-organized plan that may allow them to compete on equal ground with their teammates and competitors without diabetes.

Body weight

Total energy intake must be raised to meet the increased energy expended during training. Maintenance of energy balance can be assessed by monitoring body weight, body composition, and food intake.

Weight gain

For those athletes who wish to gain body weight, caloric intake should exceed energy expenditure. Increased muscle mass, from physical training, can lead to increased body weight even with a reduction in body fat percentage.

Weight loss

For those athletes who wish to lose weight, caloric intake should not exceed energy expenditure. The caloric deficit will dictate the amount of weight that can be lost. To maximize the loss of fat and minimize the loss of lean tissue, weight loss should be limited to 500–1000 g per week. This would require an energy restriction of 2–4 megajoules (MJ) per day.

When body weight needs to be reduced, this should be done gradually and not immediately before competition. The use of diuretics and laxatives should be discouraged.

Fluid status will affect body weight. Volume depletion will show "weight loss" whereas hyperhydration can present with body-weight gain. These fluid gains and losses are transient and can be detrimental to health if carried out for the wrong reasons (i.e., "making weight" in sports that require weight classes for competition).

Body mass index (BMI)

BMI is generally used as a descriptive tool for assessing health risks. BMI can be calculated with imperial or metric units.

Weight in pounds / [(height in inches)^2] × 703

or

Weight in kilograms / [(height in meters)^2]

Energy requirements

The main component of daily energy turnover in an average person is the basal metabolic rate (BMR).

BMR represents the *minimum* amount of energy expenditure needed for ongoing processes in the body in the resting state, when no food is digested and no energy is needed for temperature regulation. The most variable component of daily energy turnover is the energy expenditure for activity (EEA), which can range between 15% and 25% of the BMR in moderately active persons.

For sports such as gymnastics, dancing, diving, and running, in which a lean physique is desired, athletes will routinely restrict their caloric intake to achieve a leaner body composition. This practice reduces the metabolic rate and may lead to conditions such as menstrual dysfunction (amenorrhea), iron deficiency (anemia), and a decrease in bone density (osteoporosis or osteopenia).

A chronic negative energy balance will result in a loss of fat-free (muscle) mass as well as a loss of body fat. Lethargy from the excessive loss of lean body mass and depletion of glycogen stores generally limits performance and the ability to train properly, making an athlete more susceptible to illness and injury.

An increase in lean body mass will increase energy requirements for basal activities and visa versa. Athletes who sustain hard and vigorous activity for prolonged periods of time must supplement their caloric needs by ingesting more energy-dense foodstuffs to sustain exercise and match energy demands during exercise. While increased energy consumption can be achieved by ingesting primarily more carbohydrate-rich solid food or liquid carbohydrate formulas, increases in fat and protein ingestion are also part of a healthy mixed diet.

The higher the intensity of the exercise and the more muscle groups that are activated, the more the energy requirements of that activity are increased.

Food and exercise

Physically active individuals must meet their energy requirements by ingesting a variety of foodstuffs before, during, and after exercise. For most individuals, the consumption of a normal mixed diet consisting of 50% carbohydrate and 10%–30% fat, with the difference made up with protein, is adequate.

The only reason to consume protein or fat several hours before exercise or exercise performance is to provide satiety, which can influence performance by promoting a sense of well-being. If carbohydrate stores are adequate, the choice of food before exercise should be based on the past experience of the athlete—the food choice should minimize hunger, yet not interfere with the exercise mode and duration.

Habituation to a high-fat diet decreases the amount of muscle glycogen used during exercise by increasing the body's ability to use and mobilize fat. The increased ability to oxidize fat for fuel may enable an athlete to continue exercising for longer periods at intensities of 70% of VO_2max or less. However, habituation to a high-fat diet is associated with a reduced performance ability during high-intensity exercise performance, such as when attempting to elevate power output during hill climbing in endurance cycling or running events.

Carbohydrate needs

The carbohydrate (CHO) needs of individuals vary depending on their mass and the level of physical activity. Larger and more active individuals will require generally more energy and therefore more CHO. However, in the normal exercising population the CHO needs will be met by consuming a normal mixed diet as described above.

Protein needs

The protein needs of individuals also vary with mass and activity level, but are also generally met when one is consuming a normal mixed diet. Although the RDA for protein is 0.8 g/kg of body mass, highly active endurance athletes may require up to 1 g/kg of body mass, while those striving to build large amounts of muscle mass may require in excess of 1.5 g/kg of body mass.

Usually these requirements are adequately covered by the increased energy intake stimulated by physical activity, and it is often unnecessary to increase actively the protein content of the diet by eating selectively protein-rich foodstuffs.

Pre-event diet

Carbohydrate loading has been shown to increase muscle glycogen content before exercise and delay the time at which low muscle glycogen concentrations are reached. The main effect of this practice is to decrease the amount of fat oxidized during exercise.

Carbohydrate loading is achieved by eating a high-carbohydrate diet (75%–90%) for 3 days prior to the competitive event. To achieve this, athletes should consume approximately 8 g CHO or more per kg of body mass.

Pre-event meal

The pre-event diet aims to optimize muscle glycogen and liver glycogen stores that maintain blood glucose levels during exercise. The ingestion of carbohydrate before an event will stimulate carbohydrate oxidation and inhibit fat oxidation.

Evidence suggests that performance is improved when 200–300 g CHO is consumed 3–4 hours before prolonged exercise, compared to when no food is ingested.

Immediately prior to the event

Foods that are consumed immediately prior to an event should be low in fat, protein, and fiber, and should not cause gastrointestinal distress.

Foods ingested 4–6 hours before an event should be of a low to moderate glycemic index to minimize the insulin response. If the muscles are not fully stocked with glycogen (because of recent exercise or a low CHO diet), however, then foods with a moderate to high glycemic index are preferred prior to an athletic event.

Food supplements

Numerous well-controlled studies have concluded that individuals eating a well-balanced diet do not need to supplement their diet with vitamins, minerals, or trace elements when undertaking an exercise program. The ingestion of these supplements on physical performance has not been clearly shown to have benefits.

Vitamins

Vitamins are divided into water- and fat-soluble categories. Water-soluble vitamins such as thiamin, riboflavin, B_6, niacin, pantothenic acid, biotin, and vitamin C are involved in mitochondrial metabolism. Folate and vitamin B_{12} are primarily involved in DNA synthesis and red blood cell development.

Fat-soluble vitamins include vitamins A, K, E, and D, with vitamin E being the most widely studied as an ergogenic aid. Vitamin E has antioxidant properties, as do vitamins C, A, and beta-carotene. There is a linear relationship between energy intake and vitamin intake, thus vitamin intake should exceed the RDA, provided that a varied diet is consumed.

Mega-doses of both fat- and water-soluble vitamins have been shown to have toxic effects.

Minerals

Minerals are divided into macrominerals and microminerals (trace minerals). Macrominerals include calcium, magnesium, phosphorous, sulfur, potassium, sodium and chloride with calcium, phosphorus, and calcium, each constituting 0.01% of total body weight.

Trace minerals include iron, zinc, copper, selenium, chromium, iodine, fluorine, manganese, molybdenum, nickel, silicon, vanadium, arsenic, and cobalt, with each constituting <0.001% of total body weight. Iron, zinc, copper, selenium, and chromium have been proposed to enhance physical performance and may improve physical performance if an athlete is deficient in that certain mineral, or if an increased level of this mineral would boost the body's natural response to enhance performance.

Amino acids, electrolytes, and herbal supplements have not been shown to improve physical performance in well-controlled scientific studies.

Iron

Iron is a necessary component of hemoglobin and myoglobin and facilitates the transport of oxygen through the bloodstream as well as the transfer of electrons in the electron transport chain system. Between 60% and 70% of iron is found in hemoglobin, with the remainder found in bone marrow, muscle, liver, and spleen.

Organ meats, black strap molasses, clams, oysters, dried legumes, nuts and seeds, red meats, and dark leafy vegetables are good exogenous sources of iron. Symptoms of an iron deficiency include generalized fatigue and anemia. Liver damage can occur from iron excess.

Iron deficiency anemia in athletes may result from a poor diet, excess blood loss (through menstruation in females), and footstrike hemolysis, and through sweat loss. Although numerous studies have documented that athletes, particularly endurance athletes, are iron depleted, the degree and percentage of iron depletion are similar between athletes and non-athletes.

Pseudoanemia occurs in athletes secondary to an increase in plasma volume, which occurs as an adaptation to training. This increase in plasma volume "dilutes" an otherwise normal red blood cell count into falsely low levels. Hence, this is an artificial lowering of hemoglobin rather than a true anemic response, which is a common laboratory finding in endurance athletes.

The recommended daily allowance for iron intake for males is 10–12 mg/day and 15 mg/day for females.

Calcium

Calcium is required for the formation and maintenance of hard bones and for the conduction of nerve impulses. Calcium activates enzymes responsible for the transmission of membrane potentials and for muscle contraction. The skeleton contains 99% of calcium, with the remainder found in extracellular fluid, intracellular structures, and cell membranes.

Dairy products, sardines, clams, oysters, turnips, broccoli, and legumes are good exogenous sources of calcium. Osteoporosis and fractures can occur from a deficiency in calcium intake over decades. Constipation, kidney stones, and chelation with antibiotics and other nutrients (such as iron and zinc) can occur with calcium excess.

Weight-bearing exercise has been shown to increase bone density, especially when undertaken at critical growth periods (8–14 years of age). Estrogen has been shown to reduce urinary calcium excretion, increase intestinal absorption of calcium, and increase the secretion of calcitonin, which reduces bone resorption.

Calcium also can be lost through sweat, which may increase an athlete's total daily requirement if exercise is regularly performed in hot and humid environments. The recommended daily allowance for calcium is 800–1200 mg/day for both men and women.

Creatine

Creatine is a naturally occurring compound in the body, specifically in the muscles. Creatine supplementation is widely practiced by professional and recreational athletes. The benefits and side effects are varied and debatable. Purported benefits include increased mass, improved rate of recovery after exercise, and increased power or speed. Side affects incluce cramping and water retention.

Although much research has been devoted to creatine anc its effects, the real value of creatine supplementation remains uncertain Untrained persons undertaking a weight training program for the first time appear to benefit the most. Elite athletes who eat diets with adequate protein intake may benefit less.

Recovery after exercise

Recovery after exercise is most important if another bout of physical activity will shortly follow. Full recovery after exercise is also important in reducing the risk of overtraining, although the training volumes required to produce overtraining are usually achievable only by highly trained individuals.

Recovery is also an important part of adapting to exercise training, because the physical adaptations that are stimulated by exercise training occur during the rest and recovery phase.

Recovery appears to be aided by the ingestion of carbohydrate- and protein-rich foodstuffs within 30–60 minutes after the termination of exercise.

Exercise and the environment

Different environmental conditions will affect exercise tolerance and capacity in different ways. There are three overriding environmental factors to which athletes may be exposed in either training or racing, or both—heat, cold, and reduced oxygen content in the inspired air as occurs at increasing altitude.

In order to survive, humans need to regulate their body temperatures between 35° and 41°C and to maintain the partial pressure of oxygen in their blood in excess of about 40 mmHg.

Environmental conditions, in particular the environmental temperature, the wind speed, and the water content of the air (humidity), determine the rate at which heat is lost from the body. The normal average human skin temperature is 33°C. At any lower environmental temperature, heat will be lost from the skin to the environment in the process of heat conduction. The rate at which this heat will be lost by conduction from the body will, in turn, be determined by the magnitude of the temperature gradient—the steeper the gradient, the greater the heat loss—and the rapidity with which the cooler air in contact with the skin is replaced by colder air.

Continual replacement of warmed air by cooler air causes loss of heat from the body, by means of convection. Convective heat loss rises as an exponential function of the speed at which air courses across the body, in effect, the prevailing wind speed. With high humidity, sweat loss by evaporation is reduced.

Body temperature

At rest, humans regulate their body temperatures within a narrow range of between 36.5° and 37.5°C. During exercise, this safe thermoregulatory range is increased to up to 41.5°C. Heat-acclimatized human athletes have a superior capacity to exercise without apparent distress even up to body temperatures of 41.5°C.

The human body temperature represents a balance between the rate of heat production by, and heat loss from, the body. Hence, changes in the rates of either heat production or heat loss or, more commonly, both, determine whether an abnormal rise in body temperature (hyperthermia leading to heatstroke) or an excessive fall (hypothermia) is likely to develop and under what conditions.

The principal physiological challenge that athletes face during exercise is how to lose the excess body heat produced by muscle contraction.

Hypothermia

When environmental conditions are particularly cold, for example, (1) during winter conditions at latitudes above about 50° in either hemisphere, (2) when cold is associated with windy and especially wet conditions, or (3) when athletes exercise in cold water for prolonged periods, the risk arises that athletes will lose heat faster than they can produce it. Under these conditions, the body may be unable to maintain its core body temperature, which may fall progressively, leading to *hypothermia* (core temperature <35°C) and the risk of death from the exposure/exhaustion syndrome.

Low body temperatures of 35°C occur frequently in swimmers exposed to cold water temperatures for many hours, for example, in long-distance English Channel swims. This occurs because water is an excellent conductor of heat, approximately 30 times more effective than air. As a result, the naked body exposed to a body of water that is colder than the normal body temperature of 37°C is unable to produce heat as rapidly as it is lost by conduction to the surrounding water.

If exposed for sufficiently long, the human body will be cooled to the temperature of the surrounding water, which is seldom more than 20°C except at the tropics. Wearing more appropriate clothing, in particular, dry or wet suits that maintain a layer of insulating water or air heated to body temperature, is the only way to prevent the ultimate development of a fatal hypothermia when exposed to cold water for any protracted period (hours).

Prevention of hypothermia

When exercising in cold conditions, hypothermia can be prevented by continued activity, adequate clothing, and the presence of insulating layers. There is a high rate of heat production during exercise. Thus, as a general rule, continuing to move reduces the risk that hypothermia will develop. However, once athletes become too exhausted to continue, their rate of heat production falls sharply and the risk of hypothermia rises dramatically.

The important practical point to make here is that continuing to exercise will protect against hypothermia if it maintains the rate of heat production that equals or exceeds the heat loss. In contrast, once the hiker, runner, or mountain climber starts to walk or stops walking altogether, the rate of heat production falls dramatically, providing the necessary conditions for hypothermia.

The change from running to walking, for example, has a marked effect on the clothing needed to maintain body temperature, even at relatively mild temperatures. Clothing with at least four times as much insulation is required to maintain body temperature at rest at an effective air temperature of 0°C, as when running at 16 km per hour. Thus, extra clothing should always be available if there is any possibility that fatigue will develop when exercising in cold conditions.

Whereas air is a poor conductor of heat and hence a good insulator, water is a very poor insulator. The thin layer of air trapped next to the skin by clothing is rapidly heated to the skin temperature, thereby producing a layer of insulation. But the saturation of clothing with water removes this insulating layer and essentially exposes the skin to whatever the external temperature is.

Under these conditions, the exposed human must either find dry, warm clothing and a warm shelter, or they will cool to the prevailing environmental temperature. This loss of insulation caused by water explains why saturated, wet clothing on runners, climbers, or hikers in windy, wet conditions or, alternatively, swimmers in cold water, predisposes them to the development of hypothermia.

Experience with the English Channel swimmers has shown that body build, especially the body muscle (but also the body fat) content, is a critical factor determining the rate at which a swimmer will cool down during a long-distance swim in water temperatures below about 24°C. The same principle probably applies in out-of-water activities: subjects who are more muscular and fatter are likely to cool down more slowly when exposed to very cold conditions.

Thus, appropriate fitness, proper clothing including water-repellent outer garments, adequate nutrition to prevent premature fatigue, early recognition of danger, and avoidance of extreme environmental conditions are crucial to ensure that exercise can be safely undertaken in cold, wet, and windy conditions.

Diagnosis of hypothermia

- Rectal temperature <37°C (usually much lower)
- Exposure to cold conditions for prolonged periods
- Fatigue
- Muscle weakness and loss of coordination
- Desire to stop exercising
- Disorientation, leading to coma

Treatment of hypothermia

- Removal from the cold environment, application of dry clothing and/or blankets
- External heating in the form of hot water bottles, warm water bath, radiant heat, convective heat, or even the body heat of other humans
- In severe hypothermia, consider using heated intravenous fluids or extracorporeal blood-warming techniques.
- Warming efforts should continue until the body temperature exceeds 35°C, since a person with hypothermia is not "cold and dead" until they are shown to be "warm and dead."

NOTE: Be aware that ventricular fibrillation is a common complication of treatment for hypothermia, especially during rapid re-warming, and should be treated appropriately.

Hyperthermia

Hyperthermia describes an increase in body temperature above the normal resting upper limit of 37.5°C. Elevated body temperatures of up to 41.5°C are frequently measured in healthy winners of short-distance (5–15 km) running events contested in hot, humid, windless environmental conditions. Such high body temperatures occur because the rate at which elite athletes produce heat when running at their maximum pace can exceed the capacity of the hot environment to absorb that heat.

Fortunately, the brain also has protective mechanisms that reduce the allowable rate of energy production (exercise intensity/speed) during exercise in the heat. As a result, incidences of severe heat injury (heat-stroke) are remarkably uncommon in sports despite the frequency with which sports are played in severe environmental conditions.

During exercise, the chemical energy stored in the muscles in the form of adenosine triphosphate (ATP) is converted into the mechanical energy of motion. However, this process is inefficient, so that only 25% of the chemical energy used by the muscles produces motion; the remaining 75% is released as heat that must be lost from the body if the body temperature is to be safely regulated.

Thus, when elite ultra-marathon runners run at an average pace of about 16 km per hour during races of 90–100 km, they use approximately 56 kJ of energy every minute, or about 18,480 kJ in the 5.5 hours that they require to complete these races. But, of the total amount of kilojoules used, only about 4000 kJ actually transport them from the start to the finish of their races. The remaining 14,480 kJ serve only to overheat the runners' bodies. To prevent their temperatures from rising to over 43°C and causing heatstroke, these athletes have to lose more than 90% of the heat they produce.

The humidity of the air determines the extent to which heat can be lost to the environment in the form of sweat, which evaporates from the skin surface and, to a lesser extent, from the respiratory membranes. This process of evaporation is the predominant source of heat loss in exercising humans, especially in the heat since each gram (mL) of water so evaporated removes 1.8 kJ from the body. As the humidity of the air rises, the efficiency of heat loss by evaporation falls so that the ease of maintaining heat balance becomes increasingly difficult as the humidity rises above 60%–70%.

Sweating is an extremely efficient mechanism for heat loss. Thus, provided the humidity is low, well-trained and heat-acclimatized humans can regulate their body temperatures and prevent dangerous hyperthermia even when they exercise at high intensities in hot environmental conditions (up to 34°C).

The brain provides the final mechanism that protects humans from unsafe hyperthermia when exercising in hot, warm, and humid conditions. Feedback from sensors throughout the body to a central regulator in the brain monitor both the extent of the environmental stress to which the body is exposed and the rate at which the body stores heat during exercise in those environmental conditions.

Since it is safe to exercise only to a body temperature of <42°C, immediately on exposure to the prevailing environmental conditions at the onset of exercise, and on the basis of the rate at which heat will be stored and the expected duration of the exercise, the brain calculates the rate at which work can be safely performed under those specific environmental conditions.

This central governor, therefore, presets the number of motor units in the active muscles that can be recruited in order to ensure that a safe rate of heat production is allowed for the expected duration of the exercise. At the same time, the brain presets the rate at which the perception of effort increases during the period of exercise so that the perceived effort of continuing to exercise becomes intolerable before the body temperature is elevated to dangerous levels.

In this way, the brain ensures that dangerous hyperthermia including heatstroke occurs uncommonly during exercise. When heatstroke does occur during exercise, the presence of pathological precursors must be considered. These include the presence of a pre-existing medical condition, such as a muscle disorder that predisposes to excessive heat production during exercise (exercise-induced malignant hyperthermia), any condition that elevates the body temperature before the onset of exercise, or the use of drugs, especially amphetamines, that prevent the normal function of the central-governor mechanism by reducing the sensations of discomfort during exercise.

Exercise in the heat

Hot (>30°C) and humid (>50% relative humidity) environmental conditions will reduce exercise capacity and performance, although they represent no immediate danger to an individual.

Acclimatization and the heat

In addition to the general adaptations that occur with exercise training, individuals can also adapt to exercise in hot and humid environments. This is referred to as heat acclimatization and can be achieved with a specific program of exercise and conditions.

General terminology

Wet bulb

The temperature value derived from a specialized thermometer used to measure the amount of water vapor pressure in the air is commonly referred to as the wet bulb (WB) or relative humidity (RH). WB is less than the dry bulb (DB) in proportion to the environmental humidity. When the RH is 100%, the WB and DB are the same.

Dry bulb

The temperature value derived from a normal thermometer and from which the ambient temperature is obtained is commonly referred to as the dry bulb (DB).

Black globe

A black globe is a specialized thermometer to measure the radiant heat load. It consists of a dry bulb thermometer enclosed inside a black, metal sphere. Its value is commonly referred to as the globe temperature (GT).

Wet bulb globe temperature (WBGT)

This an index system used to rate the combined environmental variables of temperature, radiation, and humidity, as measured with the above terms. WBGT is calculated with the following equation:

$$WBGT = 0.7\ WB + 0.2\ GT + 0.1\ DB$$

Heat acclimatization

Complete heat acclimatization requires 7–10 consecutive days of low- to moderate-intensity exercise of 60–120 minutes in ambient temperatures above 30°C and 50% relative humidity. A large proportion of the adaptations occur within the first 5 days, but 7–10 days are required for full acclimatization. The general adaptations that occur with heat acclimatization are described in p. 395.

Earlier onset of sweating
Sweating begins at an earlier core temperature, representing an increased ability to dissipate heat.

Decreased sweat sodium concentration
To conserve Na^+, the body produces more dilute sweat. Unacclimatized sweat Na^+ concentration is approximately 75 mmol Na^+ per liter. After acclimatization this can decrease to 20–30 mmoL Na^+ per liter of sweat.

Cardiovascular adaptations
After acclimatization, the heart rate and core temperature at the same given exercise intensity will be lower than pre-acclimatization levels.

Fluid retention
The amount of fluid in blood (plasma volume) increases.

Heat-related illness in children

Children are at a disadvantage compared with adults when exercising in the heat.

Reasons for children's increased susceptibility

- Higher surface area to body mass ratio means that children absorb more heat from the environment in hot conditions.
- They are less efficient exercisers, i.e., they produce more heat for a given work load.
- They have lower cardiac output, therefore, they are less able to divert blood to the skin for cooling.
- They have a lower sweat rate.
- They have a higher sweating threshold.
- They are slower to acclimatize.

Signs and symptoms of heat-related illness

The signs of heat-related illness represent a continuum from heat exhaustion (at the early stage) to heatstroke (a medical emergency).

Early signs of heat exhaustion include the following:
- Headache
- Dizziness
- Nausea
- Muscle fatigue

The signs of heatstroke include the following:
- Tachycardia
- May or may not be sweating
- Altered mental state (confusion l seizures l coma)
- Rectal temp >41°C

Children at particular risk

- Obese children
- Children with a previous history of heat-related illness
- Children with diabetes, cystic fibrosis, and cardiac conditions
- Children taking certain medications, including antihistamines, phenothiazines, and anticholinergics

Treatment of heat-related illness

- Remove the child to a shady area and remove unnecessary clothing.
- Measure the rectal temperature.
- Give cool fluids if the child is conscious.
- If there is altered consciousness or rectal temperature is >41°C, this is a medical emergency and child should be immediately transferred to a hospital.
- Cooling and rehydration, however, should commence immediately.
- Early treatment is important for a favorable outcome.

Prevention of heat-related illness

- Avoid scheduling events during the heat of the day.
- Ensure adequate hydration by providing cool drinks with flavoring as these appear to be associated with increased consumption.
- Wear appropriate clothing, i.e., light-colored, permeable materials.
- Early identification of symptoms

Guidelines for organizers of events (see Table 11.4)

Table 11.4 Guidelines for organizers of children's events

WBGT*		Restraint on activities
°C	°F	
<24	<75	All activities allowed, but be alert for symptoms of heat-related illness in prolonged events
24.0–25.9	75.0–78.6	Longer rest periods in the shade; enforce drinking every 15 minutes
26–29	79–84	Stop activity of unacclimatized persons and other persons with high risk; limit activities of all others (disallow long-distance races, cut down duration of other activities)
>29	>85	Cancel all athletic activities

*Wet bulb globe temperature (WBGT) is an index of climatic heat stress. It combines air temperature, humidity, and radiation and is measured with a special apparatus.

Committee on Sports Medicine and Fitness, American Academy of Pediatrics (1991). *Sports Medicine: Health Care for Young Athletes*, 2nd ed. Elk Grove Village, IL: American Academy of Pediatrics; p. 98.

Exercise at altitude

Altitudes exceeding 1500 m above sea level will have an effect on exercise tolerance and capacity by reducing the maximal oxygen consumption in a curvalinear fashion. High altitude poses two distinct physiological challenges for the human body:

1. Increasingly lower amount of O_2 in the air as one ascends to higher altitudes

As the altitude above sea level increases, the barometric pressure falls. As a result, the number of oxygen molecules in each liter of air falls. In order to compensate for this, humans breathe more often and more deeply at altitude. But as the altitude increases, the partial pressure of oxygen in the blood falls, reaching values that are not compatible with sustained human life at altitudes much above about 7000 m. That some humans are able to reach the summit of Mount Everest (8840 m) attests to the phenomenal biology of some humans, the value of oxygen inhalation for others, and the quite remarkable ability of most humans to adapt to the stresses to which they are exposed for weeks to months.

Originally it was argued that exercise performance at altitude was "limited" by the production of excessive amounts of lactic acid by the oxygen-starved muscles. However, early studies showed that this could not be the case, since blood lactic acid levels during maximal exercise are as low at the summit of high mountains as they are at rest at sea level.

This finding is paradoxical since, according to the traditional understanding, exercise in the increasing levels of hypoxia that occur at altitude should cause an increased skeletal muscle anaerobiosis with an increased production of lactic acid. Elevated lactic acid concentrations would then explain why the capacity to exercise is substantially reduced at increasing altitude. In addition, the maximal cardiac output is much reduced during exercise at altitude.

This too is paradoxical, since a higher cardiac output should be advantageous. It would increase blood and oxygen delivery to the exercising muscles to offset the effects of the progressive reduction in the amount of oxygen stored in each unit of arterial blood.

2. Increasingly harsh ambient conditions due to the cold and wind

Fortunately, at the temperatures at high altitude, water exists in the form of ice and snow so the environment is usually dry. As a result, it is easier to keep clothes dry than it is in the cold and wet conditions that predominate at lower altitudes.

The presence of high winds at altitude, however, markedly increases the coldness of the environment by increasing the wind chill factor and promoting heat loss by convection to the environment. Many deaths at altitude occur not as a result of fatal falls but from hypothermia.

Studies show that the ability of the brain to recruit the muscles is regulated by a number of variables, including, at increasing altitude, the partial pressure of arterial oxygen (PaO_2), which is a direct function of the barometric pressure. Thus, as the barometric pressure falls, the brain reduces the mass of muscle that it will allow to be activated during exercise. The end result of this control is to reduce the maximal exercise capacity at altitude specifically to prevent a reduction in the PaO_2 to levels that cannot sustain normal brain function.

Hypoxia

As humans ascend to increasing altitude, they are exposed to a progressively lower partial pressure of oxygen in the inspired air. As a result, the partial pressure of oxygen in the blood supplying their brains also falls. While there are a number of physiological adaptations that increase this pressure, ultimately each human will reach an altitude at which they are no longer able to survive, since their blood oxygen pressure falls below that required for those crucial brain functions necessary for sustaining life.

Exercise at altitude is also "limited" by the brain to ensure that no exercise intensity is undertaken that will produce a blood oxygen partial pressure at which unconsciousness develops.

Altitude acclimatization

Acclimatization to altitude can be achieved with a gradual ascent to higher altitudes over a number of days or weeks. The regulator of exercise at altitude appears to be the partial pressure of oxygen in the arterial blood (PaO_2).

When the PaO_2 falls below some critical value (which is different between individuals, perhaps on the basis of genetic factors or the extent of the adaptation to altitude), the brain prevents the continuing recruitment of motor units in the exercising limbs so that exercise must terminate.

Effective adaptations to altitude must increase the PaO_2 at any altitude (barometric pressure), maintain higher PaO_2 during exercise, and adapt the brain so that it is able to maintain the recruitment of an appropriate muscle mass at the same or lower PaO_2, without risking brain damage from hypoxia.

Specific adaptations to altitude

- Increase ventilation rate
- Rise in arterial pH as arterial CO_2 is reduced (due to hyperventilation that drives the reaction ($H^+ + HCO_3^- \rightarrow H_2O + CO_2$) to the right)
- Kidney retention of H^+ compensates for this respiratory alkalosis.
- Increased PaO_2 (due to hyperventilation)
- Increase in blood hemoglobin concentration due to an initial fall in blood volume
- Increased excretion of erythropoietin (EPO) by the kidneys in response to the reduction in PaO_2
- Progressive increases in the red cell mass (for up to 3–12 months) with more prolonged exposures above about 3250 m. This is due to increased EPO production at altitude.
- Oxygen dissociation curve of hemoglobin shifts to the left, favoring increased hemoglobin oxygen saturation at any PaO_2
- No change in pulmonary diffusing capacity at moderate altitude but becomes impaired at very high altitudes

- Increased pressure in the pulmonary circulation due to pulmonary arteriolar vasoconstriction; develops in proportion to the reduction in PaO_2
- Potential right ventricular hypertrophy when pulmonary hypertension is sustained
- Increased cerebral blood flow in response to the reduction in PaO_2 (The extent to which cerebral blood flow increases is limited by the cerebral arteriolar vasoconstriction that occurs in response to the fall in $PaCO_2$ induced by hyperventilation.)
- Increased secretion of adrenal cortical hormones and activation of the sympathetic nervous system
- Increase in the blood concentrations of sodium and water conserving hormones (renin, aldosterone, and ADH) especially in response to exercise. These hormones favor increased fluid retention.
- Increased respiratory water losses in response to hyperventilation and the low humidity of the air at altitude

As a result of these adaptations, exercise performance capacity at altitude improves but is always less at altitude than at sea level.

Altitude sickness

Altitude sickness occurs in about 25% of persons unacclimatized to moderate altitude on acute exposure to altitudes in excess of about 2500 m. In about 5%, symptoms will be sufficiently severe to require bed rest. The incidence of symptoms, including incapacitation requiring bed rest, increases with increasing altitude and may be 100% in those who ascend rapidly to above 3000 m.

Although acute altitude sickness is usually no more than an illness of inconvenience, progression to high-altitude pulmonary edema or cerebral edema can occur. Thus, all persons with the condition must be observed until symptoms disappear.

Symptoms

Symptoms are most intense for the first 48 hours after arrival at altitude, lessening thereafter and disappearing within 5–8 days. Symptoms are worse in the morning, perhaps as a result of increased hypoxemia during sleep.

Headache, insomnia, lassitude, and anorexia are often associated with nausea and vomiting.

Etiology

The etiology is unknown but may be related to cerebral hypoxia and an increased cerebral blood flow.

Prevention

- Avoid rapid ascension to altitudes above 2000–2500 m.
- Ascend slowly with stops at intermediate altitudes.
- Avoid vigorous exercise on the first few days of arrival at altitude. Emphasize rest during that period.

- The use of acetazolamide (125–250 mg twice daily) beginning 48 hours before ascent to altitude and continued for the first 5 days after arrival at altitude is the only proven efficacious medication.
- Low-flow oxygen at night may be helpful if available.

Treatment
- Treat mild symptoms with appropriate medications.
- If symptoms progress, oxygen at high flow should be administered.
- If available, a hyperbaric bag can be used.
- If symptoms progress further despite these interventions, urgent evacuation to a lower altitude is essential.
- Descent to a sufficiently low altitude cures the symptoms.

Cerebral or pulmonary edema

This is a potentially fatal but preventable condition that develops rapidly and with little warning in persons who are unacclimatized to altitude but ascend rapidly to altitudes in excess of about 2500 m and, on arrival at altitude, often partake of vigorous exercise.

Easier access to high altitudes for unacclimatized mountain climbers, skiers, and trekkers has increased the incidence of the condition with about 20 deaths per year reported annually around the world.

Etiology (pulmonary edema)
The etiology is uncertain but probably involves hypoxic pulmonary arteriolar vasoconstriction with thrombotic obstruction of some parts of the pulmonary vascular bed.
- Overperfusion of nonobstructed capillaries increases capillary shear forces.
- Increased shear forces injure capillaries, causing leakage of red cells and protein into the alveoli.
- Individual susceptibility (as repeat attacks occur in some individuals)

Etiology (cerebral edema)
Increased cerebral blood flow with capillary damage induces leakage of edema fluid into the brain.

Symptoms (pulmonary edema)
- Dyspnea, cough, weakness, chest tightness, and occasionally hemoptysis, usually within the first 3 days of arrival at altitude
- In more severe cases, alterations in consciousness may occur.

Symptoms (cerebral edema)
Symptoms of central nervous system dysfunction, including ataxia, headache, lethargy, and irrational behavior, indicate the impending development of high-altitude cerebral edema. Coma indicates advanced cerebral edema.

Signs (pulmonary and cerebral edema)
- Cyanosis, tachycardia, tachypnea, and pulmonary rales
- Papilledema
- Abnormal reflexes
- Altered level of consciousness

Treatment
- Oxygen at high flow rates
- Use of a hyperbaric bag if available
- Immediate evacuation to lower altitudes
- Bed rest, oxygen, and nifedipine should be given at lower altitudes if rapid clinical improvement does not occur.
- Descent to lower altitude cures the condition.

Deaths usually occur only when the initial diagnosis is delayed; the emergency nature of the condition is not appreciated and descent to lower altitude either does not occur, or occurs too late in the course of the illness.

Cardiovascular

Preparticipation screening

Students

Introduction

Accurate detection of underlying cardiovascular abnormalities in young athletes is difficult because of the large populations involved, inconsistent screening measures and quality standards, and a very low prevalence of disease state in the young athletic population.

The strongest clinical risk factor is exertion-related syncope.

American Heart Association (AHA) recommendation

There are 12 elements of the preparticipation screening process to detect potential cardiac-related abnormalities in competitive athletes.

Personal history

1. Exertional chest pain
2. Unexplained syncope or near-syncope, particularly exertional
3. Excessive exertional dyspnea or fatigue
4. History of a heart murmur
5. Systemic hypertension

Family history

6. Early cardiac-related death (<50 years old)
7. Cardiac-related disability in close relative <50 years old
8. Presence of hypertrophic or dilated cardiomyopathy, long QT syndrome or other ion channelopathy, Marfan syndrome, other clinically relevant arrhythmia

Physical examination

9. Heart murmur; auscultation in supine and standing positions or with Valsalva
   - Murmurs in children and adolescents are common and usually benign.
   - Murmurs that should be further evaluated prior to sport participation clearance include any diastolic murmur, systolic murmurs higher than grade 2/6, or any murmur that increases with standing or with Valsalva's maneuver.
10. Femoral pulses for screening of aortic coarctation
11. Physical stigmata of Marfan syndrome
12. Blood pressure; readings in both arms
    - Measurements should be evaluated in reference to age, gender, and height; available at http://www.nhbli.nih.gov/guidelines/hypertension/child_tbl.htm

Use of electrocardiogram (ECG)

This is a subject of controversy; there are no current AHA guidelines recommending or requiring use in the United States Government-mandated screening of all athletes in Italy includes an ECG (Lausanne criteria).

Limitations in implementing ECG as part of the preparticipation exam (PPE) include the large athlete population, cost, accessibility, low specificity, and a rate of false positives estimated at 10%–25%. The false-positive rate has been shown to be closer to 5% when common and training-related ECG findings are excluded. These include sinus bradycardia, 1° AV block, incomplete RBBB, early repolarization, and isolated QRS voltage criteria for LVH.

ECG abnormalities may be found in 10%–40% of athletes with such changes as bradycardia, ventricular hypertrophy patterns, incomplete right bundle branch block, and ST-segment elevation patterns referred to as "benign early repolarization."

Adults

Preparticipation screening of adults is controversial, with relatively limited data. The American College of Sports Medicine (ACSM) recommends symptom-limited exercise testing before vigorous exercise (>60% VO_{2max}) is undertaken by men ≥45 years and women ≥55 years. Those with two or more major cardiac risk factors; persons with any signs or symptoms of coronary artery disease; or those with known cardiac, pulmonary, or metabolic disease should also undergo such testing.

According to a 2003 AHA report, exercise testing is not necessary for all people beginning a moderate-intensity physical activity program.

Symptomatic persons or those with any cardiovascular disease, diabetes, other active chronic disease, or any medical concern should consult a physician or health-care provider prior to any substantive increase in physical activity, particularly vigorous-intensity activity.

Sudden cardiac death in athletes

Incidence
- Prevalence of cardiac abnormalities raising the risk of sudden death is likely <0.3%.
- The rate of sudden cardiac death (SCD) in high school athletes is approximately 1 in 200,000 participants per year.
- Only 3% of athletes with SCD were previously suspected of any cardiac abnormality on PPE, with none having been disqualified.

Etiology
The most prevalent causes of SCD in young athletes, in decreasing order, are as follows (see Fig. 12.1):
- Hypertrophic cardiomyopathy (HCM) (36%)
- Coronary artery anomalies (CAA) (17%)
- Indeterminate left ventricular hypertrophy (possible HCM) (8%)
- Myocarditis (6%)
- Arrhythmogenic right ventricular cardiomyopathy (ARVC) (4%)
- Mitral valve prolapse (MVP) (4%)
- Tunneled left anterior descending artery (LAD) (3%)
- Coronary artery disease (CAD) (3%)
- Aortic stenosis (AS) (3%)

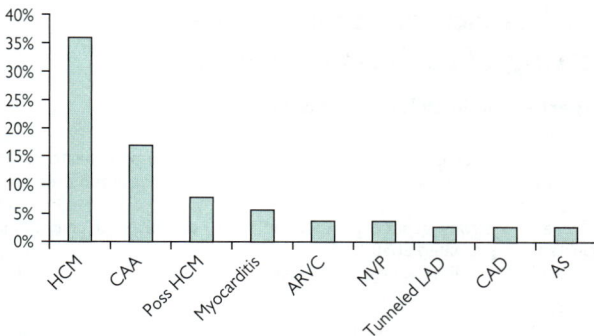

Figure 12.1 The most prevalent causes of sudden cardiac death (SCD) in young athletes.

Cardiovascular abnormalities in the setting of athletic participation

Hypertension in children and adolescents

Epidemiology

Childhood obesity is a strong risk factor for early-onset hypertension. Race may also play a role, with Black children having higher blood pressure than Caucasians.

There is a strong genetic component, with heritability of childhood hypertension estimated at 50%.

Breastfeeding is likely a negative risk factor for childhood hypertension.

Etiology

Essential hypertension is a diagnosis of exclusion in children younger than 10 years old. Secondary causes should be considered in all children and adolescents with hypertension.

By age group, the most common etiologies for hypertension are as follows:

- *1–6 years old:* renal parenchymal disease, renal vascular disease, endocrine disorders (e.g., pheochromocytoma, hyperthyroidism), coarctation of the aorta, essential hypertension
- *6–12 years old:* renal parenchymal disease, essential hypertension, renal vascular disease, endocrine disorders, coarctation of the aorta, iatrogenic
- *12–18 years old:* essential hypertension, iatrogenic, renal parenchymal disease, renal vascular disease, endocrine disorders, coarctation of the aorta

Diagnosis

Blood pressure measurements should be obtained in a quiet environment while sitting, using an appropriately sized cuff. Recordings should be evaluated using age-appropriate nomograms.

If the initial reading is elevated, a recheck should follow 5 minutes of rest. With persistent elevation, a third recording should follow 10–15 minutes of rest while the patient is lying down.

Based on age-appropriate nomograms, elevated blood pressure in children is also staged.

- 90th–95th percentile is prehypertension
- 95th–99th percentile plus 5 mmHg is stage I
- >99th percentile plus 5 mmHg is stage II

Evaluation

At the time of measurement, inquire about stimulant use such as caffeine or nicotine.

Screening lab work typically includes a complete blood count (CBC); urinalysis and culture; and serum electrolyte, blood urea nitrogen (BUN), serum creatinine, calcium, and uric acid levels. Lipid analysis should be considered.

Further testing may include echocardiography; renal imaging such as ultrasonography, radionuclide scan, Doppler ultrasonography and angiography; and renal and peripheral plasma renin activity.

Treatment options

For prehypertension or stage 1 hypertension, family-centered lifestyle changes include weight control, regular exercise, a low-fat and low-sodium diet, and avoidance of alcohol or tobacco.

Pharmacological treatment should be considered in children and adolescents with symptomatic hypertension, end-organ damage (e.g., LVH, retinopathy, proteinuria), secondary hypertension, stage 1 hypertension that does not respond to lifestyle changes, and stage 2 hypertension.

If there is no end-organ damage and no comorbid conditions, the goal is blood pressure <95th percentile for age, height, and gender. If end-organ damage or coexisting illness is present, the blood pressure goal is <90th percentile.

Diuretics and beta-blockers have documented safety and effectiveness in children. Angiotensin-converting enzyme (ACE) inhibitors may be considered in children with diabetes or proteinuria. See Treatment options under Hypertension in adults (p. 412) for details regarding physiological effects of commonly used antihypertensive medications.

The legality of use according to the appropriate sports governing body also needs to be considered.

Sport participation

Stage I hypertension requires further evaluation but no disqualification.

Stage II hypertension results in disqualification from sport participation until further testing and treatment, if necessary.

End results

Left ventricular hypertrophy (LVH) is the most prominent clinical evidence of end-organ damage in childhood hypertension.

Severe cases of childhood hypertension are also at increased risk of developing hypertensive encephalopathy, seizures, cerebrovascular accidents, and congestive heart failure.

Hypertension in adults

Epidemiology

An estimated 50 million Americans have hypertension, although nearly one-third are unaware of their condition. Forty percent of Americans with hypertension are not being treated for it; two-thirds of patients are not under ideal control.

Etiology

- Genetic factors
- Increased activity of the sympathetic nervous system
- Vascular remodeling

Diagnostic Evaluation
- Screening should include 12-lead ECG; urinalysis; hematocrit; blood glucose; serum potassium, creatinine, and calcium; and a lipid analysis.
- No current recommendation regarding screening echocardiography

Treatment options

Diuretics and beta-blockers are not recommended for first-line treatment in adult athletes, particularly those engaged in competitive or high-intensity endurance exercise.

Diuretics reduce plasma volume, which may temporarily impair exercise performance and capacity. They may also cause electrolyte and fluid disturbances.

Beta-blockers reduce the maximal heart rate and thus the maximal aerobic power by an average of 7%. This is not fully compensated by increases in maximal stroke volume or peripheral oxygen extraction.

Nonselective beta-blockers reduce sustained submaximal exercise time by 40%, and cardioselective beta-blockers reduce it by 20%, likely as a result of impaired lipolysis.

Calcium-channel blockers and renin-angiotensin system antagonists are currently the preferred pharmacological options for athletes with hypertension. If a third drug is required, a low-dose thiazide-like diuretic, possibly in combination with a potassium-sparing agent, is recommended.

Sport participation

Physical activity should be encouraged as part of the lifestyle modification to treat hypertension.

Competitive sports are permitted for athletes with prehypertension, stage 1 hypertension, or controlled stage 2 hypertension in the absence of symptoms and end-organ damage. Athletes with stage 2 hypertension should be restricted from class III sports until their hypertension is well controlled. See Table 12.1 for normal, prehypertension, and stage 1 and 2 hypertension blood pressure values.

Athletes with hypertension should be monitored every 2–4 months.

Table 12.1 Normal and hypertensive blood pressure (BP) values

BP classification	Systolic (mmHg)	Diastolic (mmHg)	
Normal	<120	and	<80
Prehypertension	120–139	or	80–89
Stage 1 hypertension	140–159	or	90–99
Stage 2 hypertension	≥160	or	≥100

Hypertrophic cardiomyopathy

Introduction

The prevalence of hypertrophic cardiomyopathy (HCM) in the general population may approach 1 in 500. It is the most common cause of SCD in young American athletes. More than 400 mutations involving 12 genes have been recognized in HCM.

The hallmark feature is LVH, usually asymmetric, without cavity dilation. No specific LV wall thickness is considered diagnostic for HCM.

Normal adult maximal end-diastolic LV wall thickness is 15 mm. In children it is set as 2 or more standard deviations from the mean, relative to body surface area.

Diagnosis

Sudden death due to HCM typically occurs without prior symptoms and may transpire at rest or with mild to intense exertion.

Screening by auscultation is not sensitive, as outflow obstruction is not likely at rest, thus a systolic ejection murmur is not always present. Systolic murmur associated with HCM will increase with Valsalva maneuver.

Genetic testing may identify one of the common HCM-causing mutations, although false-negative results are possible. Genetic screening may identify family members with an HCM-causing genetic mutation but no symptoms or phenotype (i.e., LVH).

Sudden cardiac death risk factors in HCM

- Family history of HCM-related SCD
- Ventricular septum >30 mm
- Repetitive nonsustained ventricular tachycardia on ambulatory ECG
- Exertional hypotension
- Syncope that is otherwise unexplained

Sports participation

Recommendations remain conservative given the lack of reliable risk factors for HCM.

Sports participation is not restricted in an asymptomatic athlete with a normal ECG, Holter monitoring, cardiac MRI, and exertional equivalent exercise testing; testing should be done every 12–18 months.

With probable or confirmed diagnosis there should be no sports participation, with possible exception of class IA.

Placement of an implantable cardioverter defibrillator (ICD) or the availability of an automated external defibrillator (AED) does not change these recommendations.

Other congenital defects

Atrial septal defects (ASD)

These are usually asymptomatic. Commonly, they close in childhood prior to competitive sports participation.

Untreated

- Small defects, normal right heart volume, no pulmonary hypertension: no restrictions
- Large defects with normal pulmonary artery pressure: no restrictions
- Mild pulmonary hypertension: class IA
- Associated pulmonary vascular obstructive disease with cyanosis and large right-to-left shunt: no sport participation

Treated (closed by operation or device insertion)

- Chest radiograph, ECG, and echocardiogram should be performed to measure cardiac performance, pulmonary vascular resistance, and right ventricular (RV) size and to evaluate any conduction abnormalities.
- Athletes have no restrictions 3–6 months post-closure if there is no evidence of pulmonary hypertension, symptomatic arrhythmias, or myocardial dysfunction.

Ventricular septal defects (VSD)

Untreated

- Small VSD with normal cardiac size and pulmonary artery pressure: no restrictions

Treated

- Large VSD following successful repair: no restrictions after 3–6 months following surgery if normal pulmonary artery tension, cardiac rhythm, and myocardial function
- Persistent, severe pulmonary hypertension: no sport participation

Patent ductus arteriosus (PDA)

Untreated

- Small PDA with normal left heart chambers: no restrictions

Treated

- 3 months post-closure with no symptoms, normal exam, and no evidence of pulmonary hypertension or LV enlargement: no restrictions

Pulmonary valve stenosis (PS)

Untreated

- Doppler peak systolic gradient <40 mmHg and normal RV function: no restrictions, but annual re-evaluation is recommended
- Peak systolic gradient >40 mmHg: class IA and IB; usually referred for further treatment

Treated (operation or balloon valvuloplasty)

- 2–4 weeks after valvuloplasty or 3 months after operation, if asymptomatic with no or mild residual PS and normal ventricular function: no restrictions
- Persistent peak systolic gradient >40 mmHg or marked RV enlargement: class IA and IB only

Coarctation of the aorta

Untreated

- Very mild disease with normal exercise test and small pressure gradient at rest: no restrictions
- Systolic gradient >20 mmHg or exercise-induced systolic blood pressure (SBP) >230 mmHg: class IA only, until treated

Treated (operation or balloon angioplasty)

- Workup prior to final decision may include chest radiograph, ECG, exercise testing, echocardiogram, and cardiac MRI
- 3 months post-treatment with pressure gradient <21 mmHg and normal peak SBP at rest and with (asymptomatic) exercise: no class IIIA, IIIB, and IIIC sports. For first year post-treatment, activities with risk of bodily collision should be avoided.
- In presence of aortic dilation, wall thinning, or aneurysm formation: class IA, IB

Elevated pulmonary resistance in congenital heart disease

- Requires evaluation with echocardiography and/or cardiac catheterization
- Pulmonary peak systolic pressure ≤30 mmHg: no restrictions
- Pulmonary peak systolic pressure >30 mmHg: decision made on individual basis

Ventricular dysfunction after cardiac surgery

- Periodic assessment is required.
- Normal or near-normal ejection fraction (50% or more): no restrictions
- Mildly depressed ejection fraction (40%–50%): class IA, IB, IC
- Moderately to severely depressed ejection fraction (<40%): no sports participation

Cyanotic congenital cardiac disease

Untreated

- Usually participation allowed only for class IA

Treated

- Class IA allowed if arterial saturation remains >80%, no symptomatic tachyarrhythmia, and no moderate or severe ventricular dysfunction

Tetralogy of Fallot, postoperative

- Complete evaluation may require cardiac catheterization and/or exercise testing
- Excellent repair with normal or near-normal right heart pressure; no to mild right ventricular volume overload; no significant residual shunt; and no tachyarrhythmia with exercise testing: no restrictions
- Otherwise, class IA only

Transposition of the great arteries, postoperative Mustard or Senning procedures

- Complete evaluation should include a chest radiograph, ECG, ambulatory ECG, exercise testing, echocardiogram, and cardiac MRI; cardiac catheterization may be considered.
- No chamber enlargement; no atrial flutter, supraventricular tachycardia, or ventricular tachyarrhythmia; no syncope or cardiac symptoms; normal exercise test: class IA and IB
- Otherwise, the decision is made on an individual basis.

Transposition of the great arteries, postoperative arterial switch

- Normal ventricular function, normal exercise test, and no tachyarrhythmias: no restrictions
- Mild hemodynamic abnormalities or ventricular dysfunction with normal exercise test: class IA, IB, IC, and IIA

Congenitally corrected transposition of the great arteries

- Asymptomatic with no other cardiac abnormalities, no enlargement, no tachyarrhythmias, and normal exercise test: consider class IA and IIA

Post-Fontan operation

- Evaluation should include a chest radiograph, ECG, echocardiography or cardiac MRI, and exercise testing with oxygen saturations.
- Class IA allowed
- Normal ventricular function and oxygen saturation: class IA and IB

Ebstein's anomaly

- Mild cases with normal right ventricular size and no cyanosis or tachyarrhythmias: no restrictions
- Moderate tricuspid regurgitation but no arrhythmia: class IA
- Severe cases: no sport participation; selected postsurgical cases taken on an individual basis

Congenital coronary artery anomalies

- No sports participation
- 3 months after surgery with no ischemia, arrhythmia, or dysfunction during maximal exercise testing: no restrictions
- Myocardial bridging as a special consideration
  - Asymptomatic with no evidence of ischemia at rest or with exercise testing: no restrictions
  - History of myocardial infarction or evidence of ischemia: class IA
  - Following surgical resection: restricted to class IA for at least 6 months; if subsequent exercise testing is normal, no restrictions

Kawasaki disease

This is the most common cause of acquired heart disease in American children. Coronary artery aneurysms occur in ~20% of untreated cases and 4% of treated cases.

- No coronary artery abnormalities or transient ectasia that resolves: no restriction after 6–8 weeks
- Regressed aneurysms with no evidence of exercise-induced ischemia on myocardial perfusion stress test: no restrictions
- Isolated small to medium aneurysms with normal function and no arrhythmias: class IA, IB, IIA, IIB. Stress testing should be repeated every 1–2 years.
- One or more large or complex aneurysms with no ischemia, normal LV function, and no arrhythmia on stress testing: class IA and IIA. Annual stress testing is recommended.
- Patients with coronary lesions on anticoagulants or antiplatelet medication: no contact sports

Valvular disorders

Diagnosis can often be made clinically, although severity is more difficult to assess. Physical examination and Doppler echocardiography may be sufficient for workup.

Valvular regurgitation is extremely common in the general and athletic population.

Athletic participation recommendations are guidelines, based on asymptomatic cases.

Aortic stenosis (AS) in young athletes

Continuous-wave Doppler echocardiography is reliable to estimate the severity of AS. Evaluation for participation clearance should also include Holter monitoring with exercise.

Annual re-evaluation should include echocardiography.

Untreated

- Mild AS with normal ECG and full, asymptomatic exercise tolerance: no restrictions
- Moderate AS: class IA, IB, and IIA if asymptomatic, no LV strain on ECG, mild or no LVH on echocardiogram, and normal exercise test
- Presence of supraventricular tachycardia or tachyarrhythmias: class IA and IB only
- Severe AS: no sports participation

Treated (operation or balloon valvuloplasty)

- After retesting, residual AS should follow the same recommendations as untreated AS.
- Discrete subaortic stenosis and other forms of fixed AS require annual re-evaluation to assess for recurrence of LV outflow obstruction.

Aortic stenosis (AS) in adult athletes

The most common etiologies are rheumatic, congenital, and calcific/degenerative. Dyspnea, syncope, or angina are late symptoms and increase the possibility of sudden death.

Evaluation and annual re-evaluation are similar to that for AS in young athletes.

Recommendations

- Mild AS without symptoms: no restrictions
- Moderate AS: class IA
- If exertional-equivalent stress test is unremarkable: class IA, IB, IIA
- Presence of supraventricular tachycardia or tachyarrhythmias: class IA
- Moderate AS with symptoms or severe AS: no sports participation

Aortic regurgitation (AR)

The most common etiologies are congenital bicuspid valve, rheumatic, infective endocarditis, and aortic root diseases.

Severity is evaluated with physical examination, chest radiography, and echocardiography.

Recommendations

- Mild to moderate AR with normal or near-normal LV end-diastolic size: no restrictions
- Presence of moderate LV enlargement and normal exercise testing: class IA, IB, IC, IIA, IIB, IIC
- Asymptomatic nonsustained ventricular tachycardia at rest or exertional: class IA
- Symptomatic AR: no sports participation
- Severe AR with LV diastolic size >65 mm: no sports participation
- AR with dilation of proximal ascending aorta >45 mm (except patients with Marfan syndrome): class IA

Mitral stenosis (MS)

MS is usually secondary to rheumatic sequela. It is possible for patients with a mild to moderate degree of MS to be asymptomatic with exertion.

A potential effect of exercise may include pulmonary edema; its effect on development of atrial fibrillation or systemic embolization is unknown.

Echocardiography is required for accurate assessment of severity, including estimation of pulmonary artery systolic pressure during exercise testing.

Recommendations

- Mild MS with no arrhythmia and peak pulmonary artery systolic pressure during exercise <50 mmHg: no restrictions
- Moderate MS, even in atrial fibrillation, with peak pulmonary artery systolic pressure during exercise <50 mmHg: class IA, IB, IIA, IIB
- Severe MS or peak pulmonary artery systolic pressure during exercise >50 mmHg: no sports participation
- Any required use of anticoagulation therapy (e.g., history of atrial fibrillation): no contact sports or sports with risk of trauma

Mitral regurgitation (MR)

MR has a variety of causes; most common is mitral valve prolapse. These recommendations apply to primary MR.

Like MS, severity can be assessed by two-dimensional and Doppler echocardiography.

Although LV diastolic volume is commonly used to gauge the severity of chronic MR, the normal limits in elite athletes may exceed those of the general population; 60 mm may be considered the standard upper limit of LV end-diastolic volume in an athlete.

Recommendations

- Mild to moderate MR in sinus rhythm, normal LV size and function, normal pulmonary artery pressures: no restrictions
- Mild to moderate MR in sinus rhythm, normal LV systolic function at rest and mild LV enlargement (<60 mm): class IA, IB, IC, IIA, IIB, IIC
- Severe MR with LV enlargement >60 mm, pulmonary hypertension, or any LV systolic dysfunction at rest: no sports participation
- Any required use of anticoagulation therapy (e.g., history of atrial fibrillation): no contact sports or sports with risk of trauma

Mitral valve prolapse (MVP)

- Found in 2%–3% of the general population
- Favorable prognosis and a low event rate
- No restrictions if none of the following conditions are met: arrhythmogenic syncope, tachycardia or tachyarrhythmia on Holter monitoring, severe MR, LV ejection fraction <50%, prior embolic event, family history of MVP-related sudden death
- If any condition is met: class IA only

Bicuspid aortic valves with aortic root dilatation

- Bicuspid aortic valve with no aortic root dilatation (<40 mm or body surface area equivalent) and no significant AS or AR: no restrictions
- Aortic root dilatation between 40 and 45 mm: class IA, IB, IIA, IIB but no traumatic risks
- Aortic root dilatation >45 mm: class IA

Tricuspid regurgitation (TR)

- Most commonly secondary to RV dilation and failure due to pulmonary or RV hypertension
- Recommendations apply to primary TR
- Regardless of severity, if normal RV function and lack of right atrial pressure >20 mmHg and elevated RV systolic pressure: no restrictions

Tricuspid stenosis (TS)

- Commonly due to rheumatic heart disease and associated with mitral stenosis
- If no mitral stenosis, no restriction if exertional equivalent exercise testing is asymptomatic

Multivalvular disease

- Seen in rheumatic heart disease, myxomatous valvular disease, and infective endocarditis
- Generally results in full restriction from any sports participation

Prosthetic heart valves

- Abnormal response to exertion may exist even with normal hemodynamics at rest
- Bioprosthetic mitral valve with no anticoagulant use and normal valvular and normal or near-normal LV function: class IA, IB, IIA, IIB
- Mechanical or bioprosthetic aortic valve with normal valve and LV function: class IA, IB, IIA
- Athletes in class IB or IIA sports should perform exertional-equivalent exercise testing.
- Any use of anticoagulants: no sports with risk of bodily contact or trauma

Following valve repair

- After successful percutaneous mitral balloon valvotomy or surgical commissurotomy, recommendations are based on the residual degree of MS or MR with exercise testing.
- Following mitral valve repair for MR: no sports with risk of bodily contact or trauma: class IA

Arrhythmias

There are limited data on activity guidelines for affected athletes. Up to 40% of athletes may have typically benign changes such as type I second-degree atrioventricular (AV) block or single uniform premature ventricular complexes on standard monitoring.

Specific stressors involved in each sport need to be considered in deciding on level of sports participation.

Identification of arrhythmia may necessitate diagnosis for underlying structural disease.

Typical evaluation should include cardiac examination, ECG, echocardiogram, exercise test, and possible Holter monitoring with sports-specific exertion.

Regular re-evaluation is prudent. Part of evaluation for unexplained syncope is consideration of arrhythmia and structural abnormalities, especially syncope during or immediately after exertion.

Pacemakers

- No contact sports participation
- For other sports with less risk of direct trauma, protective padding is still recommended.
- Exercise testing should demonstrate appropriate function at the necessary level of exertion.

Sinus node dysfunction

- Asymptomatic sinus arrhythmia, wandering pacemaker, sinus pause, and sinus arrest <3 seconds: if asymptomatic, no further testing required
- Longer or symptomatic pauses, sinoatrial (SA) block, and sick sinus syndrome requires further testing prior to sports participation.

Premature atrial complexes

If there is no structural disease or no symptoms beyond occasional palpitation there are no restrictions.

Atrial fibrillation (no Wolff–Parkinson–White [WPW] syndrome)

- Asymptomatic, episodes of 5–15 seconds that do not prolong during exertion: no restrictions
- Asymptomatic, no structural disease, appropriately responsive ventricular rate, no therapy or therapy with AV nodal blocking medication: no restrictions
- In presence of structural disease, appropriately responsive ventricular rate, no therapy or therapy with AV nodal blocking medication: restrictions based on nature of structural disease
- No structural disease, after ablation or corrective surgery: no restrictions after 4–6 weeks without fibrillation or following reassuring electrophysiological (EP) study

Atrial flutter (no WPW)

- No structural disease, appropriately responsive ventricular rate, no therapy or therapy with AV nodal blocking medication: class IA.
  - Rapid 1:1 conduction can still occur.
  - Full participation is allowed after 2–3 months without flutter, with or without treatment.
- No structural disease, after ablation or corrective surgery: no restrictions after 2–4 weeks without flutter or several days following reassuring EP study
- In presence of structural disease, after 2–4 weeks without flutter: class IA

Sinus node re-entry, inappropriate sinus tachycardia, atrial tachycardia (no WPW)

- Asymptomatic, episodes of 5–10 seconds that do not prolong during exertion: no restrictions
- No structural disease, appropriately responsive ventricular rate: no restrictions
- No structural disease, after ablation or corrective surgery: no restrictions after 2–4 weeks without recurrence or several days following reassuring EP study

Premature AV junctional complexes

- With occasional episodes of nonsustained tachycardia: evaluation with 12-lead ECG
- No structural disease, appropriately responsive ventricular rate: no restrictions

Nonparoxysmal AV junctional tachycardia

- No structural disease, appropriately responsive ventricular rate, with or without therapy: no restrictions
- Asymptomatic, with structural disease or incompletely controlled ventricular rates: consider class IA, if appropriate for underlying disease or ventricular rate
- With or without structural disease, uncontrolled ventricular rates: no sports participation until controlled rate; after treatment and controlled rate with exertion: no restrictions

Supraventricular tachycardia (SVT), including AV nodal reentrant tachycardia

- Asymptomatic, episodes of 5–10 seconds that do not prolong during exertion: no restrictions
- Asymptomatic, no structural disease, exercise-induced SVT episodes that are prevented by therapy and confirmed with exercise testing: no restrictions

- Sporadic occurrences: following therapy, if asymptomatic with episodes of 5–15 seconds that do not prolong during exertion: sports participation consistent with cardiac status
- Symptomatic, including near-syncope: no sports participation until treated and lack of recurrence for 2–4 weeks, then limited to class IA
- No structural disease, post-ablation, asymptomatic, no inducible arrhythmia: no restrictions several days following EP testing; if no EP testing, after 2–4 weeks if no recurrence

Ventricular pre-excitation (Wolff–Parkinson–White [WPW] syndrome)

- Athletes >20 years old with no structural disease, palpitations, or tachycardia: no restrictions
- Younger athletes or those not meeting the above criteria should undergo EP testing for further evaluation and consideration of sports participation.

Premature ventricular complexes (PVC)

- No structural disease, PVC at rest and with exertion that are asymptomatic or minimally symptomatic: no restrictions
- Increased PVC with exertion that is symptomatic: class IA

Ventricular tachycardia (VT)

- No structural disease, asymptomatic nonsustained monomorphic VT: no restrictions
- No structural disease, after successful ablation: no restrictions after 2–4 weeks
- No structural disease, well controlled with pharmacotherapy for 2–3 months, noninducible with exercise testing or EP testing: no restrictions
- Presence of structural disease: class IA

Ventricular flutter and ventricular fibrillation

- Prior history treated with ICD, no episodes for 6 months: class IA

First-degree AV block

- No structural disease, asymptomatic, normal QRS: no restrictions
- Abnormal QRS or PR interval ≥0.3 seconds: further evaluation should include exercise stress test, Holter monitoring, and echocardiogram
- No structural disease, AV block does not increase with exertion: no restrictions

Type 1 second-degree AV block (Wenckebach)

- Evaluation should include ECG, exercise test, and echocardiogram; consider a Holter monitor.
- No structural disease, asymptomatic, no increase of block with exertion: no restrictions
- Exacerbation of block with exertion: further evaluation required; if pacemaker placed: class IA

Type 2 second-degree AV block (Mobitz) or acquired complete heart block

Pacemaker treatment is required before any sports participation.

Congenital complete heart block

- Evaluation should include ECG, Holter monitor, exercise test, and echocardiogram.
- No structural disease, normal function, no syncope, narrow QRS complex, no or rare PVC, no VT with exertion: no restrictions
- Ventricular arrhythmia, abnormal hemodynamics, or symptomatic: pacemaker required

Complete right bundle branch block (RBBB)

- Asymptomatic with no ventricular arrhythmias or exertional AV block: no restrictions

Complete left bundle branch block (LBBB)

- Adult athletes: same guidelines as for RBBB
- Normal HV interval and normal AV conduction response to pacing: no restrictions
- Abnormal conduction: pacemaker required

QT syndromes

Long QT syndrome (LQTS)

LQTS is an inherited disorder of ion channels resulting in increased risk of ventricular arrhythmias. A clear diagnosis can be clinically challenging.

The exact value of prolonged corrected QT interval (QTc) is unproven. A QTc ≥470 ms in males and ≥480 ms in females necessitates further workup.

Genetic testing can identify five of the genes that together account for three quarters of cases.

Ventricular arrhythmia is commonly triggered by exertion in LQT1, and auditory or emotional stimuli in LQT2, whereas LQT3 patients are at greater risk during rest.

Swimming has the highest risk of sudden death.

Recommendations
- Asymptomatic: class IA
- LQTS3: other activities may be considered
- History of cardiac arrest or LQTS-associated syncope: class IA
- Genotype (+)/phenotype (–): no restrictions, although LQTS1 precludes swimming

Short QT syndrome
- Little-known entity with QT interval <300 ms
- Consider class IA, otherwise no sports participation

Catecholaminergic polymorphic VT
- Some patients may be susceptible to exertional-related VT or ventricular fibrillation (VF).
- Commonly treated with an ICD
- Consider class IA, otherwise no sports participation
- Genotype (+)/phenotype (–): other activities may be considered

Brugada syndrome

Brugada syndrome (BrS) is an inherited disorder of ion channels resulting in increased risk of ventricular arrhythmias. There is no established relationship of BrS with exertional sudden death.

It is more prevalent in persons of Asian descent.

ECG findings may include RBBB and ST segment elevations in leads V1 through V3. Elevated body temperature may induce abnormal conduction found in BrS.

BrS is commonly treated with an ICD.

Sports participation is restricted to class IA.

Marfan syndrome

In this syndrome, mutations in a single gene affect components of the extracellular matrix, leading to a disorder of the connective tissue. Marfan syndrome is an autosomal dominant disease of connective tissue with variable penetrance. Its frequency is 1 in 20,000; 25% of cases represent new mutations.

Mutation on chromosome 15 in the fibrillin-1 gene (*FBN-1*) affects the extracellular matrix glycoprotein present in the aorta, suspensory ligament of lens, and connective tissue of tendons and ligaments.

Molecular analysis of complement deoxyribonucleic acid and deoxyribonucleic acid on the fibrillin-1 gene from skin fibroblasts culture shows reduced, absent, or structurally abnormal fibrillin.

Challenges

- Diagnosis is made on clinical grounds, with abnormalities found in two systems.
- Genetic counseling is recommended, as there may be particular problems with pregnancy.
- In the context of lifestyle advice, body habitus may allow sports participation, e.g., basketball or volleyball.
- Cardiovascular surveillance is aimed predominantly at aortic size and the mitral valve.

Diagnosis

Skeletal system

Major criteria

- Pectus carinatum, pectus excavatum requiring surgery
- Reduced upper-to-lower segment ratio or arm span-to-height ratio >1.05
- Wrist and thumb signs
- Scoliosis of >20° or spondylolisthesis
- Reduced extension at the elbows (<170°)
- Pes planus
- Protrusion acetabulae (on X-ray)

Minor criteria

- Pectus excavatum of moderate severity
- Joint hypermobility
- High-arched palate with crowding of teeth
- Typical facial appearance

Ocular system

Major criteria

- Ectopia lentis

Minor criteria

- Flat cornea (keratometry)
- Increased axial length of globe (ultrasound)
- Decreased miosis

Major criteria
- Dura
- Lumbosacral dural ectasia by CT or MRI

Family/genetic history
Major criteria
- Having a parent, child, or sibling who meets the diagnostic criteria independently
- Known mutation in fibrillin 1 gene
- Haplotype of *FBN-1* is inherited and known to be associated with unequivocal Marfan syndrome in the family

Cardiovascular system
Major criteria
- Dilatation of ascending aorta including sinuses of Valsalva
- Dissection of ascending aorta

Minor criteria
- Mitral valve prolapse
- Unexplained dilatation of main pulmonary artery <40 years
- Calcification of mitral valve annulus <40 years
- Dilatation or dissection of descending thoracic or abdominal aorta <50 years

Pulmonary system
Minor criteria
- Spontaneous pneumothorax.
- Apical blebs (chest X-ray)

Skin and integument
Minor criteria
- Unexplained stretch marks
- Recurrent or incisional herniae

Diagnostic criteria for Marfan syndrome

Negative family or genetic history
- Major criteria in at least two different organ systems and involvement of a third system, or known genetic mutations plus one major criterion and involvement of a second organ system

Positive family or genetic history
- One major criterion in an organ system and involvement of a second organ system

Cardiac problems
- Early mortality occurs, in the fourth and fifth decades.
- Children are more affected by mitral valve disease.
- Aortic problems are progressively more likely in adolescents and older people.
- Mitral complications more common in females than in males.

There is a higher risk of deterioration (25%) in this group of mitral valve prolapse than in the normal population.

Mitral valve disease

Mitral annulus dilatation stretching may occasionally rupture chordae; 10% of cases have associated calcification. Repair of the valve is often successful.

Factors influencing the results of surgery include the valve cusp being extremely redundant, marked chordal damage, and degree of calcification. There is an increased risk of dehiscence of prosthetic valve if replacement is required.

Aortic root involvement

Involvement may be dilated at birth, with rate of progression variable. Prediction of dissection is difficult. Screening with a transthoracic echocardiogram is sufficient if dilation is limited to the proximal ascending aorta. The usual rate of change is slow.

If dilatation of the descending aorta is present, transesophageal echocardiogram and serial MRI are required. Aortic valve regurgitation usually accompanies dilatation of 50 mm. Rupture of the aorta is infrequent if <55 mm.

A positive family history may influence the predisposition.

Treatment

Beta-blockers should be introduced as early as possible at the highest tolerated dose.

Valve surgery

Repair the dilated aortic root and preserve the aortic valve to avoid risks of endocarditis and anticoagulation.

Aortic root replacement

Elective root repair has low operative mortality. Emergency results are much poorer. Operate in patients with aortic roots >65 mm.

Aortic dissection

Most cases arise above the coronary ostium (type A Stanford). Some may extend the entire length (type 1 deBakey scheme), with 10% distal to the left subclavian (type B or 111). Rarely, dissection may be limited to the abdominal aorta.

Angiography, MRI, and transesophageal echocardiogram are needed for monitoring. Follow up for progression. With distal branch occlusion, there is further aortic dilatation.

Indications for monitoring

Aortic root size must be monitored with echocardiography or MRI if the echocardiographic window is inadequate.

If the aortic root diameter is 5 cm, investigation should be undertaken every 3 months. If it is 6 cm, prophylactic surgery is recommended.

If the aortic root is normal and there is no family history of sudden death, dynamic exercise may be undertaken at low to moderate levels in static or low-dynamic competitive sports, but isometric exercise should be avoided.

Sport participation

- Class IA and IIA participation is allowed if none of the following are present:
  - Aortic root dilation ($\geq$40 mm in adults or >2 standard deviations from mean for body surface area in children)
  - Moderate or severe MR
  - Family history of dissection
  - Sudden death in a Marfan relative
  - Echocardiogram should be repeated every 6 months to measure the aortic root.
- Aortic root dilatation, prior surgery on aortic root, chronic dissection, moderate to severe MR, or positive family history: class IA
- No sports with risk of bodily contact or trauma

Other cardiomyopathies

Myocarditis

This is commonly due to viral infection (Coxsackie or other enterovirus, adenovirus, parvovirus) or drug use such as cocaine. Myocardial changes create unstable electrical pathways. With probable or definite myocarditis there should be no sport participation for 6 months following the onset of symptoms.

Prior to return to sports, rest and exertional echocardiography or radionuclide studies should show normal LV function, wall motion, and cardiac dimensions, and there should be no arrhythmias on Holter monitoring and exercise testing, with normal inflammatory markers and normal ECG.

Arrhythmogenic right ventricular cardiomyopathy (ARVC)

ARVC is characterized by replacement of regular myocardium with fibro-fatty tissue. Diffuse or segmental patterns may exist. ARVC results in wall thinning.

A definitive diagnosis can be made with cardiac MRI or right ventricle biopsy. ARVC is associated with myocarditis.

With a probable or definite diagnosis there should be no sports participation, with possible exception of class IA.

Other myocardial diseases

These include dilated cardiomyopathy, primary nonhypertrophied restrictive cardiomyopathy, and systemic infiltrative diseases with cardiac involvement. No sports participation is recommended, with the possible exception of class IA.

Pericarditis

Regardless of etiology, no sports participation is recommended until there is full resolution, including normal echocardiogram and inflammatory markers. With chronic pericardial disease resulting in constriction there should be no sports participation.

Ehlers–Danlos syndrome

This rare, autosomal dominant disorder is caused by defective type III collagen. It is characterized by joint hypermobility as well as skin hyperelasticity, fragile skin and blood vessels, and poor wound healing.

There are six clinical forms. The vascular form has a high risk of aortic rupture; these patients should not participate in any sports.

Coronary artery anomalies

A variety of anomalies exist; most common is anomalous origin of the left main coronary artery from the right (anterior) sinus of Valsalva. Unfortunately, the first clinical expression is usually sudden death. Preceding symptoms may include angina, near-syncope, syncope, or myocardial infarction.

ECG and stress tests are typically unremarkable. A history of exertional syncope requires consideration of coronary artery anomaly with workup including echocardiogram, CT angiogram, or coronary arteriography.

Surgical intervention can be curative.

Coronary artery disease

Introduction

While generally protective, physical exertion transiently increases risk of cardiac events. Coronary artery disease (CAD) has been identified in approximately 75% of victims of exercise-related sudden death above the age of 35. Cardiac events may occur in arteries without previous constriction.

Standard CAD risk assessments may be difficult to translate into younger athletic populations or elite masters athletes.

Diagnosis

- History of a myocardial infarction (MI)
- History of angina pectoris with evidence of ischemia
- Presence of atherosclerosis on coronary imaging studies such as cardiac catheterization, MR angiography, electron beam CT, or cardiac CT

Evaluation

Athletes with CAD by any diagnosis should have LV function assessed.

Maximal treadmill or bicycle exercise testing should be used to approximate the demands of the activity to be undertaken, although various activities may be difficult to compare.

Risk stratification

Mild risk

- Normal resting ejection fraction
- Normal exercise tolerance
- Absence of exercise-induced ischemia or arrhythmia
- No hemodynamically significant stenosis (≥50% luminal narrowing)
- If positive surgical history, successful revascularization

Substantial risk

- Ejection fraction <50% at rest
- Exercise-induced ischemia or ventricular arrhythmia
- Significant stenosis

Recommendations for participation in competitive sports

- Mild risk group: class IA, IIA, although decisions should be evaluated on an individual basis
- Substantial risk group: class IA

Competitive sport participation in coronary vasospasm without CAD

- Restricted to class IA; annual re-evaluation should assess for remission of condition.

Commotio cordis

Commotio cordis is characterized by blunt force to the chest generating ventricular fibrillation. Survival rates are ~15% but may improve with immediate CPR and defibrillation. Some studies show increased survival if injury to defibrillation is done within 3 minutes as the heart is structurally normal.

The window of inopportunity in the cardiac electrical cycle is the 15 to 30 ms preceding the T-wave peak. Various chest protectors have not been proven effective.

There are no standard recommendations for return to play following survival of commotio cordis, although a thorough cardiac evaluation is necessary.

Implantable cardioverter defibrillators

Having an ICD generally disqualifies individuals from sports other than class IA. This is true for conditions in which ICD is used as a primary or secondary prevention.

The athlete's heart

Athletic training may result in cardiac adaptive remodeling, including increased LV wall thickness, enlarged cavities (increased LV end-diastolic size), and increased total mass. It may also result in abnormal ECG findings, which are found in up to 40% of elite athletes. Abnormal findings may be similar to those found in cardiac disease, including increased R- or S-wave voltages, Q waves, and repolarization changes.

Morphologic changes may mimic structural disease states such as HCM, dilated cardiomyopathy, and ARVC.

An LV wall thickness of 13–15 mm and LV cavity enlargement of 56–70 mm are borderline measures.

Characteristics indicating a favorable diagnosis of an athlete's heart instead of HCM are as follows:

- Symmetric enlargement
- LV cavity <45 mm in diastole
- LV end-diastolic dimension >55 mm
- Lack of left atrial enlargement
- Lack of ECG abnormalities
- Normal LV filling
- Negative family history
- Decreased LV mass in response to a period of deconditioning

Cardiac MRI may also assist in differentiation through identification of segmental hypertrophy.

Evaluation of the symptomatic athlete

Exertional chest pain

Cardiac etiology, in which oxygen demand exceeds supply resulting in ischemia, should be ruled out. Most common cardiac causes are HCM and coronary artery anomalies.

Workup includes history, examination, 12-lead ECG, echocardiogram, and usually a treadmill stress test.

Noncardiac causes are more common, with a differential diagnosis including exercise-induced asthma or bronchoconstriction, gastroesophageal reflux, or musculoskeletal pain such as costochondritis.

Exertional syncope

Although cardiac causes need to be considered and ruled out, the most common causes of exertional syncope are noncardiac. Cardiac etiologies may include HCM, coronary artery anomalies, LQTS, and other causes of ventricular tachycardia and fibrillation.

Workup also includes history, examination, 12-lead ECG, echocardiogram, and usually a treadmill stress test.

Noncardiac causes include hyperthermia, hypovolemia, postexertional collapse, hyperventilation, and hyperglycemia.

Neurocardiogenic syncope may result from increased vagal tone in the setting of hyperthermia and/or hypovolemia.

Palpitations

Cardiac workup needs to consider possible underlying structural heart disease as well as arrhythmogenic risks.

Structural issues are addressed with history, examination, 12-lead ECG, and echocardiogram, if necessary.

Arrhythmias may be detected by resting ECG, exercise stress test, or Holter monitoring, if necessary (including during exertion).

Classification of sports (see Fig. 12.2)

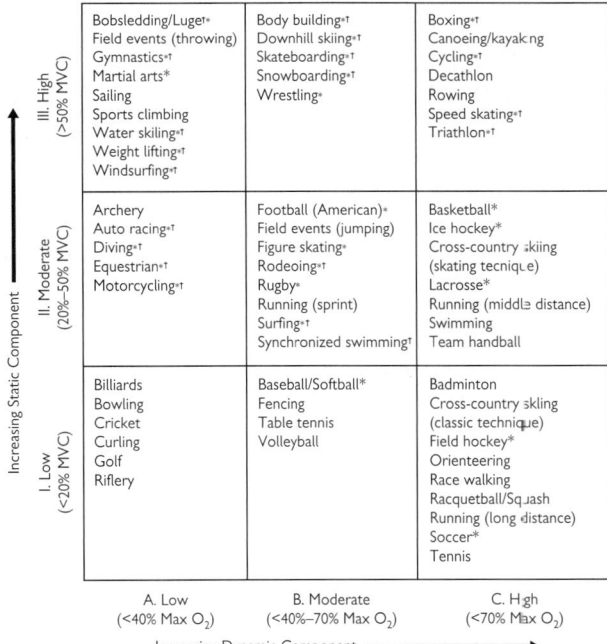

Increasing Static Component	A. Low (<40% Max O₂)	B. Moderate (<40%–70% Max O₂)	C. High (<70% Max O₂)
III. High (>50% MVC)	Bobsledding/Luge∗† Field events (throwing) Gymnastics∗† Martial arts∗ Sailing Sports climbing Water skiing∗† Weight lifting∗† Windsurfing∗†	Body building∗† Downhill skiing∗† Skateboarding∗† Snowboarding∗† Wrestling∗	Boxing∗† Canoeing/kayaking Cycling∗† Decathlon Rowing Speed skating∗† Triathlon∗†
II. Moderate (20%–50% MVC)	Archery Auto racing∗† Diving∗† Equestrian∗† Motorcycling∗†	Football (American)∗ Field events (jumping) Figure skating∗ Rodeoing∗† Rugby∗ Running (sprint) Surfing∗† Synchronized swimming†	Basketball∗ Ice hockey∗ Cross-country skiing (skating technique) Lacrosse∗ Running (middle distance) Swimming Team handball
I. Low (<20% MVC)	Billiards Bowling Cricket Curling Golf Riflery	Baseball/Softball∗ Fencing Table tennis Volleyball	Badminton Cross-country skiing (classic technique) Field hockey∗ Orienteering Race walking Racquetball/Squash Running (long distance) Soccer∗ Tennis

Increasing Dynamic Component ⟶

Figure 12.2 Max O₂, maximal oxygen uptake; MVC, maximal voluntary contraction; ∗danger of bodily collision; †increased risk if syncope occurs. Reprinted from Mitchel JH, et al. (2005). 36th Bethesda Conference. Task Force 8: Classification of sports. *J Am Coll Cardiol* **45**(8):1364–1367. Copyright (2005), with permission from Elsevier.

Automated external defibrillators

Timely access and use of an automated external defibrillator (AED) is critical in the response to sudden cardiac arrest (SCA). The rate of survival after SCA drops 7%–10% per minute of delayed defibrillation.

The AHA recommends access to an AED for the following criteria:

1. Reasonable probability of AED use (an estimated event rate of 1 sudden cardiac arrest per 1000 person-years);
2. An emergency medical system (EMS) call-to-shock time interval of <5 minutes cannot be achieved with conventional EMS services; and
3. An EMS call-to-shock time interval of <5 minutes can be achieved by training and equipping laypersons to function as first responders.

The ACSM and AHA issued a Joint Position Statement in 2002 encouraging AED access at all health and fitness facilities. Benefit of use extends beyond the involved athletes to coaches, officials, staff, and spectators.

Presence and use of an AED does not negate the use of cardiopulmonary resuscitation (CPR), which should be initiated within 1 minute of collapse.

Early studies showed that AED use on high school and college campuses are more often used in older, nonstudent persons than in student-athletes.

Survival rates of student-athletes with an SCA treated with an AED have not shown conclusive benefit.

Exercise prescription

In a 2007 statement, the ACSM and AHA issued recommendations for minimum physical activity levels for healthy adults:
- *Aerobic*: moderate-intensity aerobic activity for a minimum of 30 minutes on 5 days/week or vigorous-intensity activity for a minimum of 20 minutes on 3 days/week.
- *Resistance*: minimum of 2 days/week; 8–10 exercises focusing on major muscle groups using weight or resistance that allows 8–12 repetitions of each.

Additional health benefits and higher levels of physical fitness can be realized with increased time, intensity, and frequency of physical activity.

For individual exercise prescriptions, it is important to take into account medical history, baseline fitness level, nutrition, goals, and environmental factors. Exercise prescriptions should be written out and address the four variables of exercise: type, time/duration, intensity, and frequency.

Further reading

Haskell W, Lee I, Pate R, et al. (2007). Physical activity and public health: updated recommendation for adults from the American College of Sports Medicine and the American Heart Association. *Med Sci Sports Exercise* **39**:1423–1434.

Maron B (2007). Hypertrophic cardiomyopathy and other causes of sudden cardiac death in young competitive athletes, with considerations for preparticipation screening and criteria for disqualification. *Cardiol Clin* **25**:399–414.

Maron B, Zipes D (2005). 36th Bethesda Conference: eligibility recommendations for competitive athletes with cardiovascular abnormalities. *J Am Coll Cardiol* **45**:1312–1375.

Pigozzi F (2008). Sudden death in competitive athletes. *Clin Sports Med* **27**:153–181.

Gastroenterology and genitourinary

Abdominal injury

Abdominal injuries most often occur as a result of an unprotected unguarded blow to the abdomen. These injuries can be seen in any sport but most commonly occur in contact sports such as hockey and football. The ribs and pelvis provide some protection, but the main protection is by the abdominal musculature. In addition to the abdominal viscera, superficial structures such as skin, subcutaneous tissues, and muscle may be injured.

Children are more vulnerable to abdominal injury caused by blunt forces because they have smaller, compact torsos that provide a smaller area for the force of the injury to be dissipated. They also have relatively larger viscera, less overlying fat, and weaker abdominal musculature.

It is very important to recognize and treat these abdominal injuries because many can be life threatening.

In this chapter we will cover the most common abdominal injuries as well as some common abdominal medical problems.

History

Try to determine the type of trauma (fall, or direct trauma from contact, e.g., helmet). Location of pathology may be obscured, as pain can be referred:

- To shoulder from diaphragm (Kehr's sign)
- To shoulder blade from gall bladder
- To left chest from spleen
- To umbilicus from appendix or pancreas
- To the neck from the phrenic nerve (Seagasser's sign)
- To testis from ureter and groin

Examination

- Signs of serious intra-abdominal injury include the following:
- Absence of normal respiratory movements of chest and abdomen
- Guarding
- Rebound pain
- Absence of normal bowel sounds
- Referred pain to shoulder or back
- Falling blood pressure, increased pulse rate

Delayed or slow hemorrhage from abdominal trauma is possible, thus re-assessment over several hours to days is warranted.

Immediate management of any abdominal trauma will be assessment and appropriate treatment of hemodynamic shock.

Winded athlete

A blow to the solar plexus, with abdominal muscles relaxed, leaves the athlete temporarily unable to breathe. This is frightening for the athlete.

The sideline physician should provide confident reassurance, ensure that the airway is open and clear, loosen any restrictive clothing or equipment, and encourage a slight flexion of the trunk. After the episode has passed, the doctor should consider visceral and rib injury.

Rectus sheath hematoma

This hematoma usually occurs as a result of a direct blow to the abdominal wall. This can cause damage to the epigastric artery, which may produce a large hematoma.

The swelling may first be thought of as arising from an abdominal organ, but the later bluish discoloration gives a clue that it does not. The swelling will not cross the midline or extend beyond the lateral border of the muscle. It is relatively immovable because of the rectus sheath. Ultrasound or MRI will confirm the diagnosis if required.

Treat with protection, ice, and NSAIDs. Rehabilitation is focused on range of movement (ROM) and strength.

Splenic rupture

The spleen is a highly vascular organ located in the left upper quadrant. It is the most commonly injured organ during blunt abdominal trauma. Splenic rupture is also the most serious complication of abdominal trauma and is the leading cause of death due to abdominal injury in sports.

Because the spleen lies on the 9th to 11th ribs, it can be injured by a rib trauma. With this trauma, the abdomen usually becomes painful and tender; blood in the abdomen acts as an irritant and can cause diffuse abdominal pain and rebound tenderness. The pain is usually sharp and can be referred to the shoulder, neck, or chest.

Clinicians need a high index of suspicion for splenic bleeds. A CT scan can confirm the diagnosis. Although minor splenic injuries can be treated conservatively with ongoing observation, rapid blood loss and hemodynamic instability require a splenectomy.

In either case, if there is sideline suspicion of splenic rupture, transportation to the hospital is necessary. Return to play usually takes 3 months if treatment is nonsurgical, and 3–6 months if splenectomy is performed.

Athletes with splenomegaly are at increased risk of rupture. The most common cause of splenomegaly in athletes is glandular fever (infectious mononucleosis), which causes the spleen to be vulnerable in blows to the left upper quadrant.

Consequently, athletes should be advised against contact sports while the spleen is enlarged. Although 4 weeks is the minimum, the exact time period following the onset of glandular fever is debated. Before the athlete returns to competition, complete blood count, liver enzymes, and abdominal examination should have normalized.

Liver damage

Lacerations of the liver are rare in sports. They occur with trauma to the right upper quadrant. Injury can result in subcapsular hematoma, laceration, contusion, hepatic vascular disruption, and bile duct injury. The athlete usually complains of right upper quadrant pain, although pain can be referred to the neck or right shoulder. Nausea and vomiting can also occur.

Be aware of possible tachycardia and hypotension. Ultrasound or CT scanning may confirm the diagnosis. Most cases are treated conservatively, as most hepatic bleeding stops spontaneously.

Monitor for signs of hemodynamic instability. Intervene surgically if conservative therapy fails. Return to play varies, depending on the severity of liver damage.

Pancreatic damage

The pancreas lies deep at the back of the abdomen and is rarely injured in sports. Epigastric pain radiating to the back after severe blunt trauma, with midline tenderness, distension, and loss of bowel sounds due to reflex ileus, should lead the clinician to consider pancreatic damage. Serum amylase will be elevated and CT will confirm the diagnosis.

Bowel rupture

Rarely, the bowel may be ruptured in severe blunt trauma in sports. This occurs when a sudden force is applied to the abdominal wall and the increase in the intra-abdominal and intraperitoneal pressure is transmitted to the hollow viscera. Perforation must be suspected in cases where there is persistent abdominal pain, spasm, and tenderness, with or without nausea and vomiting.

Blood in the peritoneum may irritate the diaphragm, producing shoulder pain. Pain can also be referred to the testis.

Examination reveals tenderness, guarding, even abdominal rigidity and loss of bowel sounds. Shock may be indicated by clammy skin, tachycardia, and falling blood pressure. Peritoneal lavage may detect blood. Free air may be seen under the diaphragm in the upright plain abdominal X-ray.

The leukocyte count becomes rapidly elevated in most instances of intraperitoneal hemorrhage. The erythrocyte count is not dependable as an index of loss of blood and is often misleading.

Athletes with a history of abdominal trauma should be closely observed for up to 48 hours with repeated examinations of abdomen, pulse, respiratory rate, leukocyte count, hemoglobin, and blood pressure.

A CT scan is the preferred diagnostic examination. Prompt surgical treatment is required once the diagnosis is made.

Pancreatitis

Athletes may also develop abdominal pain due to inflammation of the pancreas. Acute pancreatitis lasts for a short period of time and usually resolves. Pancreatitis can cause serious complications such as bleeding, tissue damage, and infection. It is usually caused by heavy alcohol abuse or gallstones. Sometime the cause is never found.

Symptoms include mild to severe abdominal pain that can radiate to the back, nausea, vomiting, or fever. The pain often gets worse with eating or drinking.

Pancreatitis can cause life-threatening complications. Amylase and lipase levels are usually three times normal levels. Also check complete blood count, liver enzymes, calcium, and glucose level. An ultrasound or CT scan may be needed for definitive diagnosis.

Treatment goals are often accomplished in the inpatient setting. Goals include bowel rest and pain control. The patient can return to play once lab values have normalized and the patient tolerates a full diet.

Appendicitis

Appendicitis is thought to result from a blockage in the opening of the appendix. It results in pain that is usually located in the right lower quadrant. It can start as diffuse, poorly localized pain that progresses to pain at McBurney's point. The athlete can also have symptoms of anorexia, fever, dehydration, nausea, vomiting, and dysuria.

The physical examination usually reveals decreased or absent bowel sounds, rebound tenderness, psoas sign, and abdominal guarding. White blood cell counts are usually elevated to 12,000–18,000. Ultrasound and CT scans may be needed for definitive diagnosis.

Treat with hospitalization, antibiotics, and a surgical consultation. Return to play varies depending on severity of the case.

Diarrhea ("runner's trots")

Urgency to defecate, abdominal cramps, and diarrhea frequently occur in long-distance runners, called "runner's trots," and can be related to several factors:

- Athletes may have increased catecholamine levels.
- Athletes tend to have high-carbohydrate diets, which can increase intestinal transit time.
- Reduced visceral blood flow leading to relative ischemia of the bowel, particularly as duration of exercise increases
- Dehydration

Treatment includes staying hydrated, eating at least 4 hours prior to running, not consuming high-fiber foods before an event, limiting caffeine intake, and dairy products.

Gastroesophageal reflux disease (GERD, or heartburn)

GERD is a condition in which stomach contents regurgitate back into the esophagus. Vigorous exercise can bring this on. This happens mostly in runners. It is thought that exercise causes decreased esophageal motility. Symptoms include heartburn with or without a funny taste in the back of the throat and regurgitation.

If left untreated, ulcers, cough, and asthma symptoms can develop. Treat with H2 blockers 4 hours before exercise. Reduce caffeine intake, and monitor the timing of food intake in relation to exercise.

Renal trauma

The kidneys have some protection from blunt trauma, with aid of the 11th and 12th ribs, Psoas muscle, and surrounding fat. However, renal contusions do occur, particularly in the young, in whom the relative size of the kidney is larger.

The kidneys are the most commonly injured abdominal organ in sports. Such injuries result in many hospitalizations. The kidneys are vulnerable when the abdominal muscles are relaxed; a typical situation might be leaping high and reaching for a ball while taking a blow from another athlete.

The athlete might experience flank pain, though this may refer anteriorly and might describe hematuria. Nevertheless, the amount of blood in the urine does not correlate to the seriousness of the injury, e.g., frank hematuria may not follow a vascular pedicle injury.

Thus, after blunt trauma, the wise clinician will investigate microscopic hematuria if blood pressure is dropping (<90 mmHg systolic) or if there is any suspicion of palpable mass. Intravenous pyelogram (IVP) and CT scans are indicated, although CT has the advantage of providing information about other abdominal viscera that might be injured.

Grading of renal injury

Grade I
a. Hematuria with normal imaging studies
b. Contusions
c. Nonexpanding subscapsular hematomas

Grade II
a. Superficial cortical laceration <1 cm in depth

Grade III
a. Calix laceration
b. Cortical laceration >1 cm in depth

Grade IV
a. Vascular pedicle rupture
b. Injuries involving the main renal artery or vein with contained hemorrhage

Grade V
a. Shattered or devascularized kidney
b. Ureteropelvic avulsions
c. Complete laceration or thrombus of the main renal artery or vein

Management of renal trauma depends on the extent of injury. Few renal injuries (<10%) require surgery, although indications are as follows:
• Persistent retroperitoneal bleeding
• Urinary extravasation
• Nonviable renal tissue
• Renal vascular pedicle injury

Even for grade I injuries, return to strenuous sports should be delayed 4 weeks to reduce the risk of rebleeding (maximum at 15–21 days). Contact sport should be avoided for at least 6 weeks and follow-up should be for 6 months with repeat blood pressure readings and urinalysis.

Hypertension and hydronephrosis are late complications.

Ureteric avulsion

This is rare in sports, although is described in motor vehicle and equestrian sports. It gives rise to severe back pain and peritoneal irritation.

It is confirmed by IVP and requires surgical management.

Bladder rupture

Bladder rupture may occur with severe trauma of the abdomen or pelvis. Suprapubic tenderness and hematuria will be present with contusions, but signs of peritonism (abdominal rigidity or rebound tenderness) indicate rupture and leakage of urine. Rupture requires prompt surgical treatment.

Urethral rupture

Urethral rupture is rare in sports and tends to occur with a straddle injury, in cycling, gymnastics, or equestrian sports, or in association with pelvic fractures.

It is a more common injury in men than in women. The bulbous urethra is more likely to be injured than the penile, which can move more freely.

There will be blood at the meatus as well as signs of perineal trauma. Surgical repair and a suprapubic catheter are required.

Injuries of the scrotum and testes

External to the abdomen, the scrotum and contents are vulnerable to injury from blunt trauma. Some athletes wear protective equipment (lacrosse and baseball players).

Scrotal swelling after trauma suggests a ruptured testis or ruptured pampiniform plexus of veins. In the latter situation, a varicocele becomes a hematocele. A hematocele does not transluminate well, but if the testicular shadow is visible through the fluid a hydrocele is more likely. Ultrasound examination is effective at diagnosing the ruptured testis, which requires urgent surgery.

If trauma does not result in swelling and scrotal examination is normal, the athlete may be treated by scrotal support, NSAIDs, and return to activity when the pain subsides.

Testicular torsion

Testicular torsion should be considered whenever an athlete has scrotal pain and swelling. It is a true emergency. Excruciating testicular and abdominal pain is usually present. Physical examination should include elevation of the scrotum to see if it relieves the pain. If so, it is more likely to be epididymitis.

Elevation of the scrotum in torsion often increases the pain (Prehn's sign). If suspected, ultrasound examination should be done.

Testicular cancer

Testicular cancer is the most common malignancy in 16- to 35-year-old men. If a mass is discovered, it should be transilluminated. If it can't be illuminated, an ultrasound should be preformed.

Renal physiology and exercise

Renal parameters at rest
- Renal blood flow is 20% of cardiac output (CO) (1200 mL/min).
- Renal plasma flow is 700 mL/min.
- Glomerular filtration rate (GFR), 15% of plasma flow, is 105 mL/min.
- Smaller proteins than albumin are filtered but then reabsorbed in proximal tubules.

Renal response to exercise
- Renal blood flow decreases.
- The GFR is maintained or decreases.
- Increased filtration of macromolecules (albumin) gives rise to a "glomerular" pattern of protein loss.
- In intense exercise, reabsorption of small proteins (microglobulins) declines, giving rise to a tubular pattern of protein loss.

The decrease in renal blood flow is mediated by catecholamines and the sympathetic nervous system and is related to intensity of exercise, such that it may reduce to 25% of resting flow with strenuous activity. Plasma flow may reduce to 200 mL/min in such circumstances, yet GFR is often maintained.

With dehydration, the GFR may drop. With intense exercise, anti-diuretic hormone (ADH) and aldosterone levels increase to preserve water and sodium. During such activity, more red and white blood cells are found in the urine.

Athletic pseudonephritis
Described by Gardner (1956), athletic pseudonephritis is the presence of red and white blood cells, hemoglobin, myoglobin, protein, and casts in the urine after exercise.

This is recognized as a benign situation and has attracted various names, depending on the activity with which the findings are associated:
- Stress hematuria
- Marathoner's hematuria
- 10,000 m hematuria
- March hemaglobinuria
- Jogger's nephritis

Proteinuria
Proteinuria is common in contact and noncontact sports, and between 70% and 100% of runners are reported to have protein in their urine. This relates to intensity and not duration of event and is maximal within 30 minutes of exercise.

The pattern is glomerular (macroglobulins) for moderate exercise but glomerulotubular (macro- and microglobulins) for intense exercise. This may be due to hypoxic damage to nephrons from decreased blood flow, or efferent glomerular arteriolar constriction being greater than afferent constriction, and thus increasing filtration pressure.

However, there are other causes of proteinuria:

- Physiological proteinuria (<100 mg/L)
- Orthostatic proteinuria
- Glomerulonephritis (>0.2 g/day)
- Nephrotic syndrome (>0.05 g/kg body weight/day)
- Cystitis/pyelonephritis
- Hypertension
- Diabetes mellitus

Physiological proteinuria is common in adolescents (60%) and recurs in up to 30% of patients. It is benign.

Othostatic proteinuria clears with recumbency, thus an early-morning urine might be negative. Prognosis is good if normotensive and protein loss is 750 mg/day.

Typically, proteinuria records ++ or +++ on urinalysis corresponding to up to 300 mg/L, post-exercise. It is wise not to test an athlete's urine shortly after exercise. If urinalysis is positive for protein following exercise and there are no other symptoms to indicate another cause, repeat the urinalysis after 48 hours of rest. The urine should be negative for protein.

Hematuria

Hematuria may be macroscopic and dramatic after exercise, even with clots being passed. However, microscopic hematuria is almost universal as detected by dipstick, which may detect as few as 1 million red cells per liter. For abnormality, it is better to look for 100 million red cells per liter.

As well as being too sensitive, dipsticks look for the hem group and indicate myoglobinuria and hemoglobinuria similarly.

Hematuria has been reported in high numbers of the following athletes:

- Ice hockey players (100%)
- Swimmers (80%)
- Boxers (73%)
- Football players (60%)
- Soccer players (50%)
- Runners (10%–25%)

Proportions depend on the definitions used in studies and on the intensity of exercise, although contact also clearly plays a part in some sports.

Early cystoscopy in females showed "kissing" lesions, localized bladder contusions, and urothelial loss, in the trigone and interureteric bar,[1] leading to theories of bladder "slapping" being a cause of hematuria in sports.

However, the red cells seen in the urine of marathon runners are often dysmorphic, suggesting damage at the glomerular level. The explanation may be hypoxic damage to the nephron or increased filtration pressure (see Proteinuria, p. 452).

---

1 Blacklock NJ (1977). Bladder trauma in the long-distance runner: "10,000 metres haematuria". *Br J Urol* 49(2):129–132.

Other causes of hematuria include the following:
- Acute glomerular nephritis
- Pyelonephritis
- Acute tubular necrosis
- Urinary tract infection (UTI)
- Gallstones
- Cancer (especially >40 years old)
- Hemoglobinuria or myoglobinuria
- Spurious

History may include trauma, pain, fever, dysuria, or weight or appetite loss. Examination findings may include renal tenderness, edema, raised temperature, raised blood pressure, and cachexia. If these are not present and there is a clear relationship to exercise, it would be wise to repeat the urinalysis after 48 hours rest.

Further investigation to consider if hematuria persists would be microscopy and culture (MCS) of mid-stream sample (MSU), intravenous pyelogram (IVP), ultrasound examination of the renal tract, and cystoscopy. Clotting studies may be performed to exclude a bleeding disorder and complete blood count performed to rule out anemia.

If "athletic hematuria" is the final diagnosis, the prognosis is good and there is no need to restrict sporting activity. Adequate hydration before and during exercise may help preserve glomerular filtration and keep the bladder reasonably full to prevent "slapping."

Hemoglobinuria

The urine may be positive for blood on urinalysis, but red cells are not seen on microscopy. Hemoglobin from the breakdown of red cells is present in the urine. This was described in relation to long marches in the military and in contact sports such as karate. It is generally a benign condition.

Myoglobinuria/exercise-induced rhabdomyolysis

The presence of myoglobin in the urine indicates the breakdown of muscle, or "rhabdomyolysis." It has been recorded in both endurance sports, such as marathon running, and in contact sports, such as football. The urine appears tea or cola colored. The urinalysis is again positive for blood, but negative for red cells.

Myoglobin is broken down to hematin. Because hematin is nephrotoxic, there have been concerns that athletes with myoglobinuria may go into acute renal failure. However, the risk of acute renal failure in association with sports appears to be small.

Sinert et al.[2] proposed that a nephrotoxic factor was missing in the rhabdomyolysis of sports, unlike medical causes of rhabdomyolysis. Nevertheless, it is probably best to avoid myoglobinuria, if possible, through adequate hydration, nutrition, and conditioning.

2 Sinert R, Kohl L, Rainone T, Scalea T (1994). Exercise-induced rhabdomyolysis. *Ann Emerg Med* **23**(6):1301–1306.

Acute renal failure in sport

Although rare in sports, acute renal failure is associated with exercise to exhaustion in hot conditions. Those who are less fit and those who become dehydrated or hyperpyrexial are at risk. Prevention may include adequate hydration, nutrition, exercising in a cooler environment, and not exercising to exhaustion.

Spurious causes of red urine

Medication (e.g., rifampicin, nitrofurantoin) and diet (e.g., beetroot) give rise to red urine, but urinalysis will be negative.

Chapter 14

Infectious diseases

Effects of exercise on immunity

Benefits

Regular, moderate levels of exercise improve resistance to most infections, particularly those affecting the upper respiratory tract (URIs).

Improved resistance is possibly due to mild elevations in the following:
- T-cell lymphocytes
- Interleukins
- Macrophages
- Natural killer cells
- Endorphins

During moderate exercise, elevated immune cells circulate through the body more quickly, returning to normal levels a few hours post-exercise. Regular exercise appears to sustain these changes longer.

Adverse effects

There is good evidence that athletes undertaking more intensive training (i.e., marathon runners) are more prone to minor infections, particularly URIs. This is thought to be due to reduction of the following:
- Type 1 T-helper cells
- Salivary IgA, which plays a role in resistance to some viruses
- Immunoglobulin M (IgM)
- Natural killer cells, the number of which increases during moderate activity but drops by half after cessation of activity. With strenuous activity, the fall can begin during exercise.

Stress hormones (cortisol and adrenaline) may also contribute to suppression of the immune system in athletes with competitive training programs.

Supplementation with carbohydrate, vitamin C, glutamine, and zinc may reduce the immunosuppressive effect of heavy exercise. Training regimens should include enough rest days to allow recovery of the immune system.

Why are athletes prone to infection?

Stress, overtraining, under recovery

Symptoms may include the following:

- Decreased performance
- Decreased competitive drive
- Depressed mood, emotional lability
- Sleep disturbances, restlessness
- Loss of appetite
- Frequent URIs
- Lymphadenopathy, sore throat
- Diffuse myalgias and arthralgias
- Reduced concentration

High-level and endurance athletes are particularly at risk of training excessively because of their competitive nature.

Treatment includes rest and education about the need for increased training recovery time, optimization of nutrition, psychological monitoring and support, and gradual reintroduction of training.

Close contact with other athletes

In training and competition camps, the inevitable close contact among athletes, coaches, and support staff can encourage the spread of respiratory and gastrointestinal infections.

Sexual activity

Like the population as a whole, athletes are at risk of sexually transmitted diseases if practicing unsafe sex.

Trauma

Traumatic injury can predispose to infection, especially if wounds are open.

Foreign travel

Hepatitis B is endemic in many Third World countries, and traveling athletes should consider immunization (particularly in contact sports). Travel also carries risk of tropical diseases, such as malaria and diarrhea.

Upper respiratory infections (URIs)

Although a small proportion of URIs will be caused by group A streptococcus, most are caused by one of the following viruses:

- Rhinovirus
- Coronavirus
- Adenovirus
- Coxsackie viruses A and B
- Influenza

Investigation may include a Rapid Strep and/or a Monospot test to rule out streptococcal pharyngitis or infectious mononucleosis.

Treatment of URIs

- *Analgesia:* Acetaminophen and ibuprofen are effective and safe in correct dosages.
- *Decongestants:* Nasal sprays can help. Physicians and athletic trainers need to be aware that some decongestants are still on the World Anti-Doping Agency (WADA) banned list. If in doubt, the drug should be checked.
- *Fluids:* Adequate hydration and nutrition are necessary.

Prevention

Team groups are at risk of outbreaks of influenza, and vaccination can be offered every winter to the team members and staff.

Dangers of URIs

Coxsackie virus can cause inflammation of the heart muscle (myocarditis) and lead to sudden death. If an athlete has a combination of the following symptoms, they should be advised not to train or play:

- Resting tachycardia (>10 beats/minute above normal)
- Myalgia
- Lethargy
- Oral temperature >38°C
- Cervical lymphadenopathy

The athlete should be advised that a premature return to training and playing may delay recovery and that there is a small risk of myocarditis and cardiac arrhythmias.

"Above-the-neck" guidelines for athletes

If all symptoms are noted above the neck (i.e., stuffy or runny nose, sneezing, watery eyes, scratchy throat), athletes may train at 50% their normal intensity. If symptoms resolve after 15 minutes, intensity may be increased as tolerated.

If symptoms are noted below the neck (shortness of breath, fever, extreme fatigue, aching muscles, nausea, vomiting, diarrhea), athletes should rest until these symptoms resolve. Recovery time increases in these instances with rest.

Common infections

Otitis externa
- Also known as "swimmer's ear"
- Inflammation 9 infection in ear canal
- Common in swimmers and can be very painful
- Constant immersion during water sports produces moisture in ear canal which predisposes to the condition
- Elevated pH in ear canal decreases protective cerumen and epithelial coating
- *Pseudomonas* often grown on swab
- Treated with antibiotic 9 corticosteroid eardrops, although can sometimes require aural toilet by suction to remove debris in canal
- Athlete should refrain from water immersion until infection is cleared
- Prevention using 70% alcohol drops before and after swimming is best.

Viral gastroenteritis
- Usually self-limited and often resolves 1–2 days but may last longer
- Treated by limited dehydration with fluids and electrolytes
- The "BRAT" diet (bananas, rice, applesauce, toast) is often helpful.
- Severe cases may require IV hydration.
- The athlete may return to play if symptoms are relieved and the athlete is well hydrated.

Pneumonia
- Lung infection, often due to *Mycoplasma pneumoniae* in athletes aged 5–35 years
- Usually mild symptoms that resolve after 1–2 weeks
- Treated with macrolide antibiotics (erythromycin, azithromycin, clarithromycin)
- May also be caused by *Streptococcus pneumoniae* and various viral organisms. Symptoms may be more severe with these organisms.

Skin
- Community-acquired methicillin-resistant *Staphylococcus aureus*
- See Chapter 16, Dermatology, for other common viral, fungal, and bacterial skin infections.

Community-acquired methicillin-resistant *Staphylococcus aureus* (CA-MRSA)

Diagnosis of CA-MRSA Plus is made if diagnosed within 48 hours of admission; there is no prior history of MRSA; no c, surgeries, or dialysis in the last 12 months; and no history of catheter use.

Community-acquired MRSA (CA-MRSA) carries the Panton–Valentine leukocidin (PVL) toxin, which can cause skin necrosis leading to formation of boils and abscesses. Athletes at higher risk are football players and wrestlers.

Transmission
- Via direct contact
- Contributors to transmission include crowded conditions and poor hygiene.

Treatment
- *Incision and drainage:* If caught early, this may be the only intervention needed with frequent rechecking until resolution. A culture of drained material should be sent if possible. A larger abscess may need packing.
- *Antibiotics:* Oral trimethoprim-sulfamethoxazole double strength and/or clindamycin are first line. For more serious infections, vancomycin IV or linezolid can be used. It is important to know local bacterial sensitivies when prescribing antibiotics. Avoid fluorquinolones because of resistance and the potential to cause tendon rupture.

National Athletic Trainers Association (NATA) MRSA guidelines for prevention
- Keep hands clean by washing thoroughly
- Encourage immediate showering following activity
- Athletes should avoid use of whirlpools if they have open wounds or abrasions.
- Avoid sharing towels, razors, and daily athletic gear
- Properly wash athletic gear and towels after each use
- Maintain clean facilities and equipment
- Inform or refer to health-care personnel for active skin lesions or lesions not responding to initial therapy.
- Administer or seek proper first aid.
- Seek bacterial cultures whenever possible.
- Care for and cover skin lesions before participation.

Infectious mononucleosis

Infectious mononucleosis (IM) is also known as the "kissing disease." It is spread via saliva through close contact, airborne droplets, or sharing of utensils.

The classic triad is fever, sore throat, and cervical lymphadenopathy. It is caused by the Epstein–Barr virus.

Disease course

- 30- to 50-day incubation period
- 3–5 days prodrome of headache, malaise, myalgias
- 5–15 days of acute disease (fever, fatigue, exudative pharyngitis)
- Fatigue can last 2–6 weeks acutely
- Maculopapular rash sometimes seen
- 30% with concurrent streptococcal pharyngitis
- Recovery takes 4–12 weeks

Complications

- 5% can have significant complications
- Splenomegaly may be present (may be confirmed on ultrasound).
- Spleen fragility is greatest at 4–21 days of illness and can lead to splenic rupture (1–2 in 1000 cases).

Laboratory findings

- Leukocytosis of 10,000–20,000
- 10%–20% atypical lymphocytes
- Mild thrombocytopenia
- Liver transaminases increased, usually by 2–3×
- Monospot test: 60% positive at 2 weeks; 5%–15% false positive due to cytomegalovirus (CMV), adenovirus, or toxoplasmosis
- Epstein–Barr virus IgM positive for approximately 2 months and more accurate than Monospot

Return to play

- 21 days disqualification from onset of illness or diagnosis
- Athlete must be afebrile, have no subjective complaints, no splenomegaly or tenderness, and normal labs
- Gradual reintroduction of exercise as symptoms settle
- Chronic fatigue can continue for >3 months, especially if recovery is rushed.

Flu-like infections

These infections can be caused by several organisms, particularly the following:

- Epstein–Barr virus (infectious mononucleosis)
- Toxoplasma
- Cytomegalovirus (CMV)
- Primary HIV disease

They commonly occur in younger age groups and are linked to the development of chronic fatigue syndrome. Splenomegaly occurs, and participation in contact sports carries a risk of traumatic splenic rupture.

Toxoplasmosis

- Acquired via fecal–oral route of parasite from cats' feces or eating contaminated, undercooked meat
- Symptoms range from asymptomatic with cervical adenopathy to nonspecific flu-like symptoms (fever, hepatosplenomegaly, fatigue, generalized lymphadenopathy)
- Recent infection diagnosed on IgM serology
- 60% with positive serology have no history of illness
- Typically self-limiting. Drugs are available to treat the parasite.

Cytomegalovirus (CMV)

- Symptoms, if present, are similar to those of infectious mononucleosis and toxoplasmosis.
- Transmitted via direct contact
- Typically self-limiting but drugs are available to treat the virus

Lyme disease

- Tick-borne, spirochete infection *(Borrelia burgdorferi)*
- Most prevalent in Northeast and Midwest regions and in northwestern states where there are heavily wooded and grassy areas
- Symptoms range from "bulls-eye" rash at site of tick bite and flu-like symptoms to joint swelling and neurological problems.
- Diagnosed on serology
- Treatment usually with doxycycline or amoxicillin orally

Viral hepatitis

Hepatitis A

- Fecal–oral spread.
- Relatively common, especially in travelers
- Can be subclinical, often in childhood
- Fever, nausea, abdominal pains
- Jaundice may occur after 3–7 days.
- Hepatosplenomegaly and lymphadenopathy may be present.
- Abnormal liver transaminases and Hep A IgM positive 20+ days after exposure. Hep A IgG positive lifelong
- Treated symptomatically and full recovery ensues
- Self-limiting illness; no chronic liver disease after infection
- It is safe to return to play when clinically improved, although abnormal liver enzymes may persist.
- Effective vaccination is recommended.

Hepatitis B

- Transmitted by blood, sexual contact, IV drug use
- Endemic in Africa and parts of Asia
- Highly infectious. Incubation period is 30–180 days
- Clinical features similar to those of hepatitis A, but may have associated arthralgia and urticaria
- Abnormal liver enzymes and Hep Bs antigen positive 1–6 months post-infection. Hep Be antigen positive suggests high infectivity
- Treated symptomatically, as most patients recover spontaneously. Careful follow-up is required.
- Graded return to exercise only when liver enzymes return to normal and clinically improved
- 5%–10% of sufferers will become carriers with a high risk of transmission, especially in contact sports, and if diagnosed are excluded from boxing, wrestling, and rugby.
- Complications include chronic active hepatitis, cirrhosis and liver failure, and hepatocellular carcinoma.
- Vaccination is available and strongly advised for all participants in contact sports.

Hepatitis C

- Transmitted via contact with contaminated blood (transfustions, IV drug abuse). Less infectious than hepatitis B
- May be asymptomatic at time of infection but if symptomatic, similar to other forms of viral hepatitis
- Treated with pegylated interferon-alpha and/or ribavirin
- 85% develop chronic infection
- High incidence of cirrhosis and also hepatocellular carcinoma
- No available vaccine

Human immunodeficiency virus (HIV)

- Transmitted via blood, sexual contact, IV drug abuse
- No risk from sweat
- Present in saliva but no reports of spread by this route
- 100 times less infectious than hepatitis B
- Initial symptoms are "flu-like."
- May then be asymptomatic for months or years.
- Eventually develops into acquired immunodeficiency syndrome (AIDS)
- HIV antibodies found in blood at approximately 12 weeks after exposure and infection

Note

The risk of transmission of hepatitis B or C or HIV during sports is extremely low. The viruses cannot be transmitted via showers or shared drinks bottles. Vaccination against hepatitis B and the following infection control measures help reduce risks even further:

- Wear protective gloves when giving first aid to a bleeding athlete.
- Wipe any blood from the face or limbs of athletes.
- Bloodstained towels should not be reused. Put bloodstained clothing in a plastic bag for disposal or laundering.
- Athletes should not be allowed to continue in the game until bleeding has stopped and the wound is cleaned and covered.
- If there is concern about cross-infection, contact a physician immediately.

Travelers' diarrhea

Diarrhea of infectious origin is a major cause of morbidity in athletes who travel the world to compete. High-risk destinations for diarrheal illness include Latin America, Asia, Africa, and the Middle East.

Symptoms

- Increased frequency, volume and weight of stool during or shortly after a period of travel
- Usually four or more loose or watery stools daily
- Often accompanied by fever, nausea, vomiting, malaise, bloating, flatulence, or abdominal cramps
- Beware of dehydration

Potential causes

- Sometimes from stress of traveling and change in diet, but is often result of an infectious agent
- *Escherichia coli* (most common bacterial pathogen)
- Rotaviruses
- *Salmonella* and *Campylobacter*
- *Shigella*
- *Giardia* and *Entamoeba*

Treatment

- It usually resolves in 3–4 days with symptomatic treatment only.
- Maintain fluid and electrolyte balance.
- Stick to simple starchy foods.
- Seek medical advice if diarrhea is bloody, accompanied by high fever or signs of severe dehydration, or lasts more than 14 days. Further investigations may be necessary.
- *Loperamide* and *Lomotil* are antimotility agents that can reduce stool frequency and ease muscle cramps and spasms. Do not use if there is bloody diarrhea, fever, or symptoms for more than 48 hours.
- *Bismuth subsalicylate* can decrease the frequency of stools. Do not use if patient is <12 years, pregnant, or allergic to aspirin.
- *Antibiotics* may be used with severe symptoms.

Prevention

- Wash hands thoroughly before eating or handling food and after going to the toilet.
- Use only sealed bottled water or boiled water for drinking and brushing teeth.
- Avoid ice in drinks, shellfish, salads, and cold vegetables.
- Peel all fruits and vegetables if uncooked.
- Avoid food at room temperature or that has been kept warm.
- Avoid food from street vendors.
- Eat only hot, well-cooked food.
- Do not swim in water that may be contaminated and keep mouth closed while showering.

Rheumatology

Arthritis overview

Arthritis is defined as a group of conditions that involve damage to the joints. *Arthralgia*, which is often the cause of musculoskeletal pain, differs from arthritis in that there is pain with no swelling or effusion. Arthritis is the leading cause of disability in older adults and is a major public health concern.

More than 21% of U.S. adults (46.4 million people) have arthritis. It is projected that over the next 25 years the number of people affected will increase by 40%.

Arthritis can be defined as monoarticular, affecting one joint; oligoarticular, affecting five or fewer joints; or polyarticular, affecting more than five joints. Arthritis can be inflammatory or noninflammatory, and acute or chronic. Extra-articular features such as tenosynovitis or skin lesions can help with classifying a particular type of arthritis. The history and physical examination are critical in diagnosing arthritis.

In sports medicine practice it is common to evaluate patients with acute musculoskeletal symptoms, in which case it is helpful to have an approach to the preliminary evaluation of acute presentations of arthritis. As a preliminary step, "red flags" that should trigger a search for serious medical issues are hot, swollen joints; constitutional symptoms; focal or diffuse muscle weakness; neurogenic pain; and claudication. Diagnostic clues that suggest a systemic rheumatic disease include severe and prolonged morning stiffness, constitutional symptoms, evidence of focal inflammation, and exacerbation of symptoms after prolonged inactivity.

Another important branch-point in the evaluation of a patient with acute arthritis symptoms is the distribution of involved joints. After trauma is ruled out or X-rays are normal in a patient with one or a few involved joints, the most important step is to assess for signs of joint effusion or inflammation.

Signs of inflammation should prompt joint aspiration in search of infection, leukocytosis, crystals, or hemarthrosis. Potential diagnoses in this setting can include unsuspected trauma, gout, pseudogout, infectious arthritis, or a systemic rheumatic disease. In the setting of polyarthralgia, a more complete history and physical examination are warranted in search of systemic disease.

The presence of synovitis raises the possibility of a viral arthritis or a systemic rheumatic disease. The absence of synovitis would be more consistent with noninflammatory causes of generalized musculoskeletal symptoms such as osteoarthritis, neuropathic pain, hypothyroidism, or fibromyalgia.

Osteoarthritis

Definition and etiopathology

Osteoarthritis (OA), often called degenerative arthritis, is the most common form of arthritis. Initially it was thought to be strictly a degenerative disease associated with aging. However, it is now known that OA results from interplay between "wear and tear," genetics, and other underlying conditions.

OA can be idiopathic or secondary. Secondary OA is due to conditions that can increase the risk of developing OA, such as trauma, as is often seen in athletes; inflammatory arthritis, such as rheumatoid arthritis; crystalline diseases such as gout and pseudogout; and congenital or developmental conditions such as a slipped femoral epiphysis.

The joints most commonly affected include the distal interphalangeal (DIP) joints, the proximal interphalangeal (PIP) joints, the first carpometacarpal (CMC) joints, hips, knees, cervical spine, lumbar spine, and the first metatarsophalangeal (MTP) joints. OA is considered to be non-inflammatory, but usually there is evidence for some inflammation at a microscopic level.

- 20 million people in the United States are affected.
- Knee and hand OA occur more frequently in women. Knee OA incidence is 1.5:1 female to male. Hand OA incidence is 4:1 female to male.
- Radiographic changes are present in >50% of patients >65 years of age.

Clinical features

- Joint pain that tends to worsen with activity
- Joint stiffness and loss of mobility
- Morning stiffness usually lasting 30 minutes or less
- Gelling—stiffness after limited motion, e.g., sitting
- Locking or joint instability
- Crepitus—rubbing of the bone with motion of the joint. The patient hears "cracking" on movement of the joint.
- Effusion may be present, especially in the knees
- Bony enlargement (osteophytes). On the finger joints these are known as Heberden's nodes (on the DIPs) and Bouchard's nodes (on the PIPs).
- Cervical and lumbosacral pain with spine involvement
- Misalignment of joints (e.g., hallux valgus)
- Erosions in some aggressive forms of the disease. May be confused with rheumatoid arthritis on physical exam
- Bursitis especially in the hip and knees can occur as a complication of OA (e.g., anserine bursitis).

Risk factors

- Aging is not the cause of OA, but OA is related to aging. The cartilage structure changes as patients age, leading to degeneration of the collagen fibers of the cartilage. Osteophytes form in the margins of the joints near damaged cartilage.

- Females are more likely to have rapid, destructive disease and to require total hip arthroplasty.
- Genetics can determine familial joint location for OA.
- Obesity increases stress on the joints.
- Occupation—Jobs involving repetitive stressing of one or more joints with kneeling, bending, or lifting heavy objects increases the risk for development of OA. Occupations such as floor layers, sheet metal workers, plumbers, brick layers, asphalt workers, and concrete workers are at increased risk.
- Joint injuries related to sports, occupation, or accidents, e.g., anterior cruciate ligament (ACL) tears
- Trauma leading to altered joint mechanics (meniscal tears, ACL injury, fracture)
- Inflammatory arthritis can lead to chronic injury to the joint (rheumatoid arthritis)
- Endocrine disorders (diabetes mellitus, acromegaly, hypothyroidism)
- Metabolic disorders (hemachromatosis, Wilson disease)
- Septic joint history
- Congenital conditions (slipped capital femoral epiphysis, Legg–Calvé–Perthes disease)
- In-born errors of connective tissue disease (Marfan syndrome, Ehlers–Danlos syndrome)

Diagnosis

History

Pain is the most important symptom of OA, followed by loss of function. Typically, pain is activity related but will often vary on a weekly if not daily basis. The nature and severity of pain are poorly correlated with radiographic features of OA.

Patients are more likely to report hip pain and least likely to complain of hand pain for any given severity of X-ray change. Rest and night pain is usually indicative of more severe OA. OA of the hip is commonly associated with anterior groin pain and may radiate toward the knee.

OA joint pain is multifactorial and may be influenced by the following physical factors in addition to the psychological factors:

- Altered biomechanics due to structural change (e.g., osteophytes)
- Bone pain possibly related to raised intraosseous pressure
- Synovitis; mild synovitis is common. Occasionally, patients will present with severe flares of pain related to significant inflammation which is sometimes related to the presence of calcium pyrophosphate crystals (pseudogout).
- Secondary pain from other structures (e.g., bursitis, tendinopathy)
- Referred muscular pain, usually involving muscles directly responsible for joint movement. This is particularly common in OA of the spine.

Physical examination

- *Appearance:* joint enlargement, misalignment, deformity, muscle atrophy
- *Range of motion:* assess active and passive range of motion for pain and crepitus
- *Palpation:* tenderness on palpation of the joint, assessment of effusion, rule out synovitis that may suggest an inflammatory arthritis
- *Functional assessment:* ability to walk, bend, squat, grip, reach

Laboratory

There is no laboratory test for OA. Laboratory testing is focused on ruling out other suspected conditions and assessing potential toxicity to medications used to treat OA.

- Serologies for systemic rheumatic diseases are typically negative.
- Normal erythrocyte sedimentation rate (ESR)
- Synovial fluid is noninflammatory

Imaging

Plain radiographs may be useful in assessing joint architecture. There is rarely a role for CT or MRI scanning unless another condition is suspected. Plain radiographs are usually normal in early disease. Weight bearing radiographs should be performed for knees and hips to best assess joint-space narrowing. Typical findings consistent with OA include the following:

- Osteophytes or bony spurs
- Joint-space narrowing
- Bony sclerosis
- Subchondral cysts
- Erosions are rarely seen. They are mainly in very aggressive OA, typically in the DIP and PIP joints.

Synovial fluid analysis

This is generally not indicated unless a new effusion is present or there are signs of inflammation. In the setting of OA synovial fluid features include the following:

- Fluid appearance usually clear or yellow and transparent
- Noninflammatory white blood cells (WBC) <2000/mm^2
- Negative for monosodium urate crystals (gout) or calcium pyrophosphate dehydrate crystals (pseudogout)

Management

There is no cure for OA. The goals of management should be pain control, improved health-related quality of life, and decreased disability. Methods include nonpharmacological, pharmacological, and surgical. Conservative therapy should be tried before surgery.

Nonpharmacological

- Patient education on goals of therapy and appropriateness of exercise
- Weight loss, especially in hip or knee OA
- Reduce or modify occupational risk factors

- Exercise for muscle strengthening
- Physical therapy evaluation and management to strengthen the muscles around joints and to provide assistive devices
- Occupational therapy evaluation and management to provide assistive devices and suggestions to maintain or improve activities of daily living (ADLs)
- Braces provide stability and reduce pain. Canes and walkers may be appropriate.
- Paraffin bath for hands

Pharmacological

- Acetaminophen: Use before nonsteroidal anti-inflammatory drugs (NSAIDs) unless contraindicated. It is often not as effective as NSAIDs but has a better safety profile.
- NSAIDs if acetaminophen is not effective. Patients may benefit from trying several NSAIDs in sequence to determine a better response or fewer side effects to a particular NSAID. NSAIDs should be administered with a proton pump inhibitor or misoprostol in patients with risk factors for gastroduodenal ulcers. NSAIDs may also exacerbate coronary artery disease or congestive heart failure in susceptible patients.
- Glucosamine sulfate and/or chondroitan sulfate is controversial in that results of clinical trials have been inconsistent. However, the side-effect profile is generally good.
- Opioid therapy: Clinical trials have shown modest benefit with the opioid-like drug tramadol. Stronger opioids may also provide significant improvement in pain in carefully selected patients who have not responded well or have contraindications to other pharmacological therapies.
- Intra-articular corticosteroid injection: Few systemic manifestations. Monitor the diabetic for hyperglycemia and avoid injecting into a septic joint. Beneficial effects may last 1–3 months.
- Intra-articular hyaluronic acid is FDA approved, but the benefit is debated.
- Topical capsaicin or topical NSAIDs

Surgical intervention

Surgical interventions should be performed when nonpharmacological and pharmacological measures have been ineffective. Surgical options include the following:

- Debridement has been shown to be of questionable benefit in recent clinical trials.
- Total or partial joint arthroplasty results in marked improvement in pain and often function in properly selected patients.

Crystal arthropathy

Gout

Definition and epidemiology

Gout is a monosodium urate deposition disease of the joints and soft tissues. Urate underexcretion and/or overproduction lead to increased body burden of urate and ultimately gout. Typical presentation is acute onset of a painful intermittent monoarthritis, which may evolve to more chronic arthritis and formation of urate deposits called *tophi*.

Gout is more common in men than in women. Peak age is 40–50 years in men and >60 years in women, with a prevalence in men of 5–28 per 1000 and in women, 1–6 per 10,000. Gout is the most common inflammatory arthritis in men and is more common than rheumatoid arthritis in women over age 60. The annual incidence in men is 1–3 per 1000 and in women, 0.2 per 1000.

Genetic association includes mutations in genes involved in purine metabolism. More recently, polymorphisms in urate transporter genes have also been associated with gout.

There are also environmental associations with diet, chronic kidney disease, medications such as diuretics, and, less commonly, toxins such as lead.

Clinical features

Initial presentation is usually an acute arthritis with erythema, swelling and intense tenderness. During a flare involving the foot or ankle, tenosynovitis is common and can be mistaken for cellulitis.

Normally flares are monoarticular (90%) but may be oligo- or polyarticular in more advanced disease. In early disease patients are usually asymptomatic between flares.

The lower extremities are most commonly affected in early disease. The first MTP joint is affected eventually in up to 90% (referred to as *podagra*). However, gout can affect any joint. Bursa and tendon sheaths can also be sites of acute flares.

Flares are self-limited and will often resolve within several days. Occasionally, acute flares can be associated with systemic features such as fever and leukocytosis that raise concern for infection or a systemic rheumatic disease.

In the setting of uncontrolled disease, patients may develop more frequent flares. Deposits of urate, or tophi, may develop in "wear-and-tear" locations such as the Achilles tendon insertion, the dorsum of the hands and fingers, and the elbow. Patients may also develop an erosive, deforming, chronic arthritis in advanced gout.

Diagnosis

The gold standard of diagnosis is an arthrocentesis with detection of monosodium urate crystals using polarized microscopy. Arthrocentesis is often indicated in order to rule out a septic joint. Uric acid levels cannot be used to diagnose gout in a patient with acute arthritis.

Lack of expertise in arthrocentesis of small joints and availability of a polarizing microscope are often impediments to accurate office-based diagnosis of gout. In these settings, empiric therapy is reasonable in patients without any risk factors for an infected joint.

Management

Acute flare

The goal of therapy is to reduce symptoms and accelerate the resolution of the flare. This usually requires a period of rest and pharmacological therapy.

NSAIDs

The treatment of choice for acute gout flares is a 7- to 10-day course of NSAIDs at maximum recommended doses. Any NSAID may be used. Patients should be carefully screened to identify relative contraindications to NSAID use such as chronic kidney disease, peptic ulcer disease, uncontrolled hypertension, bleeding risk, or congestive heart failure.

Corticosteroids

Either a single intra-articular injection or 7–10 days of a systemic corticosteroid (0.5–1.0 mg/kg/day) is very effective. Intra-articular injection is beneficial in the patient with renal failure or one or two joints involved, or postsurgically with evidence of a nonseptic joint.

ACTH

Give 25–40 USP units, may repeat q12h for 1–3 days. Therapy is effective, but expensive and may not be readily available except in hospital settings.

Colchicine

Give 0.6 mg orally every hour to a maximum of 3–6 doses. Many or most patients will experience gastrointestinal side effects after several doses, making this a second-line choice for treating acute flares. Patients with renal failure need to be monitored closely to make dose adjustments and prevent toxicity.

Consider providing narcotic analgesics for pain management in the acute setting. Splinting of the affected joint may provide comfort to the patient as the flare resolves.

Chronic gout

In patients with recurring flares, chronic gouty arthritis, or tophi, the goal is to lower the urate level to <6 mg/dL. Sustained reduction of serum urate levels will ultimately resolve excess tissues stores of urate and will result in resolution of the clinical manifestations of gout.

Reduction in serum urate levels may be approached through a variety of lifestyle and pharmacological interventions. Management of chronic gout should be undertaken by a physician who plans to provide ongoing care to the patient as this is a lifelong undertaking for the patient. Important considerations in managing chronic gout include the following:

- Lifestyle modifications such as weight loss, reduction of excessive alcohol consumption, and control of hypertension

- Initiate urate-lowering therapy such as probenecid or allopurinol. Titrate dose upward to achieve a stable serum urate level of <6 mg/dL. Therapy should be continued indefinitely. Frequent monitoring of serum urate levels is necessary to ensure maintenance of a therapeutic target.
- Do not initiate therapy until after an acute flare has resolved.
- Administer colchicine 0.6 mg daily or twice daily, or an NSAID daily, to prevent gout flares that may temporarily increase in frequency during the first several months of urate-lowering therapy.

Calcium pyrophosphate dihydrate disease (CPPD) or pseudogout

Definition and epidemiology

CPPD is a crystal-induced disease that causes deposition of calcium pyrophosphate crystals into the connective tissue. Often the disease is asymptomatic and is diagnosed after calcium deposition (chondrocalcinosis) is noted as linear and punctuate linear radiodensities in the cartilage in radiographs. Pseudogout, which occurs when the CPPD crystals cause an inflammatory reaction, has features similar to those of gout.

CPPD is usually associated with underlying osteoarthritis or metabolic diseases (hemachromatosis, hypophosphatasia, possibly hyperparathyroidism).

Disease onset usually occurs after age 60. Women are affected about as often as men. Initial symptoms of pseudogout often present in the knee.

Clinical features

- Acute flares of mono- or oligoarticular arthritis (pseudogout) similar to those seen in gout
- Chronic arthropathy, and may cause osteoarthritis in "unusual" joints such as the shoulder, elbows or wrists

Diagnosis

Diagnosis is by arthrocentesis with analysis of synovial fluid using polarized microscopy. Calcium pyrophosphate crystals are seen as small, rod-shaped, weakly positively birefringent crystals when oriented parallel to the axis on the polarizer.

Radiographs show chondrocalcinosis, typically seen in larger joints such as the meniscus and articular cartilage of the knee, and the triangular fibrocartilage of the wrist.

Serum urate levels should be normal except in patients with coexisting gout.

Consider evaluation of secondary causes of CPPD (e.g., hemachromatosis).

Management

Treatment is focused on managing acute flares in a manner identical that in gout. There is no treatment for alleviating calcium pyrophosphate deposition. It may be possible to prevent progression of the disease by treating underlying conditions.

Rheumatoid arthritis

Definition and etiopathology

Rheumatoid arthritis (RA) is an inflammatory, peripheral, symmetric, polyarthritis of unknown etiology. Synovium becomes inflamed and proliferates, forming a pannus that can lead to erosion, deformity, and destruction of bones and cartilage. RA is associated with extra-articular features and an increased risk for mortality that is primarily due to cardiovascular disease.

The etiology is multifactorial, due most likely to genetic and environmental factors. RA is strongly associated with major histocompatibility (MHC) alleles of the HLA-DR4 gene.

RA affects 1.3 million adults. There has been a progressive decline in RA incidence since the 1960s, and in evaluating prevalence there is an increase in the age of RA patients from 63.3 years in 1965 to 66.8 years in 1995. RA is more common in women than men by 3:1.

The advent of new biological therapies has transformed the management and prognosis of this condition. Accordingly, the sports medicine physician's focus should be on recognition of possible RA and prompt referral to a rheumatologist for definitive diagnosis and therapy.

Clinical features

Typical presentation is peripheral joint pain with joint swelling. Morning stiffness is common and may last for hours or all day. Most patients also describe significant fatigue. Onset may vary from indolent to explosive. The pattern of joint involvement is helpful.

Common joints affected include MCPs, PIPs, wrists, MTPs, and knees. Other joints that may be involved are the cervical spine, shoulders, elbows, hips, and knees. Established disease is typically a symmetric polyarthritis. However, initial onset may be in just a few joints and symptoms are sometimes migratory.

Deformities are a feature of advanced disease and are usually avoided with early aggressive therapy. Common types of deformities are as follows:

- Ulnar deviation of fingers with MCP subluxation
- Swan-neck deformity (MCP joint flexion contracture, PIP hyperextension, DIP flexion)
- Boutonniere deformity (PIP flexion, DIP hyperextension)
- Hammer toe or claw toe (due to subluxation of the metatarsal heads from inflammation of the MTPs)

Cervical spine involvement occurs in 30%–50% of patients and usually affects C1 and C2. Patients with long-standing erosive disease are at risk for anterior C1 on C2 subluxation, which can lead to spinal cord compression. It is important to obtain cervical spine radiographs with flexion and extension views before surgeries requiring intubation.

Extra-articular manifestations of RA may occur in up to 35% of patients but are often avoided with timely disease-modifying therapy.

Examples of extra-articular disease features are as follows:

- Anemia of chronic disease
- Elevated platelets in active disease

- General—fever, fatigue, weight loss
- Cardiovascular—atherosclerosis, pericarditis, nodules on valves (rare)
- Pulmonary—interstitial lung disease, nodules
- Hematological—Felty's syndrome (RA with splenomegaly, leukopenia), lymphomas
- Neuromuscular—mononeuritis multiplex, entrapment and peripheral neuropathy, carpel tunnel syndrome
- Dermatological—subcutaneous nodules (20%–35% of patients, on extensor surfaces, vasculitis)

Diagnosis

Patient history and physical examination are key to the diagnosis of RA. Laboratory studies support a clinical suspicion of RA. Diagnosis is not based on just labs but includes clinical findings and radiographic findings.

A diagnosis of RA should be considered in a patient with a history of joint pain in three or more areas for more than 6 weeks. Morning stiffness is common.

Physical examination should include a systematic assessment of all joints for signs of tenderness to palpation and synovial thickening.

Patients with a history and physical examination suggesting RA should have laboratory studies done, include rheumatoid factor (RF), anti-cyclic citrullinated peptide (anti-CCP) antibody, erythrocyte sedimentation rate (ESR), C-reactive protein (CRP), complete blood count (CBC), and serum chemistries. Keep in mind that up to 30% of patients with RA will also have a positive anti-nuclear antibody, but this study is not helpful in diagnosing RA.

Imaging

Radiographs of the hands and feet should be obtained in patients with suspected RA. Characteristic findings in RA are marginal erosions, joint-space narrowing, and juxta-articular osteopenia.

It is unusual to find erosive changes in very early disease, but the presence of erosions in this setting is a potential marker for aggressive disease. The absence of erosions does not obviate the need for early aggressive therapy to control disease activity.

Management

The objectives of RA management are to relieve symptoms, restore function, and prevent joint damage. Optimal outcomes are realized when coordinated application of patient education and nonpharmacological and pharmacological interventions are deployed by an experienced physician.

The complexity of pharmacologic therapy of RA generally requires consultation with a rheumatologist.

Pharmacological therapy

It can be stated unequivocally that pharmacological therapy with disease-modifying antirheumatic drugs is the most important intervention in RA. Objectives of pharmacological therapy are to modify the disease course and reduce the signs and symptoms of disease.

Disease-modifying therapies usually include methotrexate as a foundation drug, although sulfasalazine and leflunomide may also function as first-line agents. In patients who do not achieve disease remission with methotrexate, addition of a biological agent is indicated. The combination of methotrexate and a biological agent have been shown to be superior to either drug alone.

Oral corticosteroids may play an important role in achieving optimal disease control. These are usually employed in low doses and in combination with methotrexate and/or biological agents.

Current biological therapies include drugs that specifically target tumor necrosis factor, interleukin-1, the CD20 molecule on B lymphocytes, co-stimulatory molecules on T lymphocytes, and interleukin-6.

Symptom-modifying therapy in RA is also important. The most commonly used agents are NSAIDs, but may also include other opioid and nonopioid analgesics. NSAIDs are not disease modifying and are employed primarily to control pain.

Nonpharmacological therapy

- Patient education
- Exercise, to prevent and reverse loss of joint motion, muscle atrophy, contractures
- Physical and occupational therapy

Seronegative spondyloarthropathies

Overview

The seronegative spondyloarthropathies are a group of inflammatory arthritis/enthesitis disorders that includes ankylosing spondylitis (AS), psoriatic arthritis (PsA), reactive arthritis (ReA), enteropathic arthritis, and undifferentiated spondyloarthritis.

A common feature of these disorders is inflammatory arthritis of peripheral and axial joints, enthesitis, and extra-articular manifestations such as uveitis and dermatitis. These disorders are often associated with inheritance of human leukocyte antigen-B27 (HLA-B27). These diseases are considered to be seronegative because rheumatoid factor, anti-CCP antibody, and antinuclear antibody are absent.

Approximately 0.6 million to 2.4 million adults in the United States are affected.

Ankylosing spondylitis

Definition and etiopathology

Ankylosing spondylitis is a chronic inflammatory disease that affects mainly the axial skeleton, resulting in back pain, stiffness, and loss of flexibility. The typical patient is young <40 years of age with a peak incidence in the 20s to 30s, male, and Caucasian, although the disease is seen in other ethnic groups.

Ninety percent of patients with ankylosing spondylitis are HLA-B27 positive.

Clinical features

A typical presentation is the insidious onset of low back pain that has "inflammatory" characteristics, including morning stiffness >30 minutes and symptoms that worsen with rest and improve with activity. As disease advances, ankylosis of the spine and sacroiliac joints can reduce mobility of the spine, sometimes severely. Peripheral joints may also be involved as in psoriatic arthritis (see next page).

Diagnosis is difficult because the disease is insidious. On musculoskeletal examination assess range of motion of the spine (Schober test, head-to-wall measurement). Evidence of uveitis should be sought. There are no laboratory studies that are diagnostic. Sedimentation rate may be normal or elevated.

X-ray of the pelvis (30° tilt or Ferguson view) may reveal changes in the sacroiliac joints. Squaring of the vertebral bodies and bridging syndesmophytes may be seen on spine X-rays. However, plain radiographs are usually normal in early disease. MRI of the pelvis may demonstrate bone edema and effusion in the sacroiliac joints in early disease.

Management

Patients with suspected ankylosing spondylitis should be evaluated by a rheumatologist for treatment. Therapy involves patient education, physical therapy, NSAIDs, and disease-modifying therapies such as sulfasalazine, methotrexate, and tumor necrosis factor inhibitors.

Psoriatic arthritis

Definition and etiopathology

Psoriatic arthritis is an inflammatory arthritis that can occur in up to 25% of patients with psoriasis. Arthritis follows the onset of psoriasis, but may rarely precede onset of rash. Men and women are affected equally, and onset is usually in the fourth or fifth decade. Prevalence is about 1 per 1000.

Clinical features

Psoriatic arthritis is characterized by five different patterns of joint involvement: mono- or oligoarthritis, polyarthritis (distribution similar to that of RA), classical with involvement of distal joints of the fingers and toes and nail dystrophy, and axial disease that can mimic ankylosing spondylitis.

Psoriatic lesions should be sought on skin examination. Special attention should be given to the extensor surfaces, scalp, umbilicus, and gluteal cleft. Pitting of the nails with onycholysis and subungual hyperkeratosis is common. Eye inflammation is present in 30% of patients.

Diagnosis is based primarily on history and physical examination. Radiographs may be helpful only in more advanced disease.

Management is similar to that of ankylosing spondylitis and includes NSAIDs, methotrexate, and biologics such as etanercept, infliximab, and adalimumab.

Reactive arthritis

Definition and etiopathology

Reactive arthritis is a seronegative arthritis that develops 10–30 days after a genitourinary or gastrointestinal infection such as *Shigella, Salmonella, Yersinia, Campylobacter, Klebsiella, Clostridium difficile, Chlamydia,* or *Ureoplasma.*

Clinical features

Reactive arthritis usually presents in an asymmetric mono- or oligoarticular pattern. Nonarticular manifestations may include urethritis, uveitis, conjunctivitis, balanitis circinata (shallow, painless ulcers of the glans penis and the urethral meatus), and keratoderma blenorrhagica (scaling skin lesions on the soles of the feet, palms, trunk, and scalp).

Diagnosis is made on clinical grounds in association with a history of infectious illness.

Therapy is adjusted according to the duration and severity of illness. In many cases NSAIDs alone are sufficient. In more severe disease, treatment similar to that of RA is required.

Other seronegative spondyloarthropathies

Spondyloarthritis in the absence of a defining illness such as ankylosing spondylitis or psoriasis may be seen. Often the sacroiliac joints are involved. Diagnosis and treatment are similar to that for other spondyloarthropathies. Enteropathic arthritis occurs in the setting of inflammatory bowel disease such as Crohn's or ulcerative colitis. The arthritic features are similar to ankylosing spondylitis. Treatment is directed toward controlling the underlying bowel disease.

Infectious arthritis

Arthritis can also be associated with actual infection of the joint with bacteria, viruses, mycobacteria, and fungi. It is imperative to perform an arthrocentesis on a joint with possible infection because of the risk for rapid joint destruction.

Bacterial

Bacterial infections associated with septic arthritis are often separated into nongonococcal and gonococcal. The bacteria enter the joint usually through the blood supply, deposit into the synovium, and cause an inflammatory reaction.

Nongonococcal septic arthritis

This is the most dangerous and destructive type of acute arthritis. Destruction of cartilage can occur within days, and the in-hospital mortality is as high as 7%–15%. Usually patients have significant comorbid illnesses and risk factors for bacteremia.

The most common pathogens are staphylococci and streptococci. However, in hospitalized or immunocompromised patients, gram-negative bacteria may also cause infection of the joint.

Risk factors include age >80 years, diabetes mellitus, rheumatoid arthritis, recent joint surgery, knee or hip prosthesis, skin infections, and HIV.

Monoarticular arthritis affects the large joints such as the knees. Associated fever occurs in approximately 60% of patients, with pain, swelling, and warmth.

Arthrocentesis is critical for diagnosis. Positive cultures are seen in >95% of patients.

Send synovial fluid for Gram stain and culture, cell count and differential, and crystals. There is concern for a septic joint if WBCs >50,000, but lower numbers do not rule out infection. Crystals in the fluid do not rule out infection. Blood cultures are positive in 50% of patients.

Management includes broad-spectrum antimicrobials until an organism is identified. Therapy is then tailored. Joint surgery is often required.

Disseminated gonococcal septic arthritis

This arthritis is due to *Neisseria gonorrhea* and is the most common strain of bacterial arthritis. It has less morbidity than that of nongonococcal arthritis.

Women are affected 2 to 3 times more than men. The patient is typically young and in generally good health. Average duration between sexual contact and disease is around 5 days.

There is oligo- or polyarthritis with migratory synovitis. Occasionally, dermatitis can occur.

Diagnosis is made by taking cultures from the urethra, cervix, pharynx, and rectum, which are positive in 70%–90% of cases. An arthrocentesis must be performed but is not often helpful in identifying gonococcal infection. A Gram's stain is only positive in <10% of cases and synovial fluid culture is often negative.

Lyme arthritis

Lyme arthritis is caused by *Borrelia burgdorferi*, which is a spirochete transmitted via tick bite. Localized disease such as erythema migrans, arthralgias, and myalgias develop within 3–30 days after the tick bite.

Weeks to months later, there may be early disseminated disease characterized by fever, migratory arthralgias and myalgias, acute pauciarticular arthritis, and neurological features such as radiculoneuropathies and cranial nerve palsies.

Months to years later, patients may develop primarily neurological features along with monoarticular and migratory pauciarticular arthritis.

Diagnosis is made by first ordering an ELISA for IgM and IgG antibody reactivity to *B. burgdorferi*. Western blot is then used to confirm a positive or equivocal ELISA. Polymerase chain reaction (PCR) can be used to detect *B. burgdorferi* DNA in synovial fluid and cerebrospinal fluid (CSF) with a higher sensitivity in synovial fluid.

Management is typically oral amoxicillin 500 mg tid or doxycycline 100 mg bid or parenteral ceftriaxone 2 g IV once daily.

Tuberculous arthritis

Onset is insidious with stiffness, pain, and loss of function. In 15% of patients there is an acute presentation; 80% have fever, night sweats, and weight loss. There is swelling in the associated joints with the hip and then knee most affected.

Imaging can show bony erosions at the joint periphery and juxta-articular osteopenia on X-ray. MRI can identify a sinus tract formation if present, pari-articular abscesses, and any skin manifestations. Over 90% of patients have a positive PPD with neutrophil predominance. Synovial fluid from an arthrocentesis shows inflammatory fluid with WBC of 10,000–20,000. The Gram stain is often negative. A synovial biopsy is preferred. The ESR can be elevated.

Management includes 6–9 months of treatment with isoniazid, rifampin, pyrazinamide, and ethambutol for 2 months, then isoniazid and ethambutol for bone and joint involvement. Multiple arthrocenteses may be required.

Viral

Viral infections are often associated with arthritis and/or arthralgia. Most common infections are associated with hepatitis B and C, parvovirus, rubella, and alphaviruses.

Symptoms include rapid onset of symmetric polyarthralgias or polyarthritis at the time of the clinical presentation of the infection. There may be an associated rash. Most arthralgias or arthritis resolves. Occasionally, there can be chronic symptoms and it becomes necessary to rule out other causes such as rheumatic diseases.

There is no specific diagnostic test, but diagnosis is often based on clinical symptoms such as jaundice in hepatitis B and hepatitis C. Immunoassays can be used to assess for IgM antibodies, which are seen initially and then IgG which becomes present 2–3 weeks later in some viral diseases such as hepatitis B.

Rarely, the virus can be isolated from the synovium or joint fluid for a definitive diagnosis. Lab tests have very little benefit for the diagnosis of viral disease, but are more useful for ruling out other causes.

Therapy is associated with symptom relief such as with acetaminophen and NSAIDs. Corticosteroids generally have no utility.

Human immunodeficiency virus (HIV)

HIV can be associated with a reactive arthritis, septic arthritis, a painful articular syndrome that is intense but lasts 24 hours, psoriatic arthritis with the highest incidence in HLA-B27 positive patients, HIV-associated arthritis, an inflammatory myopathy, and medication-associated symptoms.

Acute rheumatic fever

This is not an infectious arthritis per se, but is a postinfectious systemic inflammatory disease that occurs after a group A streptococci pharyngeal infection. Multisystem involvement is typical.

Diagnosis is made using the Jones criteria, which includes a preceding group A streptococcal infection with two major manifestations or one major and two minor manifestations. Group A streptococcus is diagnosed with a positive throat culture or rapid streptococcal antigen test, serum anti-streptolysin-O (ASO), antideoxyribonuclease-B (antiDNAse-B), and anti-streptokinase.

Major manifestations are migratory polyarthritis, carditis, subcutaneous nodules, chorea, and erythema marginatum. Minor manifestations include arthralgia, fever, increased ESR and CRP, and a prolonged PR interval on ECG.

Acute management involves treatment with penicillin regardless of the presence of active pharyngitis. Aspirin is the treatment of choice for inflammatory manifestations of active disease. Carditis may be treated with corticosteroids, although there is no definitive evidence of benefit.

Primary and secondary prevention is the most important management objective and is focused on preventing a first or second episode because of the increased risk for a recurrence with another streptococcal infection.

Prophylaxis includes benzathine penicillin G 1.2 million units intramuscularly (IM) every 4 weeks, or penicillin V 250 mg bid or sulfadiazine based on weight. Give erythromycin stearate 250 mg bid for penicillin and sulfadiazine allergy.

Other arthritis-related conditions

Systemic lupus erythematosus (SLE)

SLE is a chronic, multifaceted inflammatory disease that can affect every organ system. Patients are more likely to have arthralgia but can have arthritis and are also at risk for myopathies and neuropathies.

The prevalence is 1 case per 2000 in the population and is typically diagnosed in patients between the ages of 14 and 65 years with a higher incidence in African Americans and women.

The diagnosis is a clinical diagnosis. A positive antinuclear antibody (ANA) is not synonymous with SLE or another rheumatological disorder. The American College of Rheumatology (ACR) criteria for research studies of SLE requires 4 of 11 items: serositis, oral ulcers, nonerosive arthritis, photosensitivity, blood disorders such as leukopenia, thrombocytopenia, hemolytic anemia, renal involvement such as lupus nephritis, positive ANA, immunological phenomena such as anti-double-stranded DNA (anti-dsDNA), neurological disorders such as seizures and psychosis, malar rash, and a discoid rash.

If SLE is suspected in a patient, order an ANA and then anti-Smith (anti-Sm) and anti-dsDNA tests, which are specific to SLE. Other studies include CBC with differential, chemistry profile, and urinalysis with microscopy to assess for proteinuria or nephritis.

Treatment often includes corticosteroids, hydroxychloroquine, methotrexate, cyclophosphamide, and azathioprine.

Inflammatory myopathies

Two major inflammatory myopathies are polymyositis and dermatomyositis.

Polymyositis (PM) is a T cell–mediated inflammatory myopathy that has a prevalence of 1 per 100,000 in the general population. It has a female-to-male ratio of 2:1 with a peak incidence between 40 and 50 years of age. Its pathology involves inflammatory cells within the individual muscle fibers.

Clinical features include symmetric, proximal muscle weakness with myalgias and muscle tenderness. A subset of patients may develop interstitial lung disease that may present with dyspnea on exertion and crackles on chest examination.

Dermatomyositis (DM) is not polymyositis with a rash, as was thought in the past. It has a similar prevalence, female-to-male ratio, and peak years. Unlike PM, however, its immunological mechanism is humorally mediated and is associated with cellular infiltration perifascicularly around blood vessels.

Clinical features include symmetric, proximal muscle weakness with myalgias and muscle tenderness; skin changes that include Gottron's papules over the PIP and MCP joints; a dusky purple "heliotrope" rash over the eyelids; a characteristic rash on the neck, chest, and back known as the shawl sign; erythroderma; periungual abnormalities; calcinosis cutis; and mechanic's hands.

Both PM and DM are associated with an increased risk of malignancy, with DM having the greater risk. The patient requires age-specific malignancy screening.

Laboratory studies include the muscle enzymes total creatine kinase (CK), aldolase, alanine transaminase (ALT), and aspartate transaminase (AST), as well as rheumatological serologies such as ANA and anti-Jo-1 for DM and PM, anti-Mi-2 for DM, and anti-SRP for PM.

Electromyography (EMG) is helpful to identify an inflammatory myopathy but is not diagnostic. Diagnosis is made by muscle biopsy.

The differential diagnosis includes inclusion body myositis, steroid myopathy, hypothyroidism, polymyalgia rheumatica, HIV, and infectious myositis.

Treatment includes corticosteroids and immunosuppressives such as methotrexate and azathioprine, IV immunoglobulin, and biologics.

Polymyalgia rheumatica (PMR)

PMR is an inflammatory condition leading to stiffness and pain in the shoulders and/or the pelvic girdle that typically affects patients over the age of 50 years. The symptoms tend to be symmetric, last longer than 1 month, and are usually associated with an ESR >40 mm/hr. The average age is 70 years and there is a female and Caucasian predominance.

Patients may report feeling weak from the stiffness and pain and may have synovitis and pitting edema. Rheumatoid factor and ANA are negative.

Temporal arteritis and PMR can occur together. Temporal arteritis can be associated with scalp tenderness, jaw claudication, headaches, and tenderness of arteries in the upper body and extremities. If temporal arteritis is suspected, the patient requires immediate initiation of prednisone at a dose of 1 mg/kg per day and urgent temporal artery biopsy.

PMR is treated with 15–20 mg/day of corticosteroids and often leads to rapid improvement in symptoms within 1–2 days. If there is no improvement after 1 month, reconsider temporal arteritis, which requires higher doses of corticosteroids. Corticosteroids should be slowly tapered over 1 year to the lowest level to maintain disease control.

PMR may require 2–4 years of treatment before resolving.

Vasculitides

Vasculitis is an inflammatory condition affecting the blood vessels, often leading to necrosis of the vessel and disruption of blood flow. The vasculitides are often classified by the size of the vessel.

The large-vessel vasculitides are Takayasu's arteritis, which is seen in young women, and giant-cell (temporal) arteritis, which is seen in patients >60 years.

The medium-vessel vasculitides include polyarteritis nodosum (PAN), which is often associated with hepatitis B, and Kawasaki's disease which is seen in children.

The small-vessel vasculitides include those associated with antineutrophil cytoplasmic antibody (ANCA)—Wegener's granulomatosis with associated sinopulmonary renal disease, microscopic polyangiitis with associated pulmonary renal disease, and Churg–Strauss syndrome with associated sinus involvement and eosinophilia, and immune complex–associated vasculitides—Henoch–Schönlein purpura, which follows a gastrointestinal illness, hypersensitivity vasculitis, and cryoglobulinemia often associated with hepatitis C.

Clinical features of a systemic vasculitis include constitutional symptoms, fever of unknown origin, and clinical manifestations that result from impaired blood flow from the involved vessels. This may include mononeuritis multiplex, vision loss, stroke, bowel ischemia, renal failure, and skin lesions such as palpable purpura, livedo reticularis, and limb or digital infarcts.

Lab testing includes CBC with differential, ESR, CRP, creatinine and urinalysis, transaminases, ANA, complements C3/C4, and anti-GBM to rule out other diseases such as Goodpasture's syndrome and SLE or to determine the vasculitis.

Vasculitis-specific labs include c-ANCA (anti-PR3) for Wegener's granulomatosis and p-ANCA (antimyeloperoxidase) for Churg–Strauss syndrome and microscopic polyangiitis.

Vasculitis is best diagnosed with a tissue biopsy.

Treatment typically involves prompt evaluation by a rheumatologist and treatment with corticosteroids and immunosuppressants such as cyclophosphamide.

Dermatology

Problems related to skin trauma

Friction blisters

Description
- Fluid-filled vesicles and bullae that form secondary to shearing forces
- Most common locations include soles, heels, palms, fingers, nipples in joggers

Risk factors
- Changes in training pattern, early in the season
- Heat, moisture
- Poorly fitted equipment, shoes
- Repetitive activity

Prevention
- Petroleum jelly, moleskin for protection of skin
- Dry socks made of synthetic wicking material. It may be useful to layer socks with a thinner base layer and thicker outer layer to maintain bulk.

Treatment
- Treat "hot spots" with ice and protection.
- If tense, drain in sterile manner and leave blister roof intact
- Antibiotic ointment or hydrocolloid dressing if open
- Wound adhesives may be beneficial.

Differential diagnosis
- Epidermolysis bullosa

Calluses

Description
- Thickening of the outer layer of skin (hyperkeratosis)
- Skin lines are maintained
- Areas with bony prominences are at risk.

Risk factors
- Repeated mechanical trauma
- Poorly fitted equipment
- Hard playing surfaces

Prevention
- Direct protection with gloves or tape, petroleum jelly, moleskin
- Orthotics for biomechanical correction
- Properly fitted shoes and equipment

Treatment
- Debride by paring after soaking in warm water
- Use of keratolytics such as salicylic acid, urea or lactic acid

Differential diagnosis
- Wart, bunion

Subungual hematoma (jogger's toe, tennis toe)

Description
- Onycholysis (separation of proximal nail plate), black discoloration and hemorrhage within the nail bed or surrounding the nail
- Most commonly involves first or second toe

Risk factors
- Sports with sudden deceleration or direction changes (i.e., racquet sports, football, distance running, soccer, dancing)
- Long or malformed toenails
- Tight shoes, especially in the toe box

Prevention
- Close trimming of toenail
- Properly fitted shoes with adequate room in toe box

Treatment
- Self-resolving
- Discoloration should grow out with the nail

Differential diagnosis
- Melanoma

Black heel and palm (talon noir, tache noir, calcaneal petechiae)

Description
- Intraepidermal hemorrhage secondary to shearing forces with sudden stopping or landing. Superficial dermal blood vessels rupture, and hemoglobin becomes trapped in epidermis
- Most commonly involves heel and edge of the foot pad

Risk factors
- Volleyball, racquet sports, running, lacrosse, basketball, gymnastics
- Poorly fitting shoes
- Repetitive trauma

Prevention
- Properly fitting shoes with thick socks
- Heel pad

Treatment
- Self-resolving

Differential diagnosis
- Melanoma, plantar warts

Onychocryptosis (ingrown toenail)

Description
- Occurs when nail plate grows into the lateral nail fold, causing pain and swelling at the lateral nail fold
- Risk of secondary infection with *Staphylococcus* or *Streptococcus*

Risk factors
- Improper trimming of the nail
- Poorly fitting shoes
- Trauma to nail plate or toe

Prevention
- Proper trimming of nails

Treatment
- Warm soaks followed by careful removal of ingrown aspect of nail. Insert cotton to keep nail plate free and repeat process until edge of nail has grown past the nail fold

Differential diagnosis
- Onychomycosis

Problems related to environmental exposure

Sunburn

Description

- Redness that develops 2–8 hours after excessive exposure to ultraviolet (UV) light
- Limited to areas of sun exposure
- Increases risk of skin cancer (basal cell cancer, scuamous cell cancer, and melanoma) and photoaging

Risk factors

- Outdoor sports, especially water sports, endurance activities, alpine sports
- Photo-sensitizing medications such as tetracyclines, sulfa drugs, phenothiazines, retinoids
- Light skin, blue eyes

Prevention

- Broad-spectrum sunscreen (UVA and UVB). Apply before exposure, 30 minutes after initial application. Reapply every 2 hours and after towel drying, swimming, or excessive sweating. A quantity of 35 mL is sufficient for entire body coverage.
- Protective clothing, hats, eyewear
- Avoidance of sun between the hours of 10 AM and 4 PM
- Provide shade near workout areas

Treatment

- Cool compresses
- Aloe vera
- Fluids
- Topical steroids to reduce inflammation
- NSAIDs taken within 1–2 hours of acute sunburn can relieve symptoms.

Differential diagnosis

- Flushing

Hyperhidrosis

Description

- Excessive perspiration
- Most common areas are palms, soles, axillae

Risk factors

- Heat exposure, physical exertion

Treatment

- Aluminum chloride, apply at bedtime and leave on 6–8 hours
- Botulinum A toxin
- Local iontophoresis, may need long-term maintenance therapy

Differential diagnosis

- Hyperthyroidism

Frostnip (first-degree frost bite)

Description
- Cold injury involving superficial layers of skin
- Redness, swelling, pain, and numbness, which are reversible
- Most common on nose, cheeks, ears

Risk factors
- Outdoor sports
- Winter sports

Prevention
- Protective clothing to cover exposed skin
- Petroleum jelly for protection of face and ears

Treatment
- Symptomatic
- Prevention is best

Differential diagnosis
- Frostbite, chillblains

Frostbite

Description
- Occurs after extended exposure to freezing temperatures. Ice crystals form in cells, causing dehydration and microvascular occlusion.
- Classified in severity from grades I (redness and edema) to IV (tissue necrosis and gangrene)

Prevention
- Recognize and avoid unsafe conditions
- Proper clothing

Treatment
- Rapid rewarming with warm water immersion (40°C/104°F). Be aware that rewarming can be painful. It is important to increase core temperature and to fluid resuscitate before rewarming a limb to avoid hypotension and shock.
- Do not rub or exercise the limb because of risk for mechanical trauma or further cold injury.
- Cleanse skin gently, dry carefully, and keep elevated to minimize edema; apply sterile cotton between digits to prevent skin maceration.
- Prevent further cold exposure
- Tetanus prophylaxis

Differential diagnosis
- Cold immersion

Chillblains (Pernio)

Description
- Chronic exposure to cold, damp, nonfreezing conditions
- Symmetric red or blue–violet macules, papules, plaques most commonly over the distal extremities, nose, ears

Risk factors
- Exposure to cold, wet conditions

Prevention
- Recognize and avoid unsafe conditions (cold, damp)
- Proper dress
- Avoid smoking

Treatment
- Gradual rewarming without direct heat, rubbing, or massaging, as this can lead to further tissue damage
- Keep dry
- Oral nifedipine
- Tends to resolve in 1–3 weeks

Differential diagnosis
- Chilblains lupus, cold-sensitive blood dyscrasias such as cryoglobulinemia

Immersion foot

Description
- Exposure of feet to continuous moisture and occlusion without drying
- Risk for permanent peripheral neuropathy
- Can happen in cold conditions if exposure is >1 week, warm conditions in 3–7 days, and tropical conditions in 1–3 days

Risk factors
- Prolonged exposure to damp conditions

Prevention
- Sandals or other open shoes that allow intermittent air drying

Treatment
- Rapid drying
- Avoid direct heating in cold-immersion foot because the presence of neuropathy can increase the risk of thermal injury.
- Silicone grease in warm water–immersion foot

Differential diagnosis
- Fungal infection, pitted keratolysis, cellulitis

Fungal infections

Tinea pedis (athlete's foot)

Description

- Red, scaling plaques on plantar surface of the foot and between toes
- Caused by multiple dermatophytes (*Trichophyton rubrum, T. mentagrophytes, Epidermophyton floccosum*)
- Can diagnose with skin scraping and potassium hydroxide (KOH), fungal culture

Risk factors

- Occlusion, moist environment
- Locker rooms and public showers

Prevention

- Remove wet socks, use breathable and wicking materials
- Keep feet clean and dry
- Drying powders

Treatment

- Topical antifungal preparations such as clotrimazole, econazole, miconazole. May combine with urea or lactic acid
- Oral antifungal

Differential diagnosis

- Pitted keratolysis, psoriasis, contact dermatitis

Tinea cruris (jock itch)

Description

- Superficial dermatophyte infection of the groin and surrounding skin (most common organisms are *Trichophyton rubrum, Epidermophyton floccosum*)
- Itchy, red, scaly plaques with sharply demarcated border and scrotal sparing

Risk factors

- Shared undergarments, towels
- Tight-fitting clothing, wet clothing
- Tinea pedis

Prevention

- Loose-fitting and absorbent clothing
- Shower and change clothing immediately after workout
- Drying powers
- Treat tinea pedis

Treatment

- Topical antifungals such as clotrimazole, econazole, miconazole
- Avoid topical steroids
- Oral antifungals

Differential diagnosis

- Intertrigo, psoriasis, candidiasis

Tinea corporis (ringworm)

Description
- Superficial dermatophyte infection of the face, neck, trunk, extremities
- Extremely itchy, red, circular plaques with central clearing that may have pustules at the periphery

Risk factors
- Sweating, warm and moist environment
- Exposure to contaminated mats, flooring, equipment

Prevention
- Treatment of mats and equipment with fungicidal cleaners after each practice and competition
- Prompt treatment and temporary isolation from activity to prevent spread of infection

Treatment
- Topical or oral antifungals

Differential diagnosis
- Contact dermatitis, atopic dermatitis, pityriasis rosea, tinea versicolor, psoriasis

Tinea versicolor (pityriasis versicolor)

Description
- Superficial fungal infection secondary to overgrowth of *Malassezia furfur, M. globosa*
- Asymptomatic light or dark patches with fine scale in areas with sebaceous glands (especially upper trunk and shoulders)
- KOH preparation shows spores and hyphae that look like "spaghetti and meatballs"

Risk factors
- Hot, humid environment
- Immune suppression
- malnutrition

Prevention
- Showering after workouts
- Weekly to biweekly use of selenium sulfide or antifungal shampoo

Treatment
- Selenium sulfide or nizoral shampoo
- Topical (econazole or ketoconazole) or oral antifungal preparation (ketoconazole)
- Postinflammatory hyper- or hypopigmentation may take several weeks to resolve

Differential diagnosis
- Pityriasis alba, nummular eczema, guttate psoriasis, secondary syphilis, pityriasis rosea, seborrheic dermatitis

Onychomycosis (tinea unguium)

Description

- Dermatophyte infection of the nail. Organisms include but are not limited to *T. rubrum, T. mentagrophytes, E. floccosum*.
- Thickened and discoloration of affected nails, may have pain with activity

Risk factors

- Abnormal nail
- Diabetes
- Poor hygiene

Treatment

- Oral antifungal
- Usually refractory to treatment with incomplete clearance and frequent recurrence

Differential diagnosis

- Psoriasis, traumatic nail injury, *Candida* infection

Intertrigo

Description

- Inflammation of skin folds with erythema and maceration secondary to friction
- Common areas include the groin, inframammary region, axillae
- Risk of secondary bacterial *(Staphylococcus,* group A *Streptococcus, Pseudomonas)* and fungal infection (dermatophyte, *Candida)*

Risk factors

- Obesity, sweating, poor hygiene

Prevention

- Absorbent powders and barrier creams (zinc oxide)
- Light absorbent clothing
- Shower immediately after sweating, keep dry
- Weight loss

Treatment

- Barrier cream
- Treat secondary infection with appropriate topical or oral antifungal or antibiotic as indicated

Differential diagnosis

- Contact dermatitis, seborrheic dermatitis, atopic dermatitis, inverse psoriasis, vitamin deficiency, Hailey–Hailey disease

Bacterial infections

Acne vulgaris

Description *(see Plate 1)*
- Common skin condition among adolescents that involves follicular plugging, excess sebum production, *Propionibacterium acnes* activity, and inflammation
- Noninflammatory open (blackhead) and closed (whitehead) comedones and inflammatory papules and pustules
- Most common on face, upper back, shoulders, upper chest

Risk factors
- Sweat and occlusion from equipment such as helmets, chin straps, shoulder pads (acne mechanica)

Treatment
- Topical use of benzoyl peroxide, salicylic acid, and topical antibiotics (clindamycin, erythromycin)
- Topical retinoids (tretinoin, adapalene)
- Oral antibiotics when inflammatory lesions are present (tetracylines are first line)
- Isotretinoin for severe nodulocystic acne or acne not responding to oral antibiotics

Differential diagnosis
- Folliculitis, rosacea

Impetigo

Description
- Superficial bacterial infection of epidermis, most commonly due to *Staph. aureus*, group A *Streptococcus*
- Red vesicles, pustules or erosions with yellow-colored crust, sometimes itchy
- Transmitted by direct contact

Risk factors
- Minor breaks in skin barrier (portal of entry)

Treatment
- May progress to invasive infection if left untreated
- Benzoyl peroxide or chlorhexidine wash
- Topical or oral antibiotics with *Staphylococcus* and *Streptococcus* coverage

Differential diagnosis
- Herpes simplex, contact dermatitis, scabies, dermatophyte infection

Folliculitis

Description
- Inflammation surrounding a hair follicle, usually secondary to bacterial infection. Can also occur with anabolic steroid use, occlusion

- Common organisms include *Staphylococcus aureus* and *Pseudomonas* (if history of hot tub exposure)
- Follicularly based papules and pustules commonly located over the face, chest, back, axillae, and buttocks

Risk factors
- Hot, humid weather
- Occlusion
- Hyperhidrosis
- Tight-fitting clothing
- Sports that promote shaving of the body

Prevention
- Shower immediately after sweating, keep dry
- Shave in direction of hair growth

Treatment
- Use of antibacterial soaps or wash (chlorhexidine), benzoyl peroxide
- Oral antibiotics is severe or refractory to topical treatment (doxycycline, minocycline)
- Hot tub folliculitis from *Pseudomonas aeruginosa* is self-resolving

Differential diagnosis
- Acne, rosacea, keratosis pilaris, pseudofolliculitis barbae, fungal or viral folliculitis, drugs (steroids, lithium, isoniazid)

Furuncle (boil, carbuncle, abscess)

Description
- Bacterial infection of one or more hair follicles with subsequent inflammatory response that forms an abscess
- Most common organism is *Staphylococcus aureus*
- Carbuncle is when many follicles are involved
- Common locations are face, neck, axillae, buttocks, thighs, perineum
- Furuncles on the face require referral to physician because of the risk of spread to the brain's venous sinuses
- Increased incidence of community-acquired methicillin-resistant *Staphylococcus aureus* (CA-MRSA) causing skin and soft tissue infections, which may affect antibiotic choice, see infectious disease for CA-MRSA.

Risk factors
- Diabetes mellitus
- Obesity
- Poor hygiene
- Immune suppression
- For community-acquired MRSA: crowded living conditions, involvement in competitive contact sports, substance abuse, child care attendance

Prevention
- Hygiene education
- Regular training-room cleaning protocols
- Consider nasal mupirocin ointment bid for 5 days for carriers
  - Recolonization may occur

Treatment
- Warm compresses
- Incision and drainage is the mainstay of treatment
- Culture for organism identification and antibiotic sensitivities
- Do not squeeze lesions
- Topical chlorhexidine
- Topical or oral antibiotics if severe
  - Consider trimethoprim/sulfamethoxizole, doxycycline, or clindamycin as first-line antibiotics, based on culture results
- Avoid contact with other athletes if lesions are actively draining

Differential diagnosis
- Inflamed cyst, hidradenitis suppurativa, cystic acne

Cellulitis
Description
- Infection of deep dermis and subcutaneous tissue most commonly by *Streptococcus pyogenes*, *Staph. aureus*
- Ill-defined red, warm, swollen plaque often associated with fever and chills

Risk factors
- Broken skin barrier
- Diabetes mellitus
- Alcoholism
- Intravenous drug use

Treatment
- Oral antibiotics with gram-positive coverage.
- Intravenous antibiotics needed if severely ill or facial involvement
- Avoid NSAIDs, as they may mask symptoms of a deeper infection

Differential diagnosis
- Deep venous thrombosis, insect bite, panniculitis, vasculitis

Pitted keratolysis (stinky foot, tennis shoe foot)
Description
- Superficial infection with *Micrococcus sedentarius* or *Corynebacterium* species, which make enzymes that digest the stratum corneum
- Small pits in weight-bearing areas of the feet

Risk factors
- Hyperhidrosis

Prevention
- Keep feet clean and dry

Treatment
- Aluminum chloride to treat hyperhidrosis
- Topical erythromycin or clotrimazole
- Keep feet dry

Differential diagnosis
- Tinea pedis, plantar warts

Erythrasma

Description
- Superficial bacterial infection with *Corynebacterium minitissimum*
- Noninflammatory well-defined scaly, wrinkled, red plaques without satellite lesions located in the groin, axillae, and inframammary and periumbilical regions
- Fluoresces coral red with Wood's lamp

Risk factors
- Occlusive clothing
- Hyperhidrosis

Treatment
- Antibacterial soap
- Topical clindamycin, erythromycin
- Oral erythromycin

Differential diagnosis
- Dermatophytosis, lichen sclerosis, candidiasis, contact dermatitis

Viral infections

Verruca vulgaris and plantaris (common wart, plantar wart)

Description
- Infection of skin with human papillomavirus (HPV)
- Flesh-colored hyperkeratotic papules or plaques that lack normal skin lines
- Thrombosed capillaries in the center look like black dots
- May occur anywhere

Risk factors
- Skin to skin contact
- Public showers and locker rooms

Treatment
- Paring, cryotherapy, salicylic acid, podophyllin, intralesional candida or bleomycin, squaric acid, topical 5-fluorouracil, laser

Differential diagnosis
- Molluscum contagiosum, seborrheic keratosis, callus/corn, squamous cell carcinoma, talon noir

Condyloma acuminata (genital warts)

Description (see Plate 2)
- HPV infection of genital region, usually types 6 anc 11
- High-risk HPV types 16 and 18 associated with cervical cancer in females
- Flesh-colored, pink, or tan flat-topped or cauliflower floret-like papules
- Most common sexually transmitted infection, highly contagious
- Transmitted by direct contact or indirectly by contact with contaminated objects

Risk factors
- Multiple sexual partners (condoms do not prevent HPV transmission)
- Multiparity
- Oral contraceptive use
- Smoking

Prevention
- HPV vaccine (Gardasil) found to decrease infection with common HPV types that cause cervical cancer and genital warts. FDA approved for females age 9 and 26 years

Treatment
- Cryotherapy, podophyllin, imiquimod (Aldara), trichloroacetic acid, laser

Differential diagnosis
- Molluscum contagiosum, condyloma lata (secondary syphilis), pearly penile papules

Molluscum contagiosum

Description (see Plate 3)
- Type of poxvirus that is transmitted through close personal contact
- Firm, umbilicated, flesh-colored papules
- May be located anywhere but have a predilection for skin folds and genital region

Risk factors
- Contact sports such as wrestling, rugby, boxing

Treatment
- Spontaneous resolution within months to years
- Can hasten resolution with cryotherapy, curettage, topical cantharidin, electrodessication, retinoids, laser

Differential diagnosis
- Warts, condyloma acuminata, basal cell carcinoma, appendageal tumors

Herpes simplex (cold sore, fever blister, genital herpes, herpes gladiatorum, herpetic whitlow)

Description
- Herpes simplex virus (HSV)-1 is responsible for most orolabial infections, and HSV-2 (see Plate 4) causes genital infections.
- Typical appearance is grouped vesicles on an erythematous base. May also see pustules, ulceration, and crusting. It can be painful or asymptomatic.
- Prodrome of local pain and tingling roughly 24 hours before eruption
- Transmitted by direct contact
- Latency in dorsal root ganglion until reactivated
- *Herpes gladiatorum*: HSV-1 infection is common in contact sports such as wrestling, soccer, and rugby. Disseminated infection after direct contact associated with lymph node swelling and fever, lethargy, headache

Risk factors
- Extensive skin to skin contact
- Consistent exposure to ultraviolet light (skiers, cycling, baseball)
- Triggers for recurrent attacks: stress, sunlight, infection, fatigue

Diagnosis
- Tzanck smear: scrape the base of a lesion and look for multinucleated giant cells (see Plate 5)
- Viral culture
- PCR or direct immunofluorescence assay (DFA), if available

Prevention
- Educate about the potential for autoinoculation and asymptomatic shedding
- Barrier protection
- Prophylactic or suppressive antiviral therapy, if indicated

Treatment
- Outbreaks are usually self-limited, but antiviral drugs (acyclovir, valacyclovir) can decrease symptoms and duration of attacks.
- Topical antiviral preparations are available (acyclovir, penciclovir) but are less effective than oral antiviral drugs.
- In herpes gladiatorum, treatment with valacyclovir will decrease viral shedding within 4 days, at which time athletes may return to activity. Need to check with governing body of athlete's sport for specific return to play time frames

Differential diagnosis
- Oral: aphthous stomatitis, herpangina, erythema multiforme, pemphigus, hand–foot–mouth disease
- Genital: trauma, syphilis, chancroid
- Herpes gladiatorum: impetigo, tinea corporis, atopic dermatitis

Varicella (chicken pox, herpes zoster)

Description (see Plate 6)
- This is an infection with varicella zoster virus (VZV), a herpes virus, which is spread via airborne route or direct contact.
- Generalized red papules evolve to vesicles and then to pustules with crusting, associated with pruritis.
- Eruption begins on the face and scalp and spreads inferiorly. As successive crops occur, lesions are present in all stages of development.
- Varicella zoster is a reactivation of VZV from dorsal root ganglion or cranial nerve sensory ganglion cells.

Risk factors
- No prior immunization or exposure

Prevention
- Varicella vaccine
- Herpes zoster vaccine to prevent shingles and associated complications

Treatment
- Symptomatic relief of itching with oral antihistamines, moisturizers
- Oral acyclovir may decrease severity of infection and secondary complications if initiated within 24 hours of onset

Differential diagnosis
- Eczema herpeticum, rickettsialpox, enterovirus infection, bullous impetigo

Common causes of dermatitis

Contact dermatitis

Description
- This is an acute or chronic inflammatory reaction of the skin to irritant (irritant contact dermatitis) or allergen (allergic contact dermatitis).
- History of exposures and timing of flares are important.
- Acute: well-demarcated itchy, red, painful plaques sometimes with vesicles. Lesions can have bizarre shapes indicating an "outside job."
- Chronic: deepened skin lines (lichenification) with excoriation and pigmentary changes
- Common causes of allergic contact dermatitis are poison ivy, oak and sumac; causes of irritant contact dermatitis include soaps and detergents.

Risk factors
- Sport-specific exposures such as equipment, unique environments

Treatment
- Topical steroids
- Patch testing to determine origin of contact allergy for future avoidance

Differential diagnosis
- Atopic dermatitis, seborrheic dermatitis, psoriasis, dermatophyte infection

Atopic dermatitis

Description
- Relapsing inflammation of skin with onset in infancy, often resolves by adulthood
- Symmetric, poorly defined red plaques with scale. If chronic, lichenification with secondary excoriation can be common. Very itchy
- Predilection for flexural areas, hands, eyelids, wrists, dorsal feet
- Exacerbated by cold, dry conditions or sweating, emotional stress, frequent bathing or hand washing (disrupts skin barrier)

Risk factors
- Family history of atopy

Treatment
- Topical steroids
- Emollients, petrolatum
- Antihistamines

Differential diagnosis
- Seborrheic dermatitis, contact dermatitis, psoriasis, dermatophyte infection

Description of terms in dermatology

See Tables 16.1 and 16.2.

Table 16.1 Primary skin lesions

Terminology	Description	Examples
Macule	Flat area that is not palpable measuring <1 cm	Vitiligo
Papule	Superficial solid raised lesion measuring <1 cm	Wart
Patch	Flat lesion measuring >1 cm	
Plaque	Palpable lesion above the skin surface >1 cm in diameter	Psoriasis
Nodule	Firm, deep papule that may be subcutaneous	Lipoma, cutaneous lymphoma
Wheal	Flat-topped pink papule or plaque	Urticaria
Vesicle	Fluid-filled elevated lesion <1 cm	Chicken pox
Bulla	Large blister >1 cm	Bullous pemphigoid
Pustule	Superficial elevated lesion with yellow fluid (pus) within	Inflammatory acne, folliculitis

Table 16.2 Secondary skin lesions

Terminology	Description	Examples
Scale	Flaking of the superficial skin layer, increased epidermal turnover	Psoriasis, dermatophyte infection
Crust	Dried serum, blood or exudate on the skin surface	Impetigo
Fissure	Crack or tear in the skin surface	
Excoriation	Excavated area dug into skin by scratching	
Erosion	Defect in epidermis that heals without scarring	Pemphigus
Ulcer	Defect extending into dermis that heals with scarring	Venous stasis or decubitus ulcers

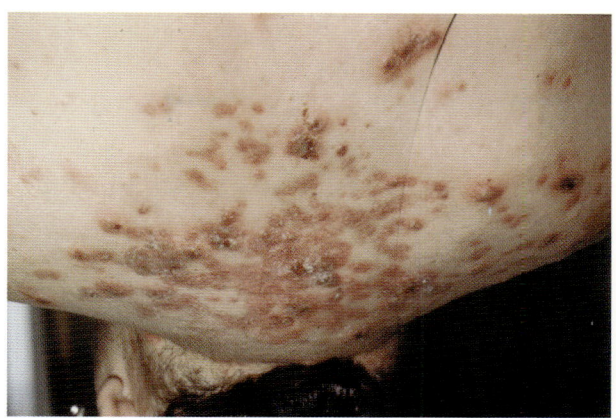

Plate 1 Severe inflammatory acne on the upper back.

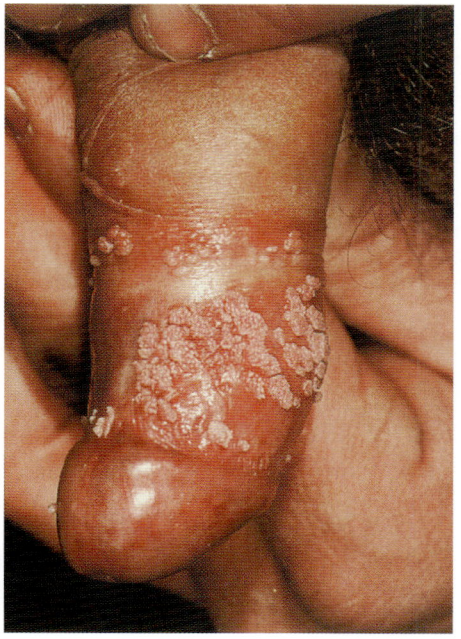

Plate 2 Condyloma acuminata, also known as genital warts, in an otherwise healthy individual.

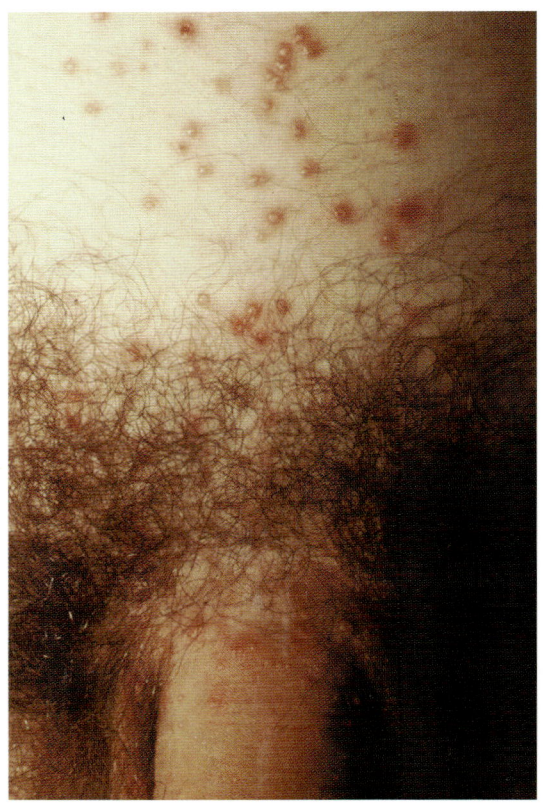

Plate 3 Characteristic domed, pearly papules in molluscum contagiosum.

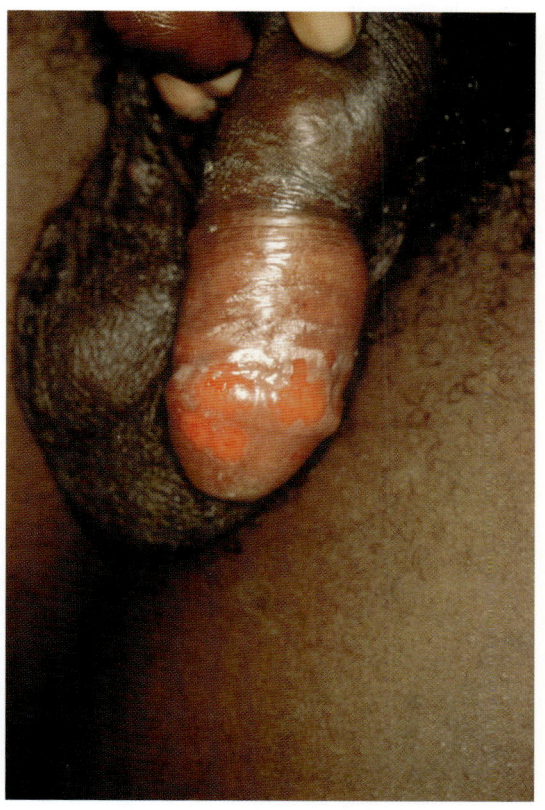

Plate 4 Punched-out ulcerations on an erythema-tous base in herpes simplex virus 2 (HSV-2) infection.

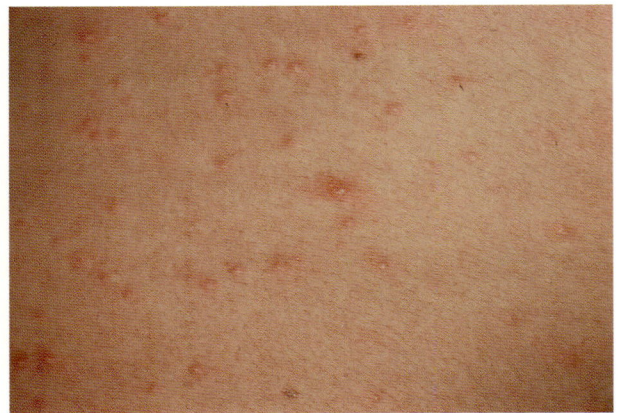

Plate 5 Positive Tzanck prep. Notice the multi-nucleated giant cells.

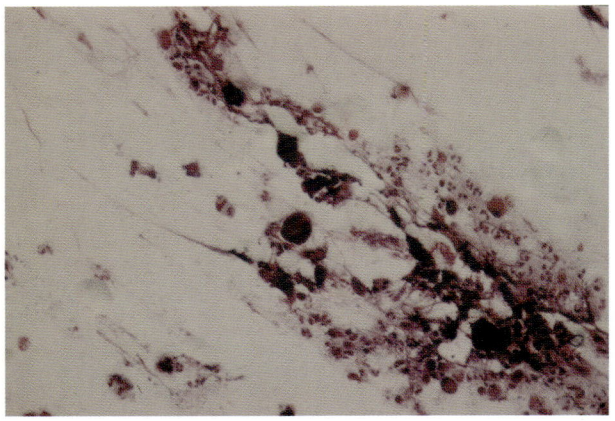

Plate 6 Varicella zoster virus (VZV) infection, commonly known as chickenpox.

Further reading

Adams BB (2004). New strategies for the diagnosis, treatment, and prevention of herpes simplex in contact sports. *Curr Sports Med Rep* **3**:277–283.

Connolly M, de Berger D (2003). Management of primary hyperhidrosis. *Am J Clin Dermatol* **4**(10):681–697.

Elston DM (2007). Community-acquired methicillin-resistant *Staphylococcus aureus. J Am Acad Dermatol* **56**:1–16.

Fatahzadeh M, Schwartz RA (2007). Human herpes simplex virus infections: epidemiology, pathogenesis, symptomatology, diagnosis, and management. *J Am Acad Dermatol* **57**:737–763.

Janniger CK, Schwartz RA, Szepietowski JC, Reich A (2005). Intertrigo and common secondary skin infections. *Am Fam Physician* **72**:833–840.

Jurkovich GJ (2007). Environmental cold-induced injury. *Surg Clin N Am* **87**:247–267.

Kockentiet B, Adams BB (2007). Contact dermatitis in athletes. *J Am Acad Dermatol* **56**:1048–55.

Lipke M (2006). An armamentarium of wart treatments. *Clin Med Res* **4**:273–293.

Levy PD, Hile DC, Hile LM, Miller MA (2006). A prospective analysis of the treatment of friction blisters with 2-octylcyanoacrylate. *J Am Podiatr Med Assoc* **96**(3):232–237.

Mailler EA, Adams BB (2004). The wear and tear of 26.2: dermatological injuries reported on marathon day. *Br J Sports Med* **38**:498–501.

Moehrle M (2008). Outdoor sports and skin cancer. *Clin Dermatol* **26**:12–15.

Palm MD, O'Donoghue MN (2007). Update on photoprotection. *Dermatol Ther* **20**:360–376.

Prentice WE (2003). Skin disorders. In *Arnheim's Principles of Athletic Training: A Competency Based Approach*, 11th ed. Boston: McGraw Hill, pp. 917–945.

Urlman CO, Gottlieb AB (2008). New viral vaccines for dermatologic disease. *J Am Acad Dermatol* **58**:361–370.

The female athlete

Gender and performance

Gender issues in sports and exercise are concerned with genetic, hormonal anatomical, physiological, psychological, and sociological aspects as well as those of sports performance and body image. World record performances in women's sports have been improved rapidly for a variety of reasons, including greater numbers of women participating and better training practices.

Female world record performances are still only 90%–95% of that of males, and in all but a minority of sports women will probably never equal or surpass male performance. Anatomical and physiological reasons for this are considered below.

Stature and body mass

Females are on average of shorter average height—1.6 m in contrast to males' average height of 1.7 m.

Girls are briefly larger and stronger between age 10 and 12 years because of an earlier growth spurt.

Skeletal differences

Women have narrower shoulders, shorter arms with a wider carrying angle, broader hips, and shorter legs.

Shoulder arm difference and smaller muscle mass in women accounts for weaker upper-body compared to lower-body strength in women than in men.

Broader hips create a greater angle of the femur to the knee (genu valgum), causing many women to throw their heels out when running.

Center of gravity

Shorter stature and differences in body shape lead to a lower center of gravity.

In adults, the center of gravity is 55% of standing height in women (S1 level) and 56%–57% in men. Consequently, women have better balance and are better suited to floor exercises and balance beam exercises in gymnastics.

Flexibility

Women have better flexibility than men, which is advantageous in gymnastics and dance.

Hypermobility of the joints can bring problems.

Body fat percentage

Females have a higher percentage of body fat (23%–28%) than males (12%–18%). This is advantageous in cold climates and during starvation and may improve performance in long-distance swimming events.

However, greater percentage of body fat is a major disadvantage in weight-bearing sports involving running and jumping.

Muscle

There is little difference in muscle quality between males and females. Strength differences in males are due to greater cross-sectional area, greater overall muscle mass (androgen effects), and longer levers.

Low-grade muscle endurance is better in females, e.g., when performing repetitions at 20%–30% of 1RM. This may benefit women in ultra-distance events, swimming, and cycling.

Cardiovascular system

Women have proportionately less blood than men (65 mL·kg^{-1} vs. 75 mL·kg^{-1}) and lower hemoglobin levels (13.9 g/dL vs. 15.8 g/dL).

Women tend to have smaller hearts, smaller left ventricular mass, and smaller stroke volume. Despite female hearts being 8% smaller than males, maximum heart rates are similar.

At maximum levels of aerobic work women need to pump 7 L of blood for every liter of oxygen consumed, whereas men require only 6 L. This affects maximum oxygen intake; highest recorded values are between 85–90 mL·kg^{-1}.min^{-1} for males and 75–80 mL·kg^{-1}·min^{-1} for females.

Motor control, vision, and hearing

Women have better fine manipulative skills but worse visual acuity than men. Women have better color discrimination especially in the blue–gray range, and are able to perceive quieter sounds.

Thermoregulation

Thermoregulation in males and females is slightly different.

- Total body water to body mass ratio is 50%–55% in females and 55%–60% in males.
- Body temperature is higher in the luteal phase of the menstrual cycle, but this is thought not to have any effect on performance.
- Men sweat more per m^2 of skin (800 mL·hr^{-1}·m^{-2} vs. 600 mL·hr^{-1}·m^{-2}).
- Women tend to lose more heat through radiation.
- Change in sweat patterns and sweat electrolytes in response to training are similar in both sexes.
- Unfit females lose heat more by radiation and onset of sweating is earlier in trained females.
- Well-trained male and female athletes respond in a similar manner in warm temperatures with low humidity.
- Women are benefited in warm, humid conditions and men in warm, dry conditions.
- Females may be able to work and survive better in the cold than males because they are better insulated.
- However, surface area to body mass ratio (SA/M) also determines heat loss and women have a larger SA/M ratio than males.
- Women lose heat more rapidly in the cold, especially if immersed in cold water.

Menstrual cycle

The normal cycle (see Fig. 17.1) lasts 21–36 days. The first day of menstruation is day 1 of the cycle.

The cycle usually includes 3–5 days of menstruation. Follicular phase is from the last day of menstruation to ovulation, which occurs at approximately 14 days, and the luteal phase lasts from ovulation to menstruation, which is approximately days 15–28.

A cycle lasting fewer than 21 days is *polymenorrhea*; a cycle lasting longer than 36 days is *oligomenorrhea*. *Secondary amenorrhea* is defined as having had no periods for 3 months.

Hormonal changes that occur during the menstrual cycle

Gonadotropin-releasing hormone (GnRH) causes the synthesis, storage, and activation release of follicle-stimulating hormone (FSH) and luteinizing hormone (LH).

During the follicular phase, levels of estrogen increase so that both LH and estrogen peak just before ovulation. Estrogen then falls and rises again during the luteal phase. Progesterone is secreted by the corpus luteum during the luteal phase, and both estrogen and progesterone levels fall if fertilization does not take place. Hormone levels should ideally be tested after the 21st day of the cycle, during the luteal phase.

Factors associated with changes to the normal menstrual cycle include the following:
- Psychological stress
- Physical exercise
- Seasonal rhythms
- Circadian rhythms

Physical exercise produces marked changes in the post-exercise pulsatile secretion of LH, FSH, estrogen, progesterone, and cortisol. The more intense and longer the duration of exercise the greater the effect, resulting in marked changes in the menstrual cycle.

Strenuous exercise causes an increase in dopamine (which inhibits GnRH), beta-endorphins, catecholamines, and estrogens. Beta-endorphins also stimulate dopamine and combine with norepinephrine receptors in the hypothalamus to further inhibit GnRH stimulation.

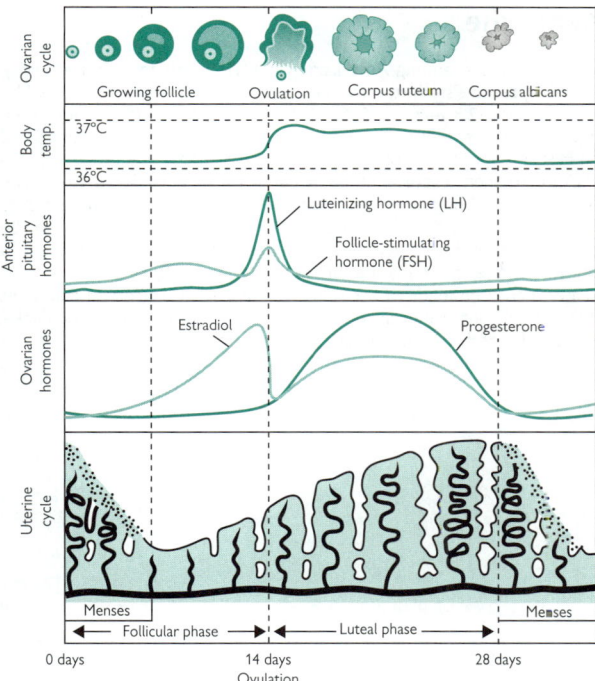

Figure 17.1 The normal menstrual cycle. Reproduced with permission from Welt CK (2008). The normal menstrual cycle. In UpToDate, Rose BD (ed.). Waltham, MA: UpToDate. Copyright 2008, UpToDate, Inc. For more information visit www.uptodate.com.

Menarche

Age of menarche among American girls varies with race and ethnicity. According to one study, the overall average age of menarche in the U.S. dropped from 12.5 years in 1988–1994 to 12.3 in 1999–2002. Among non-Hispanic whites age of menarche is 12.5, while among African Americans and Hispanic whites it is 12.1.[1]

Failure to menstruate after 16 years of age is considered to be late menarche and should be investigated. Tall, thin girls tend to have a later menarche than shorter and heavier girls. In some cases, bone age may be below the chronological age because of illness or inadequate nutrition. To determine bone age, X-ray the carpal bones of the left hand.

Later menarche tends to occur in gymnasts, ballet dancers, and athletes who start high-intensity training early. Girls who have a low caloric intake, low body fat, and high emotional stress are also affected.

1 Anderson S, Must A (2005). Interpreting the continued decline in the average age at menarche: results from two nationally representative surveys of U.S. girls studied 10 years apart. *J Pediatr* **147**(6): 753–760.

Primary amenorrhea

Any girl who hasn't menstruated by age 16, who hasn't developed secondary sexual characteristics by age 14, or who remains amenorrheic 2 years after thelarche should be evaluated for primary amenorrhea. Common causes for primary amenorrhea include central hormonal (e.g., congenital GnRH deficiency, hyperprolactinemia), peripheral hormonal (e.g., PCOS, premature ovarian failure), hormonal receptor (e.g., androgen insensitivity), congenital and developmental (e.g., imperforate hymen, uterine agenesis), and chromosomal (e.g., Turner's syndrome).

This workup should begin with a detailed medical, family, and nutritional history, complete physical exam including genitourinary exam, and a record of athletic training and competition as athletic participation has increasingly become a cause of primary amenorrhea. A pelvic ultrasound should also be performed to establish the presence or absence of the uterus as well as genitourinary anatomy.

Preliminary lab tests should include early-morning hormone levels (FSH, LH, estrogen, progesterone, testosterone, prolactin, and thyroid function tests). Further laboratory testing should be guided by the ultrasound findings. Karyotyping should be performed to look for chromosomal abnormalities.

In addition to developmental and fertility concerns, a significant concern in girls with primary amenorrhea is development of osteopenia.

Menstrual irregularities

Menstrual irregularities tend to occur among athletes with intense training schedules and with sudden increases in quantity or intensity of training, and among the longest-participating athletes. These irregularities most commonly include anovulatory cycling, irregular menstruation, oligomenorrhea, and amenorrhea.

- Vegetarians and people with a low caloric intake have the highest incidence of oligomenorrhea and amenorrhea.
- The reported prevalence of athletic amenorrhea ranges from 1% to 44% (general population range is 2%–5%). Prevalence is sport and individual dependent, e.g., 24%–26% in runners, 12% in swimmers.[1]
- One study on female varsity collegiate athletes noted an overall prevalence of menstrual irregularities of 28%, ranging from a low of 13% in basketball players to a high of 57% in cross-country runners.[2]
- Incidence depends on how the menstrual irregularities are assessed, and vary in studies by questionnaire or measured hormone levels—e.g., women with normal 28-day cycles may have abnormal serum hormone levels after day 21.
- The prevalence of menstrual irregularities among elite female athletes is now more difficult to estimate, as more elite athletes are regulating their menstrual cycles with hormone supplementation.

There is little evidence to suggest that menstruation affects performance; in fact, some data suggest that athletic participation can improve menstrual complications such as dysmenorrhea. Furthermore, women at all phases of their menstrual cycles have achieved elite athletic performances.

Multifactoral causes of menstrual irregularities

- Stress, both psychological and physical. Severe emotional stress acts above the hypothalamic–pituitary axis.
- Immature pituitary axis, late menarche, intense training prior to menarche, and irregular menstruation prior to initiating sports participation
- Inadequate nutrition for caloric expenditure, resulting in weight loss. Decreased caloric intake and a low-protein and high-fiber diet results in a high serum sex hormone binding globulin and low estrogen, both of which predispose to amenorrhea.

1 Lebrun C (2008). Menstrual cycle dysfunction. American College of Sports Medicine Current Comment. Retrieved June 2008 from http://www.acsm.org/AM/Template.cfm?Sec-tion=Current_Comments1&Template=/CM/ContentDisplay.cfm&ContentID=8621
2 Arendt E (1993). Prevalence of athletic amenorrhea. The Athletic Female. Champaign, IL: Human Kinetics, p. 45.

Progression of exercise-related menstrual changes

- *Stage 1.* Normal follicular, normal luteal phase
- *Stage 2.* Prolonged follicular and a shortened luteal phase results in luteal phase defects, which are associated with infertility and premenstrual tension.
- *Stage 3.* Euestrogenic anovulatory oligomenorrhea, hypoprolactinemia, possibility of endometrial hyperplasia adenocarcinoma if this phase persists.[1] Oligomenorrheic athletes also begin losing bone mineral density.
- *Stage 4.* Hypoestrogenic—amenorrhea leads to osteoporosis and genital atrophy.

Secondary amenorrhea

- Previously menstruating woman with no periods for 3 months
- Most likely functional secondary amenorrhea in athletes; however, may also be related to pregnancy, ovarian, pituitary, or uterine disease as well as hypothalamic dysfunction. These conditions must be ruled out before making a diagnosis of athletic amenorrhea.
- Higher incidence of skeletal demineralization (especially in setting of hyperprolactinemia) and stress fractures in amenorrheic athletes
- Workup should begin with a complete history and physical exam, as well as a pregnancy test (serum or urine β-HCG).
- If the pregnancy test is negative, consider a 10-day challenge with 10 mg medroxyprogesterone daily to test for withdrawal bleeding.
- If there is no withdrawal bleeding, then workup should include early-morning serum prolactin, FSH, LH, TSH, and T4 levels. Serum DHEA-S and testosterone levels may be considered.

Treatment of menstrual irregularities

The team approach may include the athlete, physician, nutritionist, and psychologist, and varies with the type of menstrual irregularity.
- Identify cause
- Psychological counseling if disordered eating is a concern
- Dietary advice, increase caloric intake if necessary
- Reduce training intensity, e.g., drop 1 full day of training from current regimen
- Low-dose oral contraceptive pills (OCP)
- Monophasic, biphasic, or triphasic OCP
- Further psychological counseling if unable to implement dietary and training recommendations

---

1 Shangold M, Mirkin G (1998). *Women and Exercise*, 2nd ed. New York: Oxford University Press.

Dysmenorrhea

Primary dysmenorrhea is defined as recurrent, crampy lower-abdominal pain that only occurs during menses, only during ovulatory cycles, and in the absence of pelvic pathology. This pain is thought to be related to strong uterine contractions that decrease myometrial blood flow, leading to temporary ischemia and endometrial prostaglandin release.

Studies have estimated the prevalence of dysmenorrhea among young women as high as 90%; prevalence decreases with age and with oral contraceptive use. Exercise improves dysmenorrhea, but the prevalence of dysmenorrhea appears to be the same in athletes compared to non-athletes.

Workup should include history and physical exam. In older athletes, pelvic ultrasonography will rule out secondary causes (e.g., uterine fibroid, ovarian cysts, polycystic ovarian syndrome, endometriosis).

Treatment

There is evidence to suggest that acupressure can help relieve dysmenorrhea. With the athlete lying prone, palpate for a tender point approximately 1 inch to the right of the L3 spinous process. A small, firm nodule may or may not be palpable. Begin with light pressure rotary motion for 30 seconds until the athlete begins to feel relief and continue for 3–4 minutes. Acupressure points over the first sacral openings or 1 inch lateral to either side of T8 may also provide relief.[1]

Start nonsteroidal anti-inflammatories such as 500 mg of naproxen twice a day beginning 2 days prior to onset of menses and continuing through first 1–2 days.

Consider OCP if these interventions are ineffective.

1 Prentice B (1981). Acupressure massage to relieve menstrual cramps. *Physician Sports Medicine Trainer's Corner.* **9**(3):171.

Premenstrual syndrome

The symptoms of premenstrual syndrome (PMS) include headache, fatigue, joint-pain, breast tenderness, breast swelling, and weight gain. They occur during the second half of the menstrual cycle and can interfere with athletic performance.

Prevalence estimates for PMS range from 30% to 80%, with the more severe premenstrual dysphoric disorder (PMDD) affecting 2%–6% of women.[1]

Both exercise and relaxation seem to improve premenstrual syndrome but need further evaluation in more rigorous studies.

Use of an OCP has been shown to help premenstrual syndrome by inducing ovulation. However, OCPs should ideally be started several cycles before a major competition.

Consider a selective serotonin reuptake inhibitor (SSRI) or other antidepressant if symptoms are refractory or if PMDD is suspected.

1. Casper R, et al. (2006). Clinical manifestations and diagnosis of premenstrual syndrome and premenstrual dysphoric disorder. *UpToDate*. Last updated August 3, 2006. Retrieved June 2008 from http://www.uptodate.com

Contraception

There are three major means of contraception: barrier methods, hormonal manipulation, and sterilization (see Table 17.1). Many factors can affect a woman's or a couple's choice of contraceptive method, ranging from efficacy to affordability to convenience.

One survey indicated that among all American women ages 15–44, OCPs remain the most common contraceptive at 31% of women surveyed, followed by female sterilization at 27%, condoms at 18%, and injectables, implants, and patches all at 9%.[1]

Barrier methods

Even when used ideally, barrier methods are less reliable than hormonal therapies. However, barriers generally have fewer side effects and are the only non-abstinence method of contraception that prevents many sexually transmitted infections (STIs). Barrier methods are the following:

- Condoms, the most effective protection against STIs
- Diaphragms, if correctly fitted, can be worn during exercise and protects against some STIs
- Intrauterine devices, providing no protection against STIs

Hormonal manipulation

While OCPs were the mainstay method of hormonal manipulation for decades, there are now multiple routes of hormonal contraception including transdermal patches (Ortho Evra), subdermal progestin implants, injectable depot medroxyprogesterone (Depo-Provera), intravaginal rings (NuvaRing), and a myriad of different kinds of OCPs. See Table 17.1 for more detailed descriptions.

In athletes, it is important to start any hormonal contraceptive method well in advance of any competition because of variation in individual reactions to hormonal manipulation.

Depo-Provera use is correlated with decreased bone mineral density in young women, although there is no evidence that women whose use of Depo-Provera experience higher rates of fracture than non-users.[2] Caucasians are at increased risk of osteopenia. Physicians should consider use of Depo-Provera in young athletes on a case-by-case basis.

Finally, hormonal methods of contraception often provide non-contraceptive benefits including reduced acne, reduced dysmenorrhea, menstrual cycle regulation, and reduced risk of both ovarian and endometrial cancer.

1 QuickStats: Primary contraceptive methods among women aged 15–44 years—United States, 2002. *MMWR Morb Mortal Wkly Rev* February 18, 2005 / **54**(06); 52.
2 Curtis KM, Martins SL (2006). Progestogen-only contraception and bone mineral density: a systematic review. *Contraception* **73**(5):470–487.

Surgical sterilization

Women seeking a permanent contraceptive solution may opt for bilateral tubal ligation, a minor surgery that is performed transabdominally and is >99% effective at preventing future pregnancies.

Table 17.1 Comparison of contraceptive options*

Type of contraceptive	Description	Failure rate[†]
Male condoms	Latex or polyurethane sheath applied over the penis immediately before intercourse	11
Diaphragm with spermicide	Dome-shaped rubber disk inserted immediately before intercourse that covers the cervix	17
Combined OCP	Combined estrogen–progestin pill taken daily on schedule to suppress ovulation	1–2
Progestin-only OCP	Progestin-only pill taken daily to reduce and thicken cervical mucus and prevent conception	2
91-day OCP regimen (Seasonale)	Combined pill taken in 3-month cycles (12 weeks of active pills followed by 1 week inactive pills) resulting in 1 period every 13 weeks	1–2
Patch (Ortho Evra)	Skin patch worn on lower abdomen, buttocks, or upper body that releases estrogen and progestin into bloodstream. Each patch is worn for 3 weeks followed by 1 week without a patch.	1–2
Vaginal contraceptive ring (NuvaRing)	Flexible ring inserted into the vagina that releases estrogen and progestin. Each ring remains in place for 3 weeks, followed by 1 week with no ring.	1–2
Depo-Provera injection	Injectable progestin given every 3 months to inhibit ovulation and prevent both conception and implantation	<1
Implant (Norplant)	Small levonorgestrel-releasing implants surgically placed in upper arm that can be effective for up to 5 years	<1
IUD	T-shaped device inserted into the uterus by health-care professional that can remain in place for up to 10 years	<1
Female surgical sterilization (tubal ligation)	Surgical interruption of fallopian tubes to prevent sperm from reaching egg	<1

*Adapted from FDA Birth Control Guide (12/03). Retrieved from http://www.fda.gov/fdac/features/1997/babyguide2.pdf

[†]The FDA reports failure rate as the number of pregnancies each year per 100 women.

Manipulation of the menstrual cycle

It has become increasingly possible for women to manipulate their menstrual cycles using either commercially available OCPs that cause fewer periods per year (e.g., Seasonale), by changing the cycling of regular combination OCPs through deletion of placebo pills, or by using contraceptive methods that can reduce or eliminate periods altogether (e.g., Depo-Provera).

An athlete on OCPs seeking to regulate her menses around a specific event may stop taking the pill 10 days prior, which will result in a withdrawal bleed. She may then restart a new pack of OCPs either after menses or after the event. Use of a backup method of contraception for 2 weeks after restarting OCPs is necessary.

A second option is to continue taking active pills for two cycles (42 days) or three cycles (63 days), followed by 4–7 days of placebo pills to induce menses.

Female athlete triad

- Menstrual abnormalities
- Disordered eating
- Osteoporosis or osteopenia (low bone density)

Each of these conditions can occur on their own or in combination.

Eating disorders or disordered eating patterns

Anorexia nervosa and bulimia nervosa may occur singly or together. There has been an increase in the prevalence of eating disorders in the last decade, in both the general population and among athletes. The female athlete is at greatest risk during adolescence and young adulthood. Factors contributing to the development of eating disorders include psychological, biological, and social pressures as well as inappropriate training programs.

While there is an increased incidence in participants in sports with an emphasis on leanness, e.g., gymnastics, ballet, long-distance running, synchronized swimming, and figure skating, and in weight category sports such as judo and lightweight rowing, disordered eating can occur in athletes in any sport.

It is essential to take an accurate and detailed social, medical, and menstrual history. History of stress fracture should initiate evaluation for disordered eating and/or menstrual abnormalities. If there is a history of irregular menses or amenorrhea, laboratory evaluation should be pursued as detailed earlier in this chapter.

A DEXA scan can rule out osteopenia or osteoporosis. Low bone density can result from hypoestrogenemia due to inadequate caloric intake or excessive caloric expenditure. Until normal hormone levels are restored by increasing body weight, the athlete should take OCPs to limit ongoing bone loss.

Treatment of the athlete with an eating disorder is best achieved by a team including a psychologist, physician, and nutritionist.

Osteoporosis

Osteoporosis is characterized by a decrease in bone mass and mineral density and a deterioration in microarchitecture, resulting in loss of bone strength and a greater risk of fracture.

Osteoporosis, or, in a larger number of cases, osteopenia, is associated with low levels of estrogen, hypercortisolemia, low T3 syndrome, and a deficiency in insulin-like-growth factor-1 (IGF-1). It is a silent disease that can occur at any age.

Bone is a living tissue that is constantly remodeling. The rate of turnover is determined by hormonal and local factors. Sixty percent of bone is laid down during the pubertal growth spurt. Peak bone mass occurs at around 20 years of age. Bone mass plateaus until the age of 40 and then begins declining at menopause. Peak bone mass is affected by genetic factors, environmental factors, mechanical strain, hormones, chronological age, skeletal age, and the stage of sexual maturation.

Healthy bone requires normal sex hormone levels, adequate nutrition including overall calories, 1200 mg calcium and 800 international units of vitamin D daily, and regular weight-bearing exercise. This is particularly important during the adolescent growth spurt. Low estrogen affects calcium metabolism with resultant increased bone loss, failure to accrue bone density, and low peak bone mass.

Weight-bearing activity during adolescence and early adulthood is an important predictor of peak bone mass. Mechanical stress exerts a positive effect on bone. Muscle action is the main stimulus for bone formation. Exercise should be weight bearing and produce dynamic, not static, strains. Greater loads with fewer repetitions results in greater gains in bone mass.

The osteogenic response to mechanical loading is site specific, so that professional tennis players, for example, have a 30% greater bore density in the dominant forearm. Growing bone has a greater capacity to add new bone to the skeleton than mature bone.

Bone mass

Peak height velocity for girls is between 9.5 and 13 years and peak height velocity for boys is between 11.5 and 15 years.

There is a 7%–8% gain in bone mass per year during childhood and early adolescence. Daily physical exercise has a positive effect on bone accrual. Weight-bearing aerobic exercise should be for 30 minutes daily and can be divided into 15-minute segments. Weight-bearing exercise should be continued throughout the life cycle.

Intensive endurance training and amenorrhea is associated with decreased trabecular bone density in young females. Those who have been running for the longest period of time have the highest incidence of oligomenorrhea and amenorrhea.

The best positive predictor of bone mineral density (BMD) of the lumbar spine in women in their 30s and 40s (premenopausal) are the years of regular monthly menstruation. The best negative predictor of BMD of the hip is the number of years of amenorrhea.

Pregnancy and exercise

For many women, exercise is an integral part of their lifestyle, which they wish to continue during pregnancy. When exercise is performed safely and under the monitoring of their physician, pregnant women can benefit in many areas: they are less likely to be depressed and more likely to sleep restfully, have an enhanced sense of well-being, maintain aerobic fitness, and control excess weight gain.

Pregnant women with a poor obstetrical history sedentary lifestyles, or no previous exercise experience should consult their family physician or obstetrician prior to beginning any exercise regimen.

Placental hormones

The placenta produces various hormones during the second and third trimesters of pregnancy, including estriol, progesterone, chorionic gonadotropins, and human placental lactogen (which antagonizes insulin). Exercise increases catecholamines, prolactin, endorphins, and glucagon. There is a decrease in insulin due to gonadotropins.

The placenta metabolizes amines so that only 10%–15% of maternal catecholamines reach the fetus. Excess catecholamines have an adverse effect on fetal circulation through reduced fetal breathing and reduced fetal movements.

During exercise there is a major redistribution of blood flow from the uterus to the exercising muscles and an increase n fetal heart rate within minutes. Fetal heart rate usually returns to normal 15 minutes after stopping mild or moderate maternal exercise, but may take 30 minutes to normalize after strenuous exercise.

Musculoskeletal changes

The anterior enlarging uterus causes a shift of the center of gravity posteriorly, resulting in a progressive lordosis and rotation of the pelvis. Increased gestational hormones (likely including the peptide relaxin) cause laxity of the ligaments (especially at the public symphysis and sacroiliac joints) with increased stress on the lumbar spine.

Back pain occurs in approximately 50% of pregnancies, appears to be more common in multiparous women, and may be due to sacroiliac strain, unilateral lumbarization, or unilateral sacralization. Increased anterior flexion of the lumbar spine and forward flexion of the neck may also contribute to slumping of the shoulders, which predisposes to paresthesias in the distribution of both the median and ulnar nerves.

Alterations in neck posture may also result in neck pain. Fluid retention may cause carpal tunnel syndrome.

Cardiovascular changes

There is a 30% increase in maternal blood volume during early pregnancy; this peaks mid-pregnancy, reducing cardiac reserve available for strenuous exercise. Increase in cardiac output is due to an increase in both heart rate and stroke volume. Decrease in peripheral resistance is due to vasodilation in skin, breast, uterus, GI tract, and kidneys.

Respiratory changes

Early in pregnancy, women begin experiencing relative hyperventilation secondary to significantly increased tidal volume. This hyperventilation is thought to be due to both increased sensitivity to carbon dioxide and the effect of progesterone on respiratory drive.

The increased sensitivity to CO_2 also makes pregnant women feel relatively more dyspneic than non-pregnant women with small changes in CO_2 levels. Increased tidal volume and minute ventilation result in slightly higher PaO_2 levels (110 mmHg) and slightly lower $PaCO_2$ levels (27–32 mmHg) that persist throughout the pregnancy.

Later in pregnancy, lung volumes drop as a higher diaphragm leads to lower functional residual capacity and thus lower total lung volume. Despite these changes, FEV_1 remains normal throughout pregnancy.[1]

Nutritional changes

During pregnancy, women require an additional 150 calories/day during the first trimester, 350/day during the second trimester, and 300/day during the third trimester.

Endocrine changes

Because of the greater utilization of carbohydrate, there is a greater risk of hypoglycemia. Pregnant women may also become hypoglycemic if exercise is prolonged or strenuous, and they have a higher risk of dehydration. They may become insulin resistant because of circulating human placental lactogen.

Temperature changes

Maternal body temperature is increased due to fetal and placental metabolism. Under resting conditions, the fetal temperature is 0.5°C above the maternal temperature. Trained athletes have a lower resting core temperature and more efficient thermoregulation.

During exercise their maternal temperature increase, followed by a rise in fetal temperature. Maternal temperature should not exceed 38°C. In animals a temperature of 39°C has a teratogenic effect on the neural tube in the fetus during the first trimester.

A core increase of 1–1.5°C in the non-pregnant woman may easily exceed 2–2.5°C in a pregnant woman, resulting in an increase of 2.5–3°C in the fetus. Heat production depends on the intensity and duration of exercise as well as environmental heat loads. Heat loss depends on environmental factors such as ambient temperature and humidity as well as physiological adaptations including cardiovascular conditioning and acclimatization.

Moderate or strenuous exercise in adverse conditions can increase the maternal temperature above 39°C. The risk of dehydration during exercise is increased in pregnant women.

1 Funai E, et al. (2007). Changes in the respiratory tract during pregnancy. *UpToDate*. Last updated December 4, 2007. Retrieved June 2008 from http://www.uptodate.com

Exercise

The amount and type of exercise that pregnant women can engage in depends on many factors—medical and obstetrical history, pregestational activity levels, and stage of pregnancy. Recommendations must be individual based. Recommended exercises are walking, jogging, cycling, and water aerobics. Swimming can be done throughout the pregnancy. Contraindicated sports include water skiing, downhill skiing, vigorous racquet sports, scuba diving, contact sports, and horse riding.

In 2002 the American College of Obstetricians and Gynecologists (ACOG) Committee on Obstetrics Practice outlined the following contraindications to and warning signs during pregnancy:

Absolute contraindications to aerobic exercise during pregnancy[1]

- Hemodynamically significant heart disease
- Restrictive lung disease
- Incompetent cervix/cerclage
- Multiple gestation at risk for premature labor
- Persistent second- or third-trimester bleeding
- Placenta previa after 26 weeks of gestation
- Premature labor during the current pregnancy
- Ruptured membranes
- Preeclampsia/pregnancy-induced hypertension

Relative contraindications to aerobic exercise during pregnancy[1]

- Severe anemia
- Unevaluated maternal cardiac arrhythmia
- Chronic bronchitis
- Poorly controlled type 1 diabetes
- Extreme morbid obesity *or* extreme underweight (BMI <12)
- History of extremely sedentary lifestyle
- Intrauterine growth restriction in current pregnancy
- Poorly controlled hypertension
- Orthopedic limitations
- Poorly controlled seizure disorder
- Poorly controlled hyperthyroidism
- Heavy smoker

Warning signs to terminate exercise while pregnant[1]

- Vaginal bleeding
- Dyspnea prior to exertion
- Dizziness
- Headache
- Chest pain
- Muscle weakness
- Calf pain or swelling (need to rule out thrombophlebitis)
- Preterm labor
- Decreased fetal movement
- Amniotic fluid leakage

1 American College of Obstetricians and Gynecologists Committee on Obstetric Practice. Exercise during pregnancy and the postpartum period. Committee opinion. Number 267, January 2002. Reproduced with permission.

Designing exercise programs

The intensity and amount of exercise permitted during pregnancy depends on the baseline level of fitness of the woman. If she has not exercised for some time she should start slowly, at a low intensity, always warming up and cooling down for at least 5 minutes.

She should drink adequate fluid to avoid dehydration and ensure adequate caloric intake to meet both the extra needs of pregnancy and the extra needs of exercise. She should wear the correct equipment and clothing for the type of exercise and work out in a well-ventilated room. If she is exercising on the floor, she should get up slowly to prevent postural hypotension.

Regular aerobic exercise using large muscle groups and lasting 20–40 minutes is preferable to occasional bursts of intense exercise. There is little data on strenuous exercise—if a pregnant woman wants to continue strenuous exercise during pregnancy, she must be closely monitored. Such exercise should not exceed 15 minutes (60%–90% of maximum heart rate or 50%–85% of VO_2max).

Maternal heart rate should not exceed 140 bpm and maternal core temperature should not exceed 38°C. Exercises that involve either ballistic movements or the Valsalva maneuver should be avoided. Vigorous exercise should be avoided altogether in hot and humid conditions.

The first trimester

Exercise is contraindicated in the first trimester in women with a history of spontaneous abortion; this is often associated with a luteal phase defect due to low levels of progesterone. Once the placenta takes over the production of hormones, these women may be able to exercise with close monitoring.

The second trimester

The enlarging uterus causes the center of gravity to be displaced posteriorly. Lumbar lordosis increases, resulting in stress on the sacroiliac joint, lumbar vertebrae, and supporting ligaments. No exercise should be carried out in the supine position after the fourth month, as the uterus may fall back, compressing venous return and resulting in decreased cardiac output and orthostatic hypotension.

The third trimester

Norepinephrine produced during exercise increases the frequency and amplitude of uterine contractions. Dyspnea may be more pronounced from increased displacement of the diaphragm causing a reduction in pulmonary reserve. Excessive exercise may cause fetal distress, intrauterine growth retardation, or prematurity.

Postpartum

Exercise or sport may be resumed a few weeks after a normal delivery, depending on the individual, sport, and type of delivery. Home exercise programs should include core-strengthening and hip-strengthening exercises and may facilitate postpartum recovery. Any sport should be started slowly and the amount and intensity should be gradually increased.

Pelvic pain

Although pelvic pain may be musculoskeletal in origin (e.g., pelvic stress fracture, pubalgia, sports hernia, etc.), it may arise from other sources, some of which may be gynecological. It may be acute or chronic; it may be due to a local or referred cause. Local cause may arise from the bladder, ureter, uterus (body or cervix), broad ligament, uterine tube, ovaries, rectum, vagina, or a pelvic appendix.

It is essential to take a detailed history of the pain, including the quality, type, radiation, and factors that relieve or aggravate it; its relationship to the menstrual cycle (to rule out an ectopic pregnancy, pain due to ovulation, and endometriosis); and associated symptoms such as nausea, vomiting, and diarrhea. Sexually transmitted infections should be ruled out.

Routine abdominal and gynecological examination should be performed. Referral may be appropriate for further investigation, including pelvic ultrasound.

Injuries

Women develop similar injuries as men as a result of training errors, but may be more prone to certain injuries because of anatomical differences.

Injuries to the knee and ankle are common, but injuries to the breast are rare. There is a higher incidence of anterior cruciate ligament (ACL) tears in females because of the narrow intercondylar notch of the femur. There is also a higher incidence of subluxation of the patella due to genu valgum. Back pain in females may be due to gynecological causes including ovarian cysts, endometriosis, or fibroids.

Water-skiing injuries can occur during take-off, as failure to rise from sitting position can lead to retrograde douching and hematoma of the vulva or laceration of vaginal wall.

Physicians evaluating a female athlete for recurrent stress fractures should first obtain a careful history including evaluation for eating disorders and menstrual abnormalities, followed by a complete physical exam and biomechanical evaluation.

Menstrual abnormalities should trigger investigation including prolactin, estrogen, progesterone, LH, FSH, T4, TSH, and cortisol levels. A DEXA scan should be performed; if bone mineral density is low and no other cause is found, further workup should include PTH, calcium, phosphorous, and vitamin D levels.

Further reading

Anderson S, Must A (2005). Interpreting the continued decline in the average age at menarche: results from two nationally representative surveys of U.S. girls studied 10 years apart. *J Pediatr* **147**(6): 753–760.

Arendt E (1993). Prevalence of athletic amenorrhea. *The Athletic Female*. Champaign, IL: Human Kinetics, p. 45.

Casper R, et al. (2006). Clinical manifestations and diagnosis of premenstrual syndrome and premenstrual dysphoric disorder. *UpToDate*. Last updated August 3, 2006. Retrieved June 2008 from http://www.uptodate.com

Curtis KM, Martins SL (2006). Progestogen-only contraception and bone mineral density: a systematic review. *Contraception* **73**(5):470–487.

Funai E, et al. (2007). Changes in the respiratory tract during pregnancy. *UpToDate*. Last updated December 4, 2007. Retrieved June 2008 from http://www.uptodate.com

Lebrun C (2008). Menstrual cycle dysfunction. American College of Sports Medicine Current Comment. Retrieved June 2008 from http://www.acsm.org/AM/Template.cfm?Section=Current_Comments1&Template=/CM/ContentDisplay.cfm&ContentID=8621

Pearce G, et al. (1996). Does weight-bearing exercise protect against the effects of exercise-induced oligomenorrhea on bone density? *Osteoporosis Int* 1996(6):448–452.

Prentice B (1981). Acupressure massage to relieve menstrual cramps. *Physician Sports Medicine Trainer's Corner*. **9**(3):171.

QuickStats: Primary contraceptive methods among women aged 15–44 years—United States, 2002. *MMWR Morb Mortal Wkly Rev* February 18, 2005 / **54**(06);152.

Shangold M, Mirkin G (1998). *Women and Exercise*, 2nd ed. New York: Oxford University Press.

U.S. Food and Drug Administration (2003, Dec). Birth control guide. Retrieved June 2008 from http://www.fda.gov/fdac/features/1997/babyguide2.pdf

Ergogenic aids

Ergogenic aids

Throughout history, people have competed in athletic events of all different types, and with competition there is always the desire to win. This desire to win is influenced by personal goals, media, financial rewards, and pressure from coaches, peers, and families, which can encourage a competitor to attempt to cheat by using drugs or performance-enhancing substances (or *ergogenic aids*) in an attempt to gain advantage.

A variety of ergogenic aids have been used, from mushrooms used by the Ancient Greek Olympians, stimulants taken by the Roman gladiators, strychnine used by twelfth-century boxers, to the designer drugs used by athletes today.

Many believe that most of their competitors are taking such substances and thus justify their own use as leveling the playing field. Those using such methods tend to have genuine concerns about their own health, but believe that taking the substances increase their chances of being successful.

Apart from supplements and drugs, other examples of ergogenic aids include the following:

- Psychological imagery
- Custom-fitted shoe orthoses
- Blood or gene doping

Some of the pharmaceutical and physiological aids are outlined in this chapter.

Performance-enhancing drugs

Anabolic steroids

These are natural or synthetically made derivatives of the hormone testosterone. Their ergogenic effects are as follows:
- Reduced recovery time after training
- Increased lean body mass
- Increased aggression (seen as a benefit in some contact sports)

They first came into use during WW II by the Germans to increase aggressiveness and to attempt to create the super soldier. Russian Olympians were some of the first athletes to use anabolic steroids in athletic competition during the 1956 Olympics, and steroids were later banned prior to the 1976 Olympics.

Anabolic steroids are used orally, as a cream, or injected. Needle sharing carries risks of HIV or hepatitis B or C transmission, and needle abscesses can occur from contaminated injection sites.

Despite this catalog of adverse effects (see Table 18.1), anabolic steroid abuse is still widespread; athletes and bodybuilders risk their health in the pursuit of success. Use of polypharmacy and massive doses of multiple drugs is common.

Commonly abused steroids include stanozolol, nandrolone, clembuterol, and dihydrotestosterone. Tetrahydrogestrinone (also known as "the clear"), a new synthetic "designer" steroid that was at the center of the Balco scandal, was specifically produced to be difficult to detect in urine samples and was discovered in 2003.

Testing involves urine screening for the steroids and ratio of testosterone to epitestosterone (T:E) levels.

Erythropoietin

Erythropoietin (EPO) is a glycoprotein, produced naturally in the body by the kidneys in response to hypoxia. Recombinant EPO became available in the 1980s. EPO can be prescribed to treat or be used in renal failure, some cancers, and AIDS. It is administered by subcutaneous injection.

Effects of erythropoietin

EPO exerts a direct effect on bone marrow to increase red blood cell (RBC) production, particularly in the presence of iron.

Hemoglobin levels increase, which improves aerobic performance by enhanced oxygen-carrying capacity of blood.

Ergogenic effects
- Increases VO_2max due to increased O_2-carrying capacity
- Increases buffering effect of blood because of elevated RBCs

These effects would be beneficial in endurance competition, which is why EPO has been a topic of discussion in such events as the Tour de France.

Table 18.1 Adverse effect from use of anabolic steroids

Male	Female	Both sexes
Breast enlargement	Male-pattern baldness	Acne
Testicular atrophy	Deepening of voice	↑ Blood pressure
↓ Sperm count	Enlarged clitoris	↑ LDL/total cholesterol
	↑ Facial hair	Liver abnormalities
	Irregular menses	↑ Risk of premature ischemic heart disease or death
		↑ Risk of malignancy: hepatic, renal, testicular

Adverse effects

Side effects of EPO include the following:

- Potential life-threatening thrombosis or embolism
- Cerebrovascular accidents
- Seizures and encephalopathy
- Myocardial infarction
- Iron overload causing liver or cardiac disease

Effects similar to those from using EPO can be obtained through high-altitude training, blood doping, and the use of hypoxic, hypobaric chambers at ground level.

Until 2000, EPO was undetectable. Individual sporting federations, such as cycling and triathlon organizations, have instigated blood testing, with upper limits of hematocrit levels (>50%) being deemed acceptable, leading to an indirect test "failure." Reticulocyte count has also been used as an indirect test. Although urine tests are now available, many question their accuracy.

Blood doping

Blood doping involves the intravenous transfusion of blood into an individual in order to increase red cell mass and thus improved oxygen-carrying capacity. It occurred more commonly in the 1970s and 1980s than now, and the need for this practice has been largely superseded by the abuse of EPO. Blood doping was banned by the International Olympic Committee (IOC) in 1986.

In many cases, autologous transfusions were used, which involved taking two units of blood from an athlete 6 weeks prior to competition (often while training at altitude), then reinfusing the blood on the day before competition. It is reported that this process could increase an individual's hematocrit by 5%–10%.

Growth hormone (GH)

GH is produced from the anterior pituitary and is released in a pulsatile nature. Levels are highest in childhood and adolescence and decrease throughout adulthood. The actions of GH are mediated through insulin-like growth factor 1 (IGF-1). GH acts to

- Increase protein synthesis and fat breakdown.
- Increase hepatic glucose production.
- Stimulate the liver to produce IGF-1, which helps muscle and bone growth.

GH appears to have anabolic properties; however, there have been no studies to prove that it provides benefits in performance.

Adverse effects are rare but include the following:

- Slipped capital femoral epiphysis (SCFE)
- Pseudotumor cerebri
- Fluid retention
- Increased risk of cardiovascular disease
- Hypertension
- Pancreatitis
- Joint pains
- Acromegally
- Insulin resistance

GH is now available commercially as a recombinant product, but was previously made from pituitary glands extracted postmortem. This latter process carried a risk of the recipient developing human variant Creuztfeldt–Jakob disease (CJD). GH works synergistically with testosterone. Many of its effects rely on insulin, and the two drugs are often abused in combination.

Recently, a seemingly reliable blood test for recombinant GH has allowed its direct measurement

Stimulants

Amphetamines

Athletes have abused amphetamines for over 70 years, and several high-profile deaths have been linked to their use. Amphetamines include Adderall, Dexedrine, Benzedrine, and Methedrine. The main ergogenic benefits of amphetamines are as follows:

- Increased awareness and delayed fatigue
- Enhancement of speed, power, endurance, and concentration

Adverse effects of amphetamines

- Amphetamines are highly addictive
- Delirium
- Paranoia
- Aggression
- Risk of cerebral hemorrhage

Adderall is a schedule C-II drug in the United States and is used for treatment of attention deficit hyperactivity disorder (ADHD). The National Collegiate Athletic Association (NCAA) requires documentation of this diagnosis for athletes prescribed this medication.

Modafinil

Modafinil, a stimulant licensed to treat the familial condition of narcolepsy, has recently become a drug of abuse in sports. The drug is not thought to be performance enhancing, but there is speculation that its main use is as a masking agent for new designer steroids.

Side effects include headache, nausea, insomnia, anxiety, tachycardia, and Stevens–Johnson syndrome.

Sympathomimetics

Sympathomimetics mimic the effects of epinephrine and norepinephrine and are readily available over-the-counter (OTC) remedies, used as treatments for the common cold. Many of these drugs are not performance enhancing but have been abused for years to increase energy.

Adverse effects of sympathomimetics

- Anxiety
- Agitation
- Headaches
- Hypertension
- Tremor
- Cardiac arrhythmias and myocardial infarction

Most of the drugs in this group were removed from the World Anti-Doping Agency (WADA) banned list in 2004, although ephedrine remains included.

Ephedrine was a popular herbal supplement often used in combination with caffeine to increase energy and increase lean mass. There was a strong association between ephedrine and catastrophic adverse effects such as arrhythmias, stroke, seizure, and sudden death, which lead to the FDA removing this supplement from the market.

Athletes who require a "cold cure" should be advised to always check with a doctor before taking any such drugs, even though purchased through a pharmacy. Different countries may have the same preparation on sale, but the contents can vary, which can lead to an inadvertent doping offense, particularly when traveling. Phenylephrine and pseudoephedrine are not banned.

Caffeine

Caffeine has been shown to be ergogenic at levels of 250–700 mg. However, in regular users there seems to be no significant ergogenic affect. Caffeine has been reported to decrease time to fatigue, which would be beneficial in endurance events.

Caffeine is no longer on the WADA banned list of drugs. The NCAA still monitors caffeine use and has set the maximal urine level at 15 mcg/mL.

One cup of coffee = 85 mg. Urine levels increase 1.5 mcg/mL for every 100 mg of caffeine ingested. Levels vary depending on whether the source is dietary (coffee, tea, soft drinks) or in the concentrated pill form.

Caffeine spares glycogen and thus delays the onset of fatigue. It exerts its effect by stimulating adipose tissue to release fatty acids and stimulates adrenaline production from the adrenal medulla, thus, in turn, further facilitating fatty acid release. Caffeine has also been shown to enhance motor unit recruitment.

Side effects are jitteriness and increased heart rate and blood pressure.

Beta-2 adrenoceptor agonists

- These include the drug albuterol and related compounds.
- These are potent treatments used in everyday practice to treat asthma.
- Orally, beta-2 agonists are not permitted in sports because of the anabolic benefits associated with these formulations.
- There is no evidence that these drugs, in inhaled form, are ergogenic in the nonasthmatic athlete.
- WADA does not allow the inhaled form, unless the athlete has submitted an *abbreviated therapeutic use exemption (aTUE)*. The NCAA allows the inhaled form without the requirement of special exemption forms.
- An aTUE must be completed by the usual prescribing doctor and sent to the involved sport's governing body with laboratory evidence confirming the diagnosis of exercise-induced asthma (EIA).

Tests for exercise-induced asthma

The athlete must have symptoms such as wheezing, chest tightness, or cough produced by hyperventilation or exercise that coincide with having EIA prior to being tested.

There are two approved methods by which athletes with EIA can meet the diagnostic criteria to obtain an aTUE:

- Spirometry demonstrating an increase in airway obstruction with pre- and post-exercise challenge that is reversed by inhaled beta-2 agonist
- Bronchial provocation test, which includes the following:
  - Methacholine aerosol challenge
  - Mannitol inhalation
  - The eucapnic voluntary hyperpnea (EVH) test
  - Hypertonic saline aerosol challenge
  - Exercise challenge tests (field or laboratory)

The athlete should then be treated with the lowest dose possible to achieve results. If the treatment dose results in levels >1000 ng/mL, then documentation needs to be provided to support the need for such a high treatment dose or it will be considered a positive test.

aTUE is valid for 4 years, but diagnosis needs to be clinically confirmed by a physician on a yearly basis.

Dietary ergogenic aids

Dietary supplements

Widespread use of supplements in sports is controversial. There is little evidence to support the use of supplements as ergogenic aids. The risk of contamination of supplements by banned substances is a concern.

A recent study found that as many as 19% of supplements produced in a selection of countries contained banned substances that were not mentioned on the product label.

Many high-profile sports stars have blamed their failed drug tests on a contamination of their supplements, taken in good faith. Athletes should be strongly advised to be extremely cautious about the use of any supplements, as athletes take them at their own personal risk of liability.

Carbohydrates
- The primary energy source for anaerobic activity
- Athletic diet should include 55%–70% of total calories as carbohydrate (approximately 5–10 g/kg body weight)

Proteins
- The recommended daily intake varies depending on the demands of the sport in which a person participates, with the range between 1.2 and 2 g/kg body weight.
- Strength and power athletes tend to require a larger intake than that required by athletes undertaking endurance exercise (endurance athletes: 1.2–1.4 g/kg/day; strength athletes: 1.6–1.7 g/kg/day).
- Protein supplements are useful for gaining strength during conditioning and are used post-exercise to aid recovery.
- There is no evidence that increased protein enhances performance.
- Branched-chain amino acids (BCAA) may decrease exercise-induced muscle breakdown but only in the untrained athlete. The trained athlete's body has adapted to exercise and this benefit is no longer noticed after 6–8 weeks. There is no associated ergogenic benefit.

Creatine monohydrate
- Physiologically active substance needed for muscle contraction; acts to regenerate ATP and thus serves as an energy store for short burst
- Present in the normal diet, particularly in meat
- Also synthesized in the body (liver, kidneys, pancreas)
- Increases phosphocreatine production, theoretically increasing the available energy during maximal exercise
- Some evidence that creatine enhances performance in short bursts of stationary cycling, sprints, and weight lifting when maximal efforts are being used
- Causes weight gain, although this may be due to water retention rather than muscle mass gain

Adverse effects

These include muscle cramps, GI disturbances, and a possible correlation with heat-related illnesses. It is theorized that there could be renal and hepatic damage; however, there are no short- or long-term studies to support this. Creatine monohydrate could potentially increase compartment pressures, leading to exercised-induced compartment syndrome.

Antioxidants

- They are vitamins and other compounds that occur naturally in the diet.
- They act to destroy free radicals in the body.
- Free radicals are produced as a by-product of high-intensity exercise and increased oxygen consumption, or as part of the normal process of inflammation and tissue healing.
- Free radicals are known to damage DNA and RNA and to destroy important enzymes. They are linked to arteriosclerosis, some cancers, and aging as well as exercise-associated muscle damage.
- Antioxidants such as beta-carotene (vitamin A precursor), vitamins C and E, selenium, and glutathione all are present in a normal healthy diet, which should contain at least five portions of fruit and vegetables daily. Such a diet is likely to give athletes their recommended daily allowance (RDA) of vitamins.
- Most commercial multivitamins will also contain ample antioxidants to satisfy the RDA. The potential benefits of taking a simple multivitamin probably outweigh any risks, but there is not enough evidence to recommend taking supplements to reduce post-exercise muscle damage.

Chromium

- Potentiates insulin action and thus cellular glucose and amino acid uptake
- In theory, might produce muscle mass gain, but evidence for this is lacking
- Also has the potential to induce iron and zinc deficiency through competition for binding sites and reduced absorption

Magnesium

- An essential mineral and a cofactor in many enzymatic reactions
- While a typical Western diet may be deficient in magnesium, supplementation has not been proven to be performance enhancing

L-carnitine

- Detoxifies ammonia, a by-product of metabolism associated with fatigue
- Responsible for long-chain fatty acid transport into mitochondria
- In theory, muscle glycogen will be spared and fatty acid oxidation increased, but studies are inconclusive

Beta-hydroxy-beta-methylbutyrate (HMB)

- A bioactive metabolite produced from breakdown of the amino acid leucine
- May increase fatty acid oxidation and reduce protein loss during stress by inhibiting protein catabolism
- Advertised to increase muscle mass and strength, but no studies support this
- Used by resistance-trained athletes

Glutamine

- A nonessential amino acid that is synthesized in the liver, lungs, adipose tissue, and skeletal muscle
- Stored in muscle and used for immunity, as a fuel for cells, for protein synthesis, and to maintain acid–base balance
- It has been hypothesized that intense exercise can increase demand for glutamine, leading to its depletion and thus an increased susceptibility to infection
- Although published evidence is lacking to support its use, some claim that glutamine enhances immune cell function in those at risk by undertaking high-intensity exercise

Fish and seed oils

- Athletic diets have tended to be low in these oils, which contain omega-3 oils and essential fatty acids.
- Omega-3 oils are known to have a cardioprotective effect, and it may simply be good advice for general health reasons for an athlete to include oily fish in their diet.

Lactic acid

- A by-product of anaerobic glycolysis, which builds up in muscle and blood during exercise
- Recently found to also act as a fuel during submaximal exercise, particularly by the heart, liver, and kidneys, to generate ATP
- The liver uses any remaining lactic acid for gluconeogenesis in an attempt to restore glycogen levels and maintain glucose levels

Sodium bicarbonate

- Neutralizes metabolic acids, including lactic acid
- Supplementation is said to produce an alkaline reserve to neutralize the hydrogen ions produced in anaerobic glycolysis and thus reduce the onset of fatigue

Prohibited drugs

Doping has been defined on many occasions, but in 1991 the UK Sports Council stated the following:

"Doping is the use by or distribution to a sports man (or woman) of any substance defined by (governing body, international federation, or IOC) as a banned class."

Brief history

- *1968*: Drug testing first started at the Grenoble Winter Olympics.
- *1974*: Semi-reliable tests for anabolic steroids became available.
- *1976*: Eight athletes tested positive for anabolic steroids. Rumors were rife of widespread use by athletes and swimmers despite the small number of positive tests.
- *1983*: A urine test was developed to determine the ratio between testosterone and epitestosterone.

These isomers usually exist in the body in a 1:1 ratio, so any exogenous testosterone taken would alter this. A ratio of 6:1 implies suspicion that an athlete has taken an anabolic steroid, although 10:1 is more likely to produce a guilty verdict in a court of law. Exogenous epitestosterone has also been abused in an attempt to mask any changes in the ratio caused by taking anabolic steroids.

World Anti-Doping Agency (WADA)

The banned list is no longer operated by the International Olympic Committee, and responsibility has passed to the World Anti-Doping Agency (WADA), established in 1999 after the World Conference on Doping in Sport in Lausanne recognized the need for an independent agency. The aims of WADA are to set unified standards for anti-doping work and to coordinate efforts against doping, seeking to foster a drug-free culture in sport.

Out-of-competition testing is conducted by independent parties. In 2003, the World Anti-Doping Code was accepted and most sports have agreed to implement the code.

Where can the banned list be seen?

The Banned List is available online at the WADA Web site, along with educational pages: http://www.wada-ama.org/en/t1.asp

It must be stressed that it is the athletes' responsibility to adhere to WADA regulations; ignorance is not considered a defense.

Outline of banned classes of drugs (for Olympic athletes)

Stimulants
- Amphetamines and related drugs
- Epinephrine and related drugs
- Ephedrine
- Cocaine

Narcotics
- Morphine and related drugs—note that codeine is not banned.

Cannabinoids
Hashish and marijuana are banned in competition.

Anabolic steroids
- Testosterone derivatives and related compounds

Peptide hormones and analogues
- Erythropoietin
- Growth hormone
- Insulin
- HCG

Beta-2 agonists
- Salbutamol and related drugs

Anti-estrogens (banned in males only)
- Tamoxifen
- Clomiphene

Masking agents
- Probenecid
- Diuretics
- Epitestosterone

Glucocorticosteroids
These drugs are banned orally, rectally, intravenously, or intramuscularly, though exemptions for genuine medical illness on production of evidence may be granted. Use in topical form is subject to TUE application.

Prohibited methods
- Blood doping
- Chemical manipulation
- Self-catheterization
- Gene doping

Prohibited in certain sports
- Alcohol
- Beta-blockers (shooting, archery)

Advice to doctors prescribing for athletes
Doctors who prescribe for athletes who may be liable for drug testing must be aware of the banned list of substances. The substances banned may vary depending on the sport and at what level the athlete is competing (NCAA, Olympics, NFL, MLB, NHL, NBA); therefore, physicians must be aware of the most current banned substance lists.

Most doctors will be able to access Internet resources through several valuable sites, such as the NCAA banned list at www.ncaa.org/health-safety. The banned substance list for the Olympics can be found at the WADA site at www.wada-ama.org.

Although the athlete is ultimately responsible for whatever substance is found on drug testing, incorrect prescribing by a sports doctor is a potential medicolegal issue. If in doubt, do not prescribe!

Drug testing

Drug testing varies, depending on the governing body responsible for monitoring of illegal substances (WADA, NCAA, professional or national sporting organizations, etc.). The goals of drug testing are to deter athletes from gaining an unfair advantage, to catch athletes who have taken performance-enhancing substances, and to remind them of the regulations and the inadvertent use of banned substances in an effort to eliminate any unfair advantages gained through illegal ergogenic aids.

It is imperative that athletes and physicians caring for athletes be aware that drug testing occurs in season as well as out of season. It is also important to understand the regulations set forth by the governing body for the particular sport in which the athlete is participating. It is beyond the scope of this chapter to discuss the differences in drug testing for individual sports and between the different governing bodies.

The rules, regulations, and consequences regarding ergogenic aids are usually provided to athletes at the beginning of the season and can be found online. The following Web sites can be used to find several guidelines for the NCAA, Olympics, and US sports: www.ncaa.org/health-safety, www.wada-ama.org, www.teamusa.org.

Future concerns

Designer drugs

New ergogenic aids are constantly being introduced to the sports arena. Designer drugs such as some of the recent steroids that are harder to detect make the job of regulating these agents more difficult. There must be constant monitoring and education for athletes to help prevent these newer agents from harming athletes and tarnishing the various sporting events.

Gene doping

The future of doping seems certain to involve genetic manipulation. WADA defines gene doping as "the non-therapeutic use of genes, genetic elements, or of the modulation of gene expressions, having the capacity to improve athletic performance."

Gene therapy is already used to treat muscular dystrophies, and experiments in mice show that genetic manipulation can increase muscle mass by 25%. The modified gene works via IGF-1 to increase muscle cell division. The gene is attached to an inert virus, causing "infection" in muscle cells, but no disease process in the host.

Scientists are currently working on tests to detect gene doping.

Physical therapy and rehabilitation

Physical therapy

Physical therapy

Physical therapy is a dynamic profession with an established theoretical and scientific base with widespread clinical applications in the restoration, maintenance, and promotion of optimal physical function. The role of physical therapists includes the following:

- Diagnosing and managing movement dysfunction and enhancing physical and functional abilities
- Restoring, maintaining, and promoting not only optimal physical function but also optimal wellness and fitness and optimal quality of life as it relates to movement and health
- Preventing the onset, symptoms, and progression of impairments, functional limitations, and disabilities that may result from disease, disorders, conditions, or injuries

Common interventions provided by physical therapists

- Therapeutic exercise
- Manual therapy (including mobilization and manipulation)
- Functional training (self-care, work, school, ADL, leisure integration)
- Prescription, application, fabrication of assistive devices and equipment
- Airway-clearance techniques
- Electrotherapeutic modalities
- Physical agents and mechanical

Further reading

Guide to Physical Therapist Practice, 2nd ed. *Phys Ther* 2001; **81**:9–744.

Principles of rehabilitation

The principles of rehabilitation following any injury can be broadly classified into three phases—early, middle, and late. These stages are not mutually exclusive. Short- and long-term goals should be defined for each patient and reviewed at appropriate time intervals, depending on the injury. Appropriate clinical markers should be used to define the progression of rehabilitation.

Patients should not be allowed to progress until they have, ideally, completed each stage without difficulty. Rehabilitation protocols should be used only as guidelines and each patient should have an individually negotiated rehabilitation plan.

Aerobic fitness, motor control, and coordination must be maintained where possible throughout rehabilitation.

The plan should be designed around what the patient can do, rather than what they cannot.

Early phase (protection of injured part)
- Strapping or bracing the injured part to prevent unwanted motion
- Non– or partial weight bearing with crutches may be necessary with lower-limb injury and a resultant antalgic gait.
- Relative rest
- Protect, rest, ice, compress, elevate (PRICE)

Middle phase
- Range of movement (ROM) and flexibility: aim to restore full range of joint motion (physiological and accessory) and muscle length
- Strength and conditioning (motor control and re-education, strength, power, and endurance)
- Proprioception: aim to restore normal kinesthetic awareness to the injured part
- Progression of proprioceptive exercises:
  - Static → dynamic
  - Conscious → automatic
  - Decrease the base of support
  - Decrease visual input
  - Functional

Late phase
- Agility drills: shuttle and sprint drills, cone and ladder drills. Start with straight-line work, progress to change of direction, cutting, and pivoting.
- Functional activities
- Sport-specific skills
- Power work
- Plyometric training (where appropriate)
- Identification of a safe return to full training

Prehabilitation

Physical therapy interventions are implemented prior to surgical intervention to enhance flexibility, motor control, strength, proprioception, and aerobic fitness.

The goal of prehabilitation is to promote optimal physical condition at the site of injury and throughout the body so that the patient will have a better physical base to build upon during the initial stages following surgery.

Determinants of outcome

- Age
- Preinjury activity level
- Postinjury expectation
- Motivation
- Associated injury

Physical therapy examination and screening

Four domains to an examination

1. Observation
2. Subjective/patient history
3. Differentiation
   - Red flag assessment
   - Neurological testing
   - Structural differentiation testing
4. Objective/physical examination
   - Active physiological
   - Passive physiological
   - Passive accessory
   - Confirmatory diagnostic clinical special tests

Upper quarter sequence

The upper quarter sequence functions to screen the cervical spine and upper extremities with the emphasis on differentiation between neurologically based pathology and musculoskeletal-based pathology.

- Observation/big picture: posture of spine, shoulder, upper extremities, head and neck
- Active ROM of cervical spine
- Full shoulder flexion
- Full shoulder external rotation
- Full shoulder internal rotation (behind back)
- Bilateral elbow and wrist extension
- Bilateral elbow and wrist flexion
- Resisted cervical rotation (C1)
- Resisted shoulder shrug (C2, 3, 4)
- Resisted shoulder abduction (C5)
- Resisted elbow flexion and wrist extension (C6)
- Resisted wrist flexion and elbow extension (C7)
- Resisted thumb extension (C8)
- Resisted finger abduction (T1)
- Sensory examination
- Reflex testing (biceps/brachioradialis C5–C6, triceps C7–C8)
- Upper motor neuron testing

Lower quarter sequence

The lower quarter sequence functions to screen the lumbar spine and lower extremities with the emphasis on differentiation between neurologically based pathology and musculoskeletal-based pathology.

- Observation/big picture: posture of spine, shoulder, upper extremities, head and neck
- Active ROM of the spine (flexion, extension, side bend, rotation)
- Deep squat
- Single-leg stance (L5–S1) (hip abduction sign)
- Heel walking (L4–L5)

- Toe walking (S1)
- Resisted hip flexion (L1–L2)
- Resisted knee extension or sit to stand on single leg (L3–L4)
- Resisted great toe extension (L5)
- Sensory examination
- Reflex testing (patellar tendon: L2–L3, Achilles L5–S1)
- Upper motor neuron testing

Gait analysis

Stance phase

- Heel strike to toe-off
- 60% gait cycle
- Two periods of double stance, 10% each

Swing phase

- 40% gait cycle
- Ankle dorsiflexes by the concentric contraction of anterior tibialis muscle
- Subtalar joint assumes near neutral position
- Toes dorsiflex slightly as foot prepares for next period of stance

Gait abnormality

Any variance in normal gait may result in numerous biomechanical compensations throughout the lower extremity, hip, and low back.

Weight shifting from side to side at mid-stance may indicate hip weakness.

Therapeutic modalities

A variety of these modalities are frequently used as an adjunct to treating soft tissue injury. The aim is to deliver physical energy to the tissue to help the natural healing process.

Cryotherapy

There are several ways to apply cold as a therapeutic modality. A few of the most common methods include ice pack, ice massage, compressive cold packs, and cold whirlpool.

Cryotherapy physiological processes

- Reduce the chemical mediators creating vasodilatation
- Decrease cellular metabolism (allowing cells to survive during periods of hypoxia)
- Decrease capillary permeability
- Increase threshold of afferent nerve ending, promoting pain reduction
- Decrease sensitivity of the muscle spindle, which n turn reduces the stretch reflex

Heat

Heat physiological processes

Cellular response during injury cycle

- Increase metabolic rate
- Increase waste excretion from cell
- Increase capillary flow

Blood and fluid dynamics

- Increase capillary permeability
- Increase blood flow
- Reabsorption of edema

Pain control

- Decrease muscle spindle sensitivity
- Stimulate afferent nerve endings
- Decrease muscle spasm
  - Decrease pressure on nerve ending
  - Improve blood and lymphatic flow
  - Improve ROM

Laser therapy

Laser physiological processes (theoretical)

- Increase cellular metabolism
  - Promote tissue-healing cycle
- Decrease pain
  - No thermal effect

Ultrasound

Ultrasound physiological processes

Heat production
- Sound waves create friction between molecules, which results in heat production.
- Collagen-rich tissues are preferentially heated (tendon, intramuscular fascia, bone, etc.)

Frequency parameter relates to depth of target tissue
- 1 MHz 2–5 cm (deep application)
- 3 MHz 1–2 cm (superficial application)

Research
Ultrasound seems to have some warming effect on superficial structures (1.2 cm); however, it has not been shown to have a significant warming effect at greater tissue depths (5 cm).

Electrical therapy

Electrotherapy physiological processes

Pain control
- Premodulated (constant current, 2 leads)
- Interferential (2 alternating currents, 4 leads)
- TENS (portable unit, two sets of 2 leads, constant current)

Mechanisms of pain control
- Reduce muscle spasm (mechanical pressure on nerve endings)
- Activate "gate mechanism" (high frequency)
- Release endorphins, encephalins (low frequency)

Neuromuscular (Russian)
- High frequency stimulates muscle contraction
  - Proven not to be effective alone for increasing strength
  - Combined with volitional exercise can help patient relearn how to activate a muscle

Manual therapy

Manual therapy techniques are skilled hand movements intended to improve tissue extensibility; increase range of motion; induce relaxation; mobilize or manipulate soft tissues and joints; modulate pain; and reduce soft tissue swelling, inflammation, or restriction.

Manual therapy techniques

- Mobilization and manipulation
  - Soft tissue
  - Spinal and peripheral joints
- Manual drainage
- Passive ROM
- Manual traction
- Massage
  - Connective tissue massage
  - Therapeutic massage

Joint arthrokinematics

Normal *arthrokinematics* indicate that active motion has accessory *movements* consisting of roll, glide, and spin. Without proper accessory movements, normal physiological motion cannot be safely achieved and joint hypomobility often is the result.

Joint mobilization and manipulation

Joint mobilization and manipulation techniques can be used to increase the accessory motion in hypomobile joints. Joint mobilization and manipulation increases the extensibility of tight joint capsules and ligaments that limit proper accessory motion and overall mobility of the joint. Restoration of accessory mobility is necessary to restore full physiological motion.

Further reading

Guide to Physical Therapist Practice. 2nd ed. *Phys Ther* 2001; **81**:9–744.

Stretching

Range of motion (muscle length and joint mobility)

Often the terms *stretching, flexibility,* and *mobility* are used interchangeably. Unfortunately, this can cause confusion, depending on the intent of the user, as they are truly different in their meanings.

Definitions

Range of motion (ROM) is the arc through which movement occurs at a joint or series of joints.

Muscle length is the maximum extensibility of a muscle–tendon unit. Muscle length, in conjunction with joint integrity and soft tissue extensibility, determines *flexibility*.

Joint *mobility* is the limits of ROM due to capsule–ligaments.

Stretching is an intervention to affect one's muscle length. The effects of stretching depend on whether one is trying to affect the muscle–tendon or the capsule–ligament.

Types of stretching

Passive stretching

This is externally applied force (manually or mechanically) to a muscle 30–60 seconds in duration. Appling force via an external source allows the patient's muscle to relax and elongate efficiently.

Ballistic stretching

This refers to high-intensity, short-duration stretching that results in rapid lengthening of the muscle. As a result, the muscle spindle is stimulated and facilitates a stretch reflex. Thus, the musculotendinous unit is susceptible to microtrauma with ballistic stretching.

Ballistic stretching may be beneficial immediately before performing in exercise, but only after a warm-up that includes slow static stretching.

Proprioneurofacilitation (PNF) stretching

Neurophysiological principles can be incorporated to relax muscles before elongation. This allows the contractile elements to be lengthened more easily. The two most common types are contract–relax and contract–relax–contract.

Contract–relax

During this technique, a passive stretch of the tight muscle is followed by a 5- to 10-second contraction of that same muscle. Following the contraction the patient relaxes and a passive stretch to the tight muscle is performed once again.

Neurophysiological principles state that the activation of the tight muscle via volitional contraction activates the Golgi-tendon organ, which inhibits the muscle spindle and results in decreased neurological excitation of the tight muscle group (autogenic inhibition), rendering it more susceptible to an efficient stretch.

Contract–relax–contract

This stretching technique is based on the same principle of autogenic inhibition as in contract–relax and incorporates the principle of reciprocal inhibition. Following the same process in contract–relax, a passive stretch of the tight muscle is followed by contraction of the tight muscle, then relaxation of the tight muscle. At this point, a contraction of the antagonist muscle (muscle opposing the tight muscle) is performed to the end ROM. The patient then relaxes and a passive stretch is performed once again.

Neurophysiological principles state that the activation of the antagonist muscle causes reciprocal inhibition of the agonist muscle (tight muscle), rendering it more susceptible to an efficient stretch.

Balance and proprioception

Definitions

Balance is an ability to maintain the center of gravity of a body within the base of support with minimal postural sway, in both static and dynamic positions.[1]

Proprioception is the awareness of one's posture, movement, balance, and location of various parts of the body in relation to each other, based on the sensations received by the sensors within the central (CNS) and peripheral (PNS) nervous systems.

Proprioception is modulated via afferent feedback from many areas:
- Visual and vestibular centers[2]
- *Musculoskeletal:* muscle spindles, tendon organs, joints (ligaments, disks, and menisci, pain fibers.

Biomechanics of balance

The body demonstrates postural sway in all directions. When the body's center of pressure is not immediately over its center of mass, the body moves. Resting muscle tone provides stiffness that prevents some motion. Muscles dynamically contract to restore position following perturbations.

The coupling effect of ligamentous trauma resulting in mechanical instability and proprioceptive deficits contributes to functional instability, which could ultimately lead to further microtrauma and re-injury.

Indications for balance training

- Prevention of falls and/or falls causing injury (especially in the geriatric population)
- Address fear of falling: someone with poor balance may alter behavior to avoid falls. This can have a dramatic impact on their quality of life.
- Neuromotor pathology (Parkinson's, etc.)
- Following musculoskeletal injury (sprain, strain, surgery)
- Prevention programs (ACL injury prevention programs, ankle injuries)

Role for secondary prevention

Proprioceptive deficits may predispose a patient to re-injury through decrements in the neuromuscular pathways, resulting in the limitation of complete rehabilitation.

Rehabilitation programs should be designed to include a proprioceptive component that addresses the following three levels of motor control: spinal reflexes, cognitive programming, and brainstem activity. Such a program is highly recommended to promote dynamic joint and functional stability.

1 Shumway-Cook A, Anson D, Haller S (1988). Postural sway biofeedback: its effect on reestablishing stance stability in hemiplegic patients, *Arch Phys Med Rehabil* **65**:395–400.
2 Tyldesling B, Greve J (1989). *Muscles, Nerves and Movement Kinesiology in Daily Living*. Boston: Blackwell Scientific, pp. 268–284.

Muscle performance

Definitions

Muscle performance is the capacity of a muscle or group of muscles to generate forces.

Strength is the muscle force exerted by a muscle or a group of muscles to overcome a resistance under a specific set of circumstances.

Power is the work produced per unit of time or the product of strength and speed.

Endurance is the ability of muscle to sustain forces repeatedly or to generate forces over a period of time.

The muscle force that can be generated depends on the interrelationships among such factors as the length of the muscle, velocity of the muscle contraction, and the mechanical advantage. Recruitment of motor units, fuel storage, and fuel delivery—in addition to balance, timing, and sequencing of contraction—mediate integrated muscle performance.

Principles of strength training

The fundamental principles of strength training to optimize the response are overload, specificity, and reversibility. When a muscle or group of muscles adapts to a given stimulus, additional loads must be applied for further adaptation to occur (SAID: specific adaptations to imposed demands).

During conditioning and/or rehabilitation, as adaptation to increasing workloads occurs, more loads need to be applied. This type of exercise is known as *progressive resistive exercise* (PRE).

Parameters of strength training

The parameters of a strength training program include speed, resistance, intensity, repetitions, frequency, and duration; the recovery time between bouts; the form of the exercise; and the range through which the muscle works.

Intensity

- The greater the load, the higher the intensity.
- Normally expressed as a percentage of 1 repetition maximum (1 RM)
- A resistance of 80%–95% 1 RM is optimal to maximize strength gains for most sports. This equates to 3–8 RM set.

Volume

- Volume = sets × repetitions × load
- In general, as intensity increases, volume decreases

Rest intervals and recovery

The total rest time between repetitions, sets, and exercises for the specific muscle being trained relates to the intensity of the training; 1- to 3-minute rest intervals between sets is common.

Frequency

During conditioning and rehabilitation when the emphasis is on regaining or maximizing muscle strength, this can be optimized by 2–4 sessions per week. Strength can be maintained by 1–2 sessions per week.

Mode
- Body weight
- Free weights
- Resistance machines
- Variable resistance—sport cord, Thera-Band
- Isokinetic machines

Specificity

The exercise chosen should target the specific muscle(s) with regard to its function during the specific activity or sport.

Reversibility

Any training adaptations will be reversed or reduced if training is stopped for 2–8 weeks.

Muscle training (isometric/isotonic/isokinetic)

During contraction, the internal force developed by muscle is known as *muscle tension*, and the external force acting on it is known as the *load* or *resistance*.

There are three types of muscle contraction:
- *Isometric*: Tension is generated within the muscle without a change in muscle length.
- *Isotonic*: Tension is generated within the muscle with a change in muscle length. During a *concentric* contraction the muscle shortens. During an *eccentric* contraction the muscle lengthens.
- *Isokinetic*: Tension is generated within the muscle where the velocity of contraction remains constant.

Only isometric and isotonic contractions occur naturally. Greater tension can be generated by an eccentric contraction than by a corresponding concentric contraction. Any isotonic contraction that results in a change in muscle length must initially have an isometric phase whereby enough tension is generated to overcome the load imposed.

Isokinetics can be used for assessment and training purposes. This is typically accomplished via the use of specialized equipment.

Physiological adaptation to exercise

- *Neurogenic:* responsible for early increases in strength. Occurs as a result of improved neuromuscular coordination, improved motor and activity learning, and increased activation of prime muscle movers
- *Myogenic:* occurs after ~8 weeks of consistent training. Occurs as a result of muscle hypertrophy
- Increase in muscle size, strength, and power
- Alters the mechanical properties of other connective tissues and bone

Age-related changes

As we become older we lose strength. There is debate about the effect of aging alone or disuse. Muscle mass decreases by 1% each year after the age of 60. A decrease in the number of muscle fibers (preferentially type II), results in slower contractile properties.

There is also a decrease in the number of motor units. Remaining units increase in size, but the reduction in number can compromise precision activities. However, studies consistently demonstrate the ability of the elderly to make strength gains with weight training.

Further reading

Guide to Physical Therapist Practice. 2nd ed. *Phys Ther* 2001; **81**:9–744

Plyometrics

Purpose

Plyometrics train power. Power is the ability to generate force in a very short period of time (e.g., jumping, sprinting). One study suggested that plyometrics are used by 90% of USA Division I strength and conditioning coaches, and another suggested that they are used by 94% of National Football League coaches.

Definition

Plyometrics refers to any exercise in which the muscle goes through an eccentric contraction–concentric contraction cycle repeatedly at a high rate of speed. In plyometrics the stretch–reflex is used to facilitate recruitment of additional motor units. It also loads both the elastic and contractile components of muscle.

- *Concentric exercise*: The muscle shortens as it generates force.
- *Eccentric exercise*: The muscle lengthens as it generates force because it is unable to overcome a greater force being applied to it.

Plyometric examples

- Jumping up and down from a box
- Push-ups and clapping hands when body is high
- Throwing and catching a ball against a trampoline rebounder
- High-speed resistive band concentric–eccentric exercises

Theoretical reasoning

Plyometrics is based on the SAID principle (specific adaptations to imposed demand). If one trains strength, strength is increased, but there are very small gains in power and endurance. Plyometrics are used for higher power production.

Plyometrics should be used for power jumping and throwing sports, or when acceleration is essential (sprint start).

Plyometric exercises are generally reserved for higher-level athletic programs or work-related training where these types of maneuvers need to be performed.

There are no meta-analyses or systematic reviews comparing plyometrics to other types of training. Some studies show that it is superior and some show no difference. The differing results may be due to differences in populations and/or required power output.

Safety

Plyometrics represent a high-intensity workout. As exercise intensity increases, the stress applied to muscles, tendons, and ligaments increases. If the stress applied to a tissue is greater than it can absorb, an injury can occur.

Plyometrics should typically be used in the later stages of rehabilitation and, whether in rehabilitation or conditioning, only after a solid foundation of strength and motor control has been established.

As with all exercises, the best way to prevent injury is to start slow and increase gradually.

Sports-specific fitness tests and training

Cardiorespiratory fitness tests

These tests are graded maximal exercise tests for aerobic capacity, e.g., shuttle run or beep test for VO_2 max.

Functional performance tests (FPTs)

Sporting activities require maneuvers that demand a combination of tri-planar movement and force production. In addition, sudden deceleration and change of direction are standard functional demands that must be accomplished with a high level of accuracy, often at high rates of speed.

FPTs assess a variety of musculoskeletal parameters simultaneously in order to assess patient limitations and deficits. In many FPTs the involved extremity is compared to the uninvolved extremity.

Some of the parameters assessed are as follows:
- Neuromuscular control
- Joint laxity and mobility
- Muscle extensibility (flexibility)
- Muscle strength and power
- Proprioception
- Dynamic balance
- Agility
- Pain
- Level of muscle performance conditioning
- Level of cardiovascular conditioning
- Athlete confidence

Functional tests can be performed unilaterally or b laterally, and objective parameters may be measured (repetitions, time, distance) and observed (quality of movement, body control, favoring of a injured body part, avoidance, compensatory patterns). They may be used as baseline tests (preseason), to monitor progress, or as an integral part of training.

They are used to guide rehabilitation interventions, set targets for return to sport, and determine the patient's ability to return or participate in their sport with minimal risks of injury.

These tests can include the following:
- Single-leg hop
- Single-leg triple hop
- Timed 6 m single-leg hop
- Linear crossover hop
- Lateral hop
- Rotational hops
- Vertical jump
- Stair and slope running
- Sprints
- Sprints with change of direction
- Carioca sprints
- Shuttle runs

- Figure 8 running
- Vertical squat jump
- Drop jump
- Interval running, kicking, throwing, hitting programs
- Sport-specific tasks (Lower-level sport-specific drills can be used as a component of the rehabilitation progression when a foundation of proper motor control, ROM, flexibility and mobility, and strength has been established.)

Orthotics

Indications for use

Orthotics are designed to correct abnormal foot and lower-limb biomechanics. Abnormal foot posture and biomechanics can cause abnormal lower-extremity posture and biomechanics, which can then contribute to improper muscle and joint use. Repetitive muscle and joint disuse promotes overuse injuries of the lower extremity (e.g., ITB friction syndrome, patellofemoral pain, patella tendinopathy, plantar fasciitis).

How do they work?
• Shock absorption
• Mechanical control of subtalar and midtarsal movement
• Neural control—afferent feedback from cutaneous receptors
• Muscle control—reduce muscle activation required to control the foot

Different types

Over-the-counter (OTC) heel cups or insoles are normally bought off the shelf. They generally are made of less durable material and provide less control and do not last as long as custom-made orthotics.

Custom-made orthotics follow the biomechanical assessment and plaster casting of the foot. They are generally made of more rigid material, provide more control, and last longer than OTC orthotics.

The choice of orthotics may depend on the following:
• Foot type
• The sport played and the type of footwear used
• The type of biomechanical problem
• Weight of the patient

Radiology

Imaging modalities

Plain radiograph (X-ray)
- This is typically first line for evaluation of bone injury, especially fractures and dislocations.
- A minimum of two orthogonal views should usually be obtained.

Advantages
- Fast acquisition time
- Inexpensive

Disadvantages
- Poor visualization of soft tissue
- Radiation exposure

Computed tomography (CT)
- CT provides enhanced evaluation of bony injury; it is especially useful for complex or occult injuries.
- Arthrography can aid evaluation of some joints.
- 3D reconstruction can be useful for surgical assessment.

Advantages
- Most accurate visualization of bone anatomy and some bone pathology
- Faster acquisition time than MR

Disadvantages
- Less accurate than MR for soft tissue visualization
- Significantly more radiation exposure than X-ray

Magnetic resonance (MR)
- MR provides enhanced evaluation of soft tissue injury such as muscles, tendons, ligaments, cartilage, and viscera.
- The two most fundamental sequences are T1-weighted (T1) and T2-weighted (T2).
- T1 typically provides better anatomic detail; fat appears hyperintense whereas water appears hypointense.
- T2 typically provides better pathological sensitivity; fat appears hypointense whereas water appears hyperintense.
- Arthrography can aid evaluation of some joints.

Advantages
- Most accurate visualization of soft tissue anatomy and pathology
- No radiation exposure

Disadvantages
- Less accurate than CT for bone anatomy and some bone pathology
- Prolonged acquisition time
- Expensive
- Contraindicated for patients with ferromagnetic implants or support devices

Ultrasound (US)

- Implementation varies highly with location and individual practice.
- US is useful for evaluating some anatomic relationships along with assessment of tendons and ligaments, especially the Achilles and rotator cuff tendons.

Advantages

- Images easily produced in any plane
- Fastest acquisition time
- No radiation exposure
- Inexpensive

Disadvantages

- Visualization limited by bone or gas-containing structures, as well as by depth
- Accuracy highly dependent on operator skill

Bone nuclear scintigraphy (bone scan)

- A bone scan has high sensitivity but low specificity for many bony pathologies, including stress fracture, bone contusion, avascular necrosis, and bone tumors; it is especially useful for occult pathology.
- Uptake of technetium-99m (^{99m}Tc) radiotracer occurs in three phases: perfusion phase (immediate), blood pooling phase (about 15 minutes), and the bone uptake phase (delayed, usually at least 2 hours).

Advantages

- High sensitivity for bone pathology
- Entire skeleton can be imaged simultaneously

Disadvantages

- Low specificity for most findings
- Prolonged acquisition time
- Radiation exposure

General pathology

Avulsion fracture

Modalities
- *X-ray*: first line, usually diagnostic
- *CT*: used if X-ray equivocal
- *MR*: used if X-ray is equivocal; particularly useful for nonhealing avulsion fracture of first proximal phalanx base

Views
- Vary with anatomic location
- Bilateral comparison views may be helpful

Anatomic location selected views
- *Calcaneus, anterior process*: anteroposterior (AP) foot view
- *Calcaneus, posterior tuberosity*: lateral foot view
- *Epicondyle*: AP, lateral, and oblique elbow views; consider valgus or varus stress views (for medial or lateral epicondyle, respectively) to accentuate displacement of fragment
- *First proximal phalanx base* (gamekeeper's fracture): AP and lateral thumb views
- *Fifth metatarsal tuberosity*: AP, lateral, and oblique foot views; AP and oblique ankle views if foot views are equivocal
- *Lateral malleolus*: AP, lateral, and mortise ankle views
- *Olecranon*: AP and lateral elbow views
- *Phalanx*: lateral finger view
- *Scaphoid*: bilateral PA in ulnar deviation, lateral, semipronated oblique, and scaphoid wrist views
- *Spinous process or transverse process*: AP, cross-table lateral, and oblique spine views
- *Tibial plateau, lateral* (Segond fracture): AP, lateral, and sunrise knee views; tunnel view if intra-articular fragment suspected
- *Tibial tubercle*: AP, lateral, oblique, and sunrise knee views

Findings
- Subchondral apophyseal fragment in various degrees of displacement
- Lateral tibial plateau (Segond fracture): nearly always associated with ACL tear
- First proximal phalanx base (gamekeeper's fracture): MR can identify whether the ulnar collateral ligament lies between the fragment and avulsion site (Stener lesion).
- MR: avulsed fragment and avulsion site demonstrate hypointense T1 signal. The avulsion site will also demonstrate hyperintense T2 signal.

Avascular necrosis
- Osteonecrosis resulting from ischemia

Modalities
- *X-ray*: first line; often equivocal, especially initially
- *CT*: used if X-ray equivocal and MR unavailable or contraindicated
- *MR*: most accurate and preferred modality

- *US*: adjunct
- *Bone scan*: initially more sensitive than X-ray, but low specificity

Views

- *Femoral head*: AP and frog-leg lateral hip views
- *Humeral head*: AP and axillary shoulder views
- *Lunate* (Kienböck malacia): AP, lateral, and oblique wrist views
- *Knee*: AP and lateral knee views
- *Metatarsal*: AP, lateral, and oblique foot views
- *Navicular* (Mueller–Weiss syndrome): lateral and oblique foot views, and coned-down AP view of the navicular
- *Scaphoid*: bilateral PA in ulnar deviation, lateral, semipronated oblique, and scaphoid wrist views
- *Talus*: AP, lateral, and mortise ankle views
- *Vertebral body* (Kümmell disease): AP, lateral, and oblique lumbosacral spine views

Findings

- Joint effusion, mottled density and patchy sclerosis, subchondral lucency and collapse (crescent sign), and articular surface fragmentation with variable displacement
- Femoral head may be associated with femoral neck fracture
- Lunate (Kienböck malacia): associated with negative ulnar variance
- Navicular (Mueller–Weiss syndrome): may have a comma shape from lateral collapse and medial or dorsal subluxation
- Scaphoid: associated with fracture nonunion of the proximal one-third scaphoid; proximal fragment demonstrates sclerosis and collapse
- Vertebral body (Kümmell disease): lumber vertebrae most often involved
- MR: decreased subchondral T1 signal intensity; may demonstrate a pathognomonic "double line" sign of hyperintense T2 signal adjacent and peripheral to hypointense T1 signal
- US: subchondral bony flattening
- Bone scan: area of decreased activity surrounded by area of increased activity (doughnut sign) may be demonstrated. Increased activity correlates with healing.

Chondroblastoma

- Usually benign cartilaginous tumor
- Usually occurs in the proximal tibia, proximal humerus, or distal femur

Modalities

- *X-ray*: first line
- *CT*: consider if X-ray equivocal or to determine extent of ep physeal or articular involvement
- *MR*: consider if other modalities equivocal

Views

- Vary with anatomic location, but at least two orthogonal views should be obtained

Findings

- Round lucency with narrow zone of transition, fine punctate calcifications, endosteal scalloping, and benign periosteal reaction
- Rim may be sclerotic
- CT may demonstrate calcifications, septa, and fluid–fluid level.
- MR: lesion has hypointense T1 signal intensity. T2 signal intensity is variable and heterogenous.

Chondrosarcoma

- Malignant cartilaginous tumor
- Usually occurs in the shoulder girdle, proximal humerus, spine, ribs, pelvis, or proximal femur
- Usually presents after 40 years of age

Modalities

- *X-ray*: first line; often equivocal
- *CT*: preferred modality for metastatic evaluation of thorax and for focal lesions if MR unavailable or contraindicated
- *MR*: preferred modality for focal lesions and surgical assessment
- *Bone scan*: preferred modality for metastatic evaluation of entire skeleton

Views

- Views vary with anatomic location, but at least two orthogonal views should be obtained.
- The entire extent of involved bone and adjacent joints should be imaged.

Findings

- Lucent lesion with endosteal scalloping, cortical destruction, and diffuse calcification that may be amorphic or circular
- MR: lobulated lesions that demonstrate hypointense T1 and hyperintense T2; septa demonstrate low signal intensity
- Bone scan: increased activity

Complex regional pain syndrome (reflex sympathetic dystrophy)

- Pain and sensory changes of an extremity following a noxious event

Modalities

- *X-ray*: adjunct
- *Bone scan*: adjunct
- *CT*: adjunct
- *MR*: adjunct

Views

- Vary with anatomic location

Findings

- Osteoporosis and patchy subchondral osteopenia with "Swiss-cheese" appearance
- Degenerative joint changes may occur.

- MR: contrast enhancement of soft tissues and muscle atrophy
- Bone scan: increased blood flow to affected extremity; diffuse asymmetric increased activity after approximately 6 weeks, especially at juxta-articulations of the wrist, hand, and digits

Giant cell tumor

- Usually benign multinucleated giant cell tumor
- Usually occurs in the distal femur, proximal tibial, proximal humerus, or distal radius

Modalities

- *X-ray*: first line, usually diagnostic
- *CT*: consider if X-ray equivocal, or to determine extent of epiphyseal or articular involvement
- *MR*: consider if other modalities equivocal

Views

- These vary with anatomic location, but at least two orthogonal views should be obtained.

Findings

- Nonsclerotic large, round lucency with narrow zone of transition
- Usually periosteal reaction is absent, but may demonstrate aggressive cortical destruction and soft tissue expansion with peripheral calcification
- Endosteal scalloping and septae give "soap bubble" appearance
- CT: may demonstrate fluid–fluid level
- MR: lesions demonstrate homogenous hypointense T1 signal and heterogenous intermediate-intensity T2 signal.

Myositis ossificans

- Extraskeletal ossification most often associated with trauma
- Typically will not manifest until at least 3 weeks after injury

Modalities

- *X-ray*: first line; may be incidental finding
- *CT*: used if other modalities cannot rule out malignancy
- *MR*: used if other modalities cannot rule out malignancy
- *US*: adjunct
- *Bone scan*: high sensitivity before full maturation; low specificity

Views

- Vary with anatomic location

Findings

- Soft tissue swelling initially, developing several weeks later into a homogenous lesion with peripheral lacy calcifications that are distinctly marginated and progress centrally (Fig. 20.1).
- Full maturation in approximately 6 months.
- MR: initially demonstrates hyperintense T2 signal within lesion
- US: echogenic mass
- Bone scan: extraskeletal increased activity until full maturation, then extraskeletal uptake typical of skeletal bone

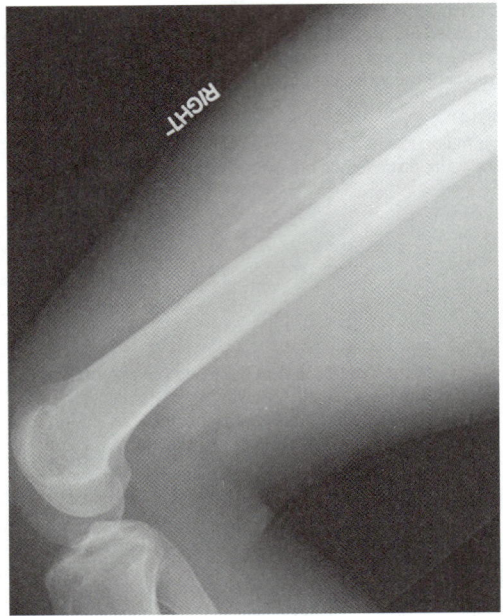

Figure 20.1 Lateral X-ray of the femur and knee demonstrating myositis ossificans within the quadriceps with characteristic lacy calcification.

Osteoarthritis (OA)

Modalities
- X-ray: first line; often equivocal initially
- CT: consider for spine assessment
- MR: used if X-ray equivocal
- Bone scan: adjunct

Views
- Vary with anatomic location
- Weight bearing views in weight-bearing joints
- Consider imaging the joints above and below the symptomatic joint.

Findings
- Joints most commonly affected include the first carpometacarpal joints, interphalangeal joints, knees, hips, subtalar joints, first metatarsophalangeal joints, and the facet joints of the cervical and lumber spine.
- Joint involvement is often asymmetric.

- Uneven joint-space narrowing, osteophyte formation, articular surface erosion, subchondral sclerosis, subchondral cysts, and subchondral collapse
- Hand: radial deviation of first metacarpal, along with bony prominences at proximal and distal interphalangeal joints (Bouchard and Heberden nodes, respectively)
- Knee: typically involves medial tibial plateau and lateral patella facet. Varus or valgus deformity may be present.
- Hip: flattening and superior migration of femoral head
- Foot: hallux valgus deformity
- Spine: associated with degenerative disc disease
- Pronounced erosions may occur at the sacroiliac, symphysis pubis, temporomandibular, and acromioclavicular joints.
- MR: cartilage thinning and fissuring may be demonstrated, as well as joint effusion. Surrounding bone edema demonstrates hypointense T1 and hyperintense T2 signal.
- Bone scan: increased activity

Osteochondral injury

Modalities
- *X-ray*: often first line, usually equivocal
- *CT*: adjunct
- *MR*: preferred modality, especially for evaluation of unstable fragment, though only rarely can it determine severity of cartilage injury
- *Bone scan*: adjunct

Views
- Vary with anatomic location

Findings
- Compression, subchondral defect, and displaced fragmentation may be demonstrated.
- MR: hyperintense T2 signal within the cartilage and surrounding bone. Completely denuded cartilage is indicated by a fluid-filled defect (Fig. 20.2).
- Bone scan: increased activity

Osteochondritis dissecans
- Osteochondral fracture with fragment detachment (complete or incomplete)

Modalities
- *X-ray*: first line; often equivocal
- *CT*: if X-ray equivocal and MR not available or contraindicated
- *MR*: detects occult lesions and correlates best with surgical staging; arthrogram may improve sensitivity
- *US*: advantageous for evaluating joint in motion
- *Bone scan*: activity correlates with healing

Views
- Vary with anatomic location

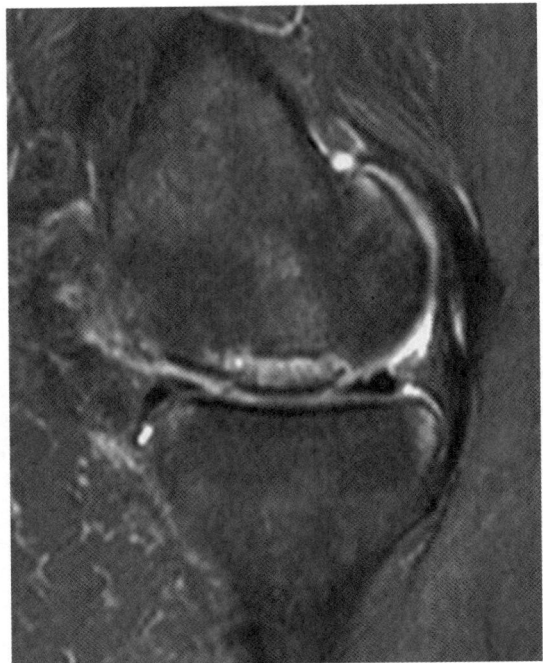

Figure 20.2 Sagittal MR demonstrating a large intra-articular osteochondral lesion of the medial femoral condyle.

- Capitellum: AP, lateral, and oblique elbow views
- Knee: AP, lateral, and tunnel knee views
- Talus: AP, lateral, and mortise ankle views

Findings
- Subchondral lucency, cysts, or compression fracture may be demonstrated.
- All modalities may reveal a subchondral fragment in various degrees of displacement.
- MR: diffuse hypointense T1 signal and hyperintense T2 signal
- US: subchondral bony flattening
- Bone scan: increased activity correlates with healing

Osteochondroma

- Most common benign bone tumor

Modalities

- *X-ray*: first line
- *CT*: used if X-ray equivocal and for surgical assessment
- *MR*: used if other modalities cannot rule out malignancy
- *US*: used to visualize the cartilaginous cap

Views

- These vary with anatomic location, but at least two orthogonal views should be obtained.

Findings

- Well-defined bony excrescence with mottled density, most often located at the metaphysis of long bones
- Cartilaginous cap may contain flakes of calcification
- MR: cartilaginous cap has hyperintenseT2 signal. Hyperintense ⁻2 signal in adjacent muscle may indicate impingement.
- US: hypoechoic cartilaginous cap covering hyperechoic bony excrescence

Osteomyelitis

Modalities

- *X-ray*: can be very useful, though often equivocal initially
- *CT*: used if other modalities equivocal and MR unavailable or contraindicated
- *MR*: most accurate modality, used if other modalities equivocal; especially useful for spine osteomyelitis
- *US*: adjunct
- *Bone scan*: preferred first line; used with dual tracer-labeled leukocyte and sulfur colloid marrow scans to increase specificity

Views

- Vary with anatomic location

Findings

- Soft tissue swelling, periosteal reaction, and cortical or medullary mottled lucencies
- Chronically, may demonstrate sclerosis, sinus tracts, new periosteal bone formation, sequestra, and involucrum
- MR: enhanced visualization of abscesses and surrounding soft tissue involvement. Marrow involvement demonstrates hypointense T1 and hyperintense T2 signal.
- US: periosteal elevation and thickening. Abscess or fluid collection may be demonstrated adjacent to bone.
- Bone scan: increased activity in all three phases with labeled leukocytes but not sulfur colloid accumulation at infection sight. Spine osteomyelitis is an exception.

Rheumatoid arthritis

- Systemic autoimmune inflammatory disease

Modalities

- *X-ray*: first line
- *MR*: used if X-ray equivocal; especially useful to evaluate cervical spine involvement
- *US*: adjunct

Views

- Vary with anatomic location
- PA of both hands and AP of both feet on initial diagnosis for baseline establishment
- Consider flexion and extension cervical spine views if assessment of instability is desired.

Findings

- Joints most often initially affected are the metacarpophalangeal joints and proximal interphalangeal joints. Other common locations include the knees, hips, feet, shoulders, and cervical spine.
- Joint involvement is often bilaterally symmetric.
- Erosion of cartilage and cortex starts at the joint margins, along with periarticular osteoporosis and cyst formation.
- Joint effusion may initially lead to joint-space widening, but cartilage destruction will eventually lead to uniform joint-space narrowing.
- Malalignment, displacement, and ankylosis of the joint spaces occur chronically.
- Hand: volar subluxation and ulnar deviation of CMC joints with radial deviation at the wrist (zig-zag deformity); nonreducible PIP joint hyperflexion and DIP joint hyperextension (boutonnière deformity) or PIP joint hyperextension and DIP joint hyperflexion (swan-neck deformity); phalangeal and metacarpal rotation and shortening (opera-glass hands); scaphoid and lunate rotational subluxation.
- Hip: axial migration of femoral head
- Knees: varus or valgus deformity may occur.
- Feet: lateral deviation of the toes, with metatarsal head plantar subluxation and phalangeal dorsal subluxation (hammertoe). Fallen arches and hallux valgus deformity may develop.
- Cervical spine: commonly affects the facet joints. Atlantoaxial subluxation or impaction may occur. Degenerative disc disease, instability, and spinal cord compression may develop.
- MR: periarticular bone edema demonstrates hypointense T1 and hyperintense T2 signal. Synovial hypertrophy and tendinopathy may be demonstrated.
- US: signs of synovitis such as proliferation and hypoechoic effusion. Rheumatoid nodules are fluid filled and have sharp margins. Tendinopathy may be demonstrated.

Septic arthritis

Modalities
- X-ray: first line; often equivocal
- CT: consider if X-ray equivocal and MR unavailable or contraindicated
- MR: most accurate modality; consider if X-ray equivocal
- US: adjunct
- Bone scan: much more sensitive then X-ray, but low specificity; especially low utility with prosthetic joints

Views
- Vary with anatomic location

Findings
- Periarticular soft tissue swelling, poorly defined cortical erosion, periarticular osteoporosis, and linear opacities due to calcium pyrophosphate deposition may be demonstrated.
- Initially effusion leads to joint-space widening, but cartilage destruction will cause chronic joint-space narrowing.
- Periarticular abscess as well as soft tissue or interarticular gas may be demonstrated.
- Transcortical sinus tracts and new periosteal bone formation are pathognomonic in the setting of a prosthetic joint; prosthesis loosening may also be demonstrated.
- US: may demonstrate periarticular abscess, joint effusion, and synovial hypertrophy
- Bone scan: increased activity
- Associated with osteomyelitis

Stress fracture

Modalities
- *X-ray:* first line; often equivocal, especially initially
- *CT:* consider if other modalities equivocal, though MR preferred if advanced imaging required
- *MR:* consider if X-ray equivocal; more specific than bone scan and perhaps even more sensitive in the setting of osteoporosis
- *Bone scan:* consider if X-ray equivocal; may be positive before onset and after resolution of symptoms; high sensitivity but low specificity

Views
- Vary with anatomic location

Anatomic location views
- *ACL* (intercondylar eminence fracture): AP and lateral knee views
- *Calcaneus:* lateral foot view
- *Epicondyle:* AP, lateral, and oblique elbow views
- *Medial malleolus:* AP, lateral, and mortise ankle views
- *Metatarsals:* AP, lateral, and oblique foot views
- *Navicular:* coned-down AP view of the navicular, though often equivocal; bone scan, CT, or MR should be considered

- *Patella:* bone scan can differentiate from bipartite patella
- *Pelvis and femoral neck:* AP and frog-leg lateral views
- *Sesamoids, feet:* AP, lateral, axial sesamoid, and medial and lateral oblique foot views
- *Talus:* AP, lateral, oblique, and talar neck views
- *Tibia:* AP and lateral lower-leg views

Findings

- Benign cortical thickening with thin lucency disrupting the cortex, or linear sclerosis
- MR: fracture demonstrated as thin, linear, hypointense T1 signal surrounded by marrow edema indicated by hyperintense T2 signal. The thickened periosteum demonstrates hypointense T1 and T2 signal.
- Bone scan: focal increased activity

Tendinopathy

Modalities

- *X-ray:* typically equivocal
- *MR:* used in the presence of treatment failure when other modalities equivocal
- *US:* adjunct

Views

- Vary with anatomic location

Findings

- Periosteal reaction at bony insertion and calcium deposits within the tendon may be demonstrated.
- MR: hyperintense T2 signal within and surrounding the tendon
- US: altered tendon morphology such as thickening. Hypoechoic or hyperechoic foci within the tendon may be demonstrated.

Hip and pelvis

Plain radiographic views of the hip and pelvis

Standard views

- *AP*: patient supine, leg rotated 15° internally; beam directed toward femoral head
- *Lateral*: patient supine, contralateral hip abducted and flexed; beam tilted 20° cephalad and directed through groin toward femoral head

Additional views

- *AP pelvis*: bilaterally demonstrates femoral head, femoral neck, greater trochanter, iliac, pubis, and sacrum
- *Flamingo*: AP centered on symphysis pubis; patient alternatively stands on each leg
- *Frog-leg lateral*: patient supine, thighs in maximum abduction, knees flexed, soles of feet together; beam directed vertically just above the symphysis pubis
- *Johnson lateral*: lateral with beam tilted 25° cephalad, 25° posterior, and directed through groin toward femoral neck
- *Inlet*: AP with beam parallel to sacrum and tilted 25° caudad
- *Internal and external oblique* (Judet views): patient supine, each hip alternately anteriorly rotated 45°; beam directed toward femoral head
- *Outlet*: AP with beam perpendicular to sacrum and tilted 35° cephalad

Acetabulum labral tear

Modalities

- *X-ray*: nondiagnostic
- *CT*: used with arthrography only if MR contraindicated or unavailable
- *MR*: preferred modality; most accurate with arthrography or with high field strength (3T)

Findings

- Fluid within the labrum or between the labrum and the bony acetabulum, detachment of the labrum from the bony acetabulum, and blunting truncation of the labrum (Fig. 20.3).
- Osteoarthritis findings may be associated.

Athletic pubalgia

- Inflammation of the pubis symphysis

Modalities

- *X-ray*: first line; often equivocal, especially initially
- *MR*: used if other modalities equivocal. Arthrography can improve accuracy.
- *Bone scan*: adjunct; positive earlier than X-ray

Additional views

- AP pelvis and bilateral flamingo hip views

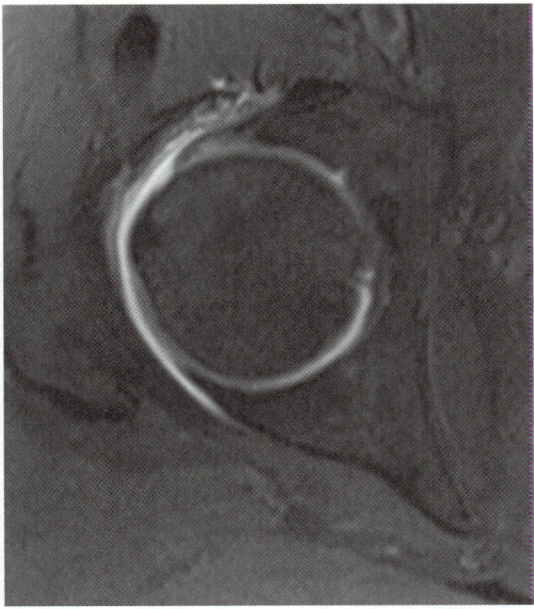

Figure 20.3 Axial MR arthrogram demonstrating extension of hyperintense contrast within and beneath the anterior acetabular labrum, characteristic of a tear.

Findings
- Periarticular sclerosis and osteolysis with widening symphysis and irregular joint contour
- >2 mm transition of superior pubic rami may be demonstrated in bilateral flamingo views
- MR: fibrocartilaginous disk inflammation and bone edema may be demonstrated. With arthrography, contrast extension within or inferior to the joint is characteristic (secondary cleft sign) (Fig. 20.4).
- Bone scan: increased activity at symphysis

Femoral head subluxation and dislocation
Modalities
- *X-ray*: first line. Pre- and post-reduction views should be obtained.
- *CT*: used to evaluate failed closed reduction and for surgical assessment
- *MR*: preferred modality for chronic screening of femoral head avascular necrosis; consider in the acute setting for an elite athlete

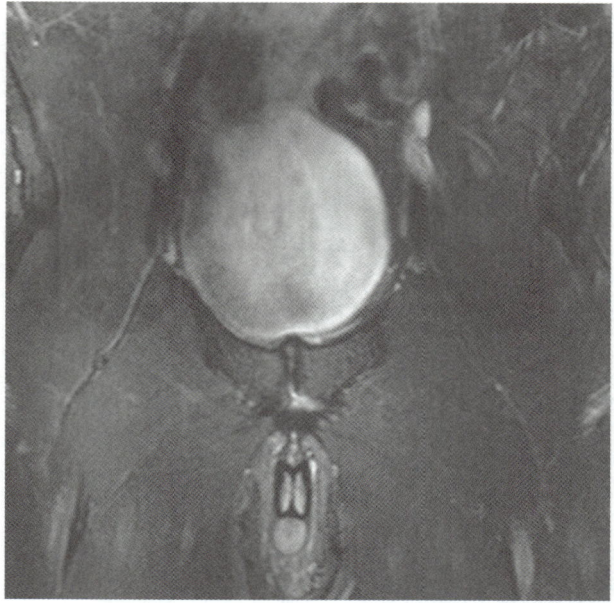

Figure 20.4 Coronal MR arthrogram demonstrating athetic pubalgia with characteristic extension of hyperintense contrast within the pubic symphysis (secondary cleft sign).

Additional views
- Internal and external oblique (Judet) hip views
- Johnson lateral hip view may be considered to avoid moving the injured hip.
- Inlet and outlet hip views may be considered to enhance evaluation of pelvic integrity.

Findings
- *Posterior dislocation*: adduction and internal rotation of femur is demonstrated. The femoral head is displaced laterally and superiorly and will appear small in the AP view.
- *Anterior dislocation*: abduction and external rotation of the femur. The femoral head is displaced medially and inferiorly and will appear large in the AP view.
- *Central dislocation*: the femoral head is forced centrally through the acetabulum, causing fracture.
- *MR*: tendon and ligament avulsion is often demonstrated, especially the ligament of head of femur.

- Widened joint space in post-reduction views indicates intra-articular bony fragment or soft tissue displacement.
- Associated with fractures of the acetabulum, pelvis, femoral head, femoral neck, and femoral shaft, as well as loose bony fragments

Femoral shaft fracture

Modalities
- *X-ray*: first line; usually diagnostic
- *CT*: used for complex or occult fractures and for surgical assessment
- *MR*: used if assessment of concomitant soft tissue injury desired

Additional views
- AP pelvis, and AP and lateral knee views that image the entire femur
- Trauma series if appropriate

Findings
- Fracture may be open, closed, spiral, transverse, oblique, or comminuted.
- Associated with other traumatic fractures, especially of the femoral neck

Sacroiliitis

Modalities
- *X-ray*: first line
- *CT*: considered if other modalities equivocal
- *MR*: considered if other modalities equivocal
- *Bone scan*: adjunct

Findings
- Bilateral irregular erosions, widening, and sclerosis of the articular surface, progressing to narrowing and fusion
- MR: hyperintense T2 signal along the SI joints demonstrated
- Bone scan: increased activity bilaterally along SI joints
- Associated with ankylosing spondylitis and other degenerative joint findings

Snapping hip syndrome

- Due to irregular tendon motion over the greater trochanter, lesser trochanter, femoral head, or iliopectineal eminence

Modalities
- *X-ray*: nondiagnostic, but usually obtained to rule out other pathology
- *MR*: used if other modalities equivocal
- *US*: advantageous to evaluate joint in motion

Additional views
- Frog-leg lateral hip views

Findings
- MR: affected tendon may be thickened, and hyperintense T2 signal may be demonstrated within the tendon and adjacent bursa.
- US: dynamic tendon subluxation may be demonstrated.

Trochanteric bursitis
- Inflamed bursa between greater trochanter and iliotibial tract

Modalities
- *X-ray*: nondiagnostic, but usually obtained to rule out other pathology
- *MR*: considered to rule out other pathology
- *US*: useful for differentiating from tendonitis

Additional views
- Standing AP pelvis

Findings
- Calcification within the bursa may be present.
- MR: bursa may demonstrate hyperintense T2 signal
- US: fluid collection may be demonstrated

Knee

Plain radiographic views of the knee

Standard views
- AP: patient supine, leg extended; beam tilted 5° cephalad
- Lateral: patient decubitus on side to be imaged, knee flexed 25°; **beam tilted 5° cephalad**

Additional views
- Internal and external oblique: lateral with beam anteriorly rotated 45° **from each side**.
- Sunrise: bilateral knees in one view; patient prone, knees flexed 115°; beam tilted 15° **cephalad and directed toward patella**
- Tunnel: AP with knee flexed 40°, beam tilted 40° caudad

Anterior cruciate ligament (ACL) tear

Modalities
- X-ray: nondiagnostic, but usually obtained to rule out other pathology
- MR: preferred modality
- US: adjunct

Additional views
- Sunrise and tunnel knee views

Findings
- Avulsion fractures of the lateral condyle or posterior lateral tibial plateau (Segond fracture) may be demonstrated
- The tibia may have abnormal anterior translocation.
- MR: ACL is absent or only remnants of disrupted fibers are seen in sagittal T2-weighted images. Bone contusions of the lateral femoral condyle and posterior lateral tibial plateau are often demonstrated with hyperintense T2 signal (Fig. 20.5).

Discoid lateral meniscus
- Can disrupt articular motion

Modalities
- X-ray: nondiagnostic, but usually obtained to rule out other pathology.
- MR: preferred modality for preoperative evaluation and only modality to evaluate concomitant tear

Findings
- Often bilateral
- Subtly widened lateral joint space, hypoplasia of the lateral tibial spine, and concavity or "cupping" of the lateral tibial plateau may be demonstrated on X-ray.
- MR: meniscal tissue slab "bow-tie" visualized in three contiguous sagittal sections

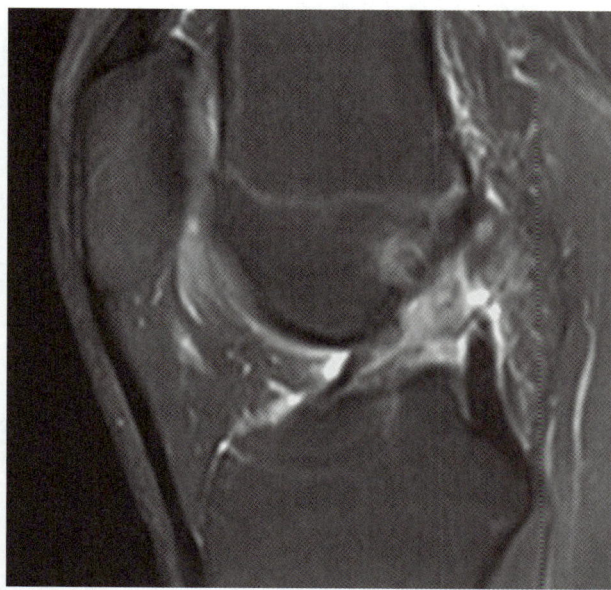

Figure 20.5 Sagittal MR demonstrating disruption of the anterior cruciate ligament (ACL) within the knee joint. The ligament would normally have a homogeneously hypointense appearance, similar to the posterior cruciate ligament that can be seen rising from the posterior tibia.

Iliotibial band friction syndrome (ITBFS)

Modalities

- X-ray: nondiagnostic, but usually obtained to rule out other pathology
- MR: used in the face of treatment failure if other modalities are equivocal.
- US: may visualize impingement during motion

Additional views

- Sunrise knee view

Findings

- Knee may have varus alignment
- MR: hyperintense T2 signal beneath the band, at the periosteal attachment, and band thickening
- US: iliotibial band impingement during motion

Jumper's knee (Sinding–Larsen–Johansson syndrome)

- Insertion tendinopathy at distal or proximal pole of patella

Modalities

- *X-ray*: nondiagnostic; used if rule out of other pathology is desired

Additional views

- Sunrise knee view

Findings

- Tendon calcification and patellar lucency at insertion site may be demonstrated.

Medial and lateral collateral ligament injury

Modalities

- *X-ray*: nondiagnostic, used to rule out other pathology
- *MR*: preferred modality

Additional views

- Sunrise and tunnel knee views

Findings

- Calcification of the ligament may occur with a chronic injury.
- MR: ligament may appear irregular or completely disrupted, hyperintense T2 signal indicates tear site.
- Avulsion fracture may be associated.

Meniscal tear

Modalities

- *X-ray*: nondiagnostic, but usually obtained to rule out other pathology
- *MR*: preferred modality

Additional views

- AP should be weight bearing
- Sunrise and tunnel knee views

Findings

- Hyperintense linear T2 signal within the meniscus that tracks to an articular surface, especially if in two consecutive images (Fig. 20.6)
- Abnormal morphology such as truncated horns that may appear square shaped instead of triangular
- Meniscal tissue slab "bow-tie" not visualized in two contiguous sagittal sections may indicate a bucket-handle tear. Displacement of the tear may appear as a second PCL ligament (double PCL sign).
- Round, hyperintense T2 signal meniscal cysts are associated, especially with horizontal cleavage tears.

Patella dislocation

Modalities

- *X-ray*: first line, usually diagnostic
- *CT*: used if X-ray equivocal; consider dynamic scanning

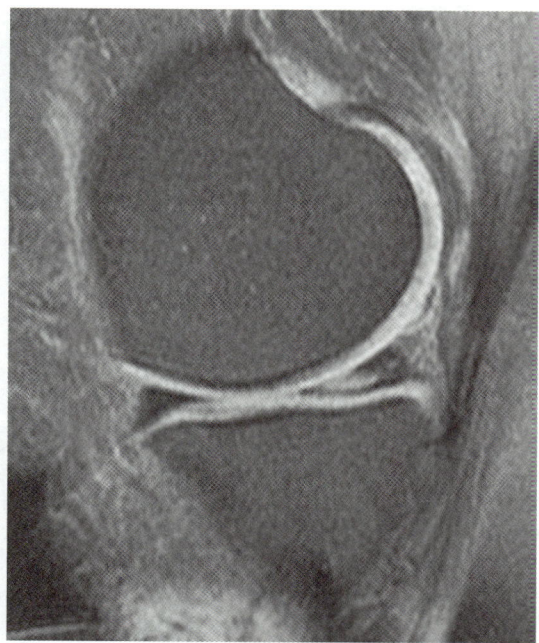

Figure 20.6 Sagittal MR demonstrating hyperintense signal within the posterior medial meniscus, characteristic of a tear.

Additional views
- Sunrise knee view

Findings
- Malalignment or tilt of patella in trochlear groove
- Associated with medial patellar facet fracture; especially with first-time dislocation
- Associated with tears of the medial patellofemoral ligament, as well as osteochondral avulsion fractures of patella and lateral femoral condyle
- Associated with patella alta and increased Q angle

Patellofemoral pain syndrome
Modalities
- *X-ray*: used if treatment refractory
- *CT*: dynamic scanning used if X-ray equivocal

Additional views
- Sunrise and tunnel knee views

Findings
- Lateral patellar subluxation with sclerosis of the lateral aspect and narrowed lateral patellofemoral joint space
- Osteoarthritic degenerative changes may be demonstrated.
- Associated with bipartite patella

Popliteal (Baker's) cyst
- Synovial cyst posterior to the medial femoral condyle, between the gastrocnemius and semimembranosus tendons

Modalities
- *X-ray*: first line; often equivocal
- *MR*: used if other modalities equivocal
- *US*: useful for diagnosis, especially to differentiate from a solid mass

Findings
- May be demonstrated as a soft tissue mass posterior to the medial femoral condyle
- Calcified loose bodies may be present within a complex popliteal cyst
- MR: homogeneous mass with joint communication and intermediate T1 signal and hyperintense T2 signal
- US: anechoic mass with posterior acoustic enhancement and joint communication

Tibial plateau fracture
- Due to impact of the femoral condyles on the medial and/or lateral tibial plateau

Modalities
- *X-ray*: first line; usually diagnostic
- *CT*: used to confirm anatomic relationship in complex fractures
- *MR*: used if other modalities equivocal, or if assessment of ligaments, tendons, and cartilage desired

Additional views
- Internal and external oblique knee views may demonstrate well the degree of compression along the lateral and medial plateaus, respectively.

Findings
- Compression fracture and lucency within the epiphysis may be demonstrated.
- Schatzker type I: wedge fracture of the lateral tibial plateau without depression
- Type II: wedge fracture of the lateral tibial plateau with depression; associated with osteoporosis
- Type III: lateral tibial plateau depression without wedge fracture
- Type IV: wedge fracture of the medial tibial plateau with or without depression
- Type V: wedge fractures through both the medial and lateral plateaus

- Type VI: wedge fractures through both the medial and lateral plateaus with distal oblique shaft fracture displacing the tibial plateau from the diaphysis
- MR: fracture appears as thin linear band of hyperintense T1 signal. The surrounding edematous bone demonstrates hyperintense T2 signal.
- Associated with injury to surrounding tendons, ligaments, and other soft tissue

Lower leg and ankle

Plain radiographic views of the lower leg and ankle

Standard views
- AP and lateral: patient supine, heal on cassette; beam directed between or through the malleoli

Additional views
- Anterior drawer stress view: lateral with traction of the foot anteriorly
- Broden's views: AP with foot internally rotated 45°; beam tilted incrementally cephalad 10°, 20°, 30°, and 40°, and directed toward lateral malleolus
- Mortise: true AP with foot internally rotated 15°; beam perpendicular to intermalleolar line
- Talar tilt: AP with foot in plantar flexion and supinated

Achilles tendon rupture

Modalities
- Diagnosis is usually clinical, but imaging can assist, especially with incomplete rupture.
- X-ray: usually equivocal
- MR: most sensitive and specific modality for complete and partial rupture
- US: first line, although may be equivocal with incomplete rupture

Findings
- Tendon calcification and soft tissue swelling may be demonstrated, as well as a poorly defined Kager's triangle.
- MR: tendon fibers will appear irregular or completely disrupted with hyperintense T2 signal at the tear site.
- US: tendon becomes hyperechoic and thickened and discontinues at the site of ruptured fibers.
- Associated with increased dorsiflexion and bony protrusion of the posterosuperior calcaneus (Haglund deformity)

Acute ankle sprain
- The most common sports-related injury; 85% are inversion injuries

Modalities
- X-ray: first line if a concomitant fracture is suspected (consider Ottawa ankle rules)
- MR: most accurate modality, but usually only considered for pain refractory to treatment. Arthrography is useful for surgical assessment, but must be performed within 1 week of injury.

Additional views
- AP and lateral ankle views should include the base of the fifth metatarsal.
- Mortise ankle view
- Bilateral talar tilt and anterior drawer stress views if instability is refractory to treatment

Findings
- Significant joint instability is indicated by 5° or more of talar tilt in the mortis view or anterior translation >3 mm compared to the uninjured side on bilateral stress views.
- MR: hyperintense T2 signal within or surrounding a ligament is indicative of injury, torn ligaments appear irregular and displaced from their insertion. Of the three lateral ligaments, the anterior talofibular ligament tears first, followed by the calcaneofibular ligament and, finally, the posterior talofibular ligament.
- Associated with concomitant fractures

Medial tibial stress syndrome (shin splints)
- Lower leg connective tissue inflammation due to repetitive loading

Modalities
- Diagnosis is often clinical.
- X-ray: often first line; usually equivocal
- MR: used if occult stress fracture a concern after other modalities equivocal; as sensitive as bone scan, but higher specificity
- Bone scan: adjunct; high sensitivity, but low specificity

Findings
- Signs of periostitis may be demonstrated.
- MR: linear hyperintense T2 signal in the tibia, most often along the medial posterior surface or along medial bone marrow adjacent to cortical bone
- Bone scan: increased activity in a linear streak on the tibia, usually the medial posterior side

Talus fracture, lateral process (snowboarder's fracture)
Modalities
- *X-ray*: first line; usually diagnostic
- *CT*: used if X-ray equivocal for occult fracture
- *MR*: used if X-ray equivocal for occult fracture

Additional views
- Mortise and Broden's views of the ankle and foot

Findings
- All modalities demonstrate fracture of the lateral talar process.

Talus fracture, posterior process (Shepherd's fracture)
Modalities
- *X-ray*: first line; usually diagnostic
- *CT*: consider if X-ray equivocal for occult fracture

Findings
- All modalities demonstrate a fracture of the posterior talar process.

Foot

Plain radiographic views of the foot

Standard views
- *AP*: patient erect with sole on cassette; beam vertical, tilted 15° posterior, and directed toward navicular
- *Lateral*: patient erect; beam directed at cuneiform

Additional views
- *Axial* (Harris–Beath): patient erect, both feet on cassette, slightly leaning forward; beam is PA, tilted 45° caudad, directed toward heels between medial malleoli.
- *Forced dorsiflexion stress view*: heel on cassette with foot in forced dorsiflexion off of cassette; beam directed perpendicular to cassette
- *Oblique*: patient supine, knee flexed, lateral foot elevated 45°, cassette against medial boarder, beam directed vertically toward fifth metatarsal base
- *Sesamoid*: foot dorsiflexed and resting on cassette, toes further dorsiflexed; beam directed vertically toward first metatarsal head

Hallux rigidus (footballer's toe)
- First metatarsophalangeal joint degeneration

Modalities
- *X-ray*: first line; usually diagnostic

Additional views
- Oblique weight bearing and sesamoid foot views

Findings
- Formation of osteophytes and irregular joint-space narrowing, subchondral sclerosis and cysts, and sesamoid hypertrophy
- Associated with Hallux valgus deformity (bunion)

Hallux valgus (bunion)
- First metatarsal lateral deviation

Modalities
- X-ray: first line; usually diagnostic

Additional views
- Oblique weight bearing and sesamoid foot views

Findings
- Hallux abductus angle >20°
- Intermetatarsal angle >10°
- Distal metatarsal articular angle >10°
- Lateral subluxation of sesamoids
- Medial displacement of tarsometatarsal articulations
- Degenerative changes of first metatarsophalangeal joint
- Bony proliferation of medial eminence of the first metatarsal head

Interdigital (Morton) neuroma

Modalities
- *MR*: most accurate modality, consider if clinical diagnosis equivocal

Findings
- Hypointense T1 and T2 signal mass with contrast enhancement between the metatarsal heads
- Typically 5 mm or larger

Kienbock disease
- Lunate osteochondrosis

Modalities
- *X-ray*: first line; often equivocal
- *CT*: used if X-ray equivocal and MR unavailable or contraindicated
- *MR*: used if X-ray equivocal

Additional views
- Oblique foot views
- Bilateral views should be obtained.

Findings
- Unilateral lunate lucency, collapse and fragmentation with possible lunate or perilunate dislocation
- MR: unilateral hypointense T1 signal
- Associated with negative ulnar variance and lunate fracture

Lisfranc fracture dislocation
- Disruption of tarsometatarsal articulations

Modalities
- *X-ray*: first line; often equivocal
- *CT*: often necessary, especially if X-ray is equivocal
- *MR*: often necessary if other modalities equivocal, or for concomitant assessment of soft tissue injury

Additional views
- Oblique weight bearing foot view
- Bilateral AP weight bearing view of the feet should be considered

Findings
- >2 mm separating the base of the first and second metatarsals (Fig. 20.7)
- Malalignment of the superior first metatarsal and medial cuneiform, medial second metatarsal and middle cuneiform, or medial fourth metatarsal and cuboid
- Avulsion fracture of the medial cuneiform or base of the second metatarsal (fleck sign) is pathognomonic.

Metatarsophalangeal dislocation (turf toe)
- Due to hyperdorsiflexion at the first metatarsophalangeal joint

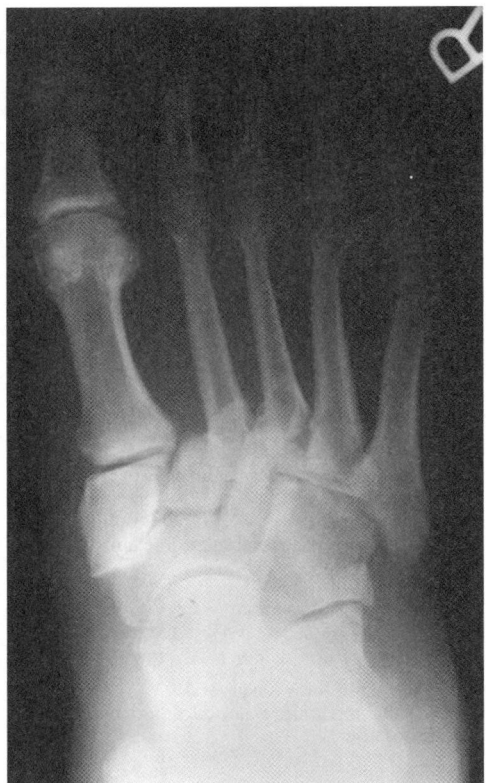

Figure 20.7 AP X-ray of the foot demonstrating widening at the base of the second metatarsal, characteristic of a Lisfranc fracture–dislocation.

Modalities
- *X-ray*: first line; usually diagnostic
- *MR*: used if X-ray equivocal, or for concomitant assessment of soft tissue injury

Additional views
- AP and lateral weight bearing foot views bilaterally
- Sesamoid and forced dorsiflexion foot views

Findings
- Joint subluxation and sesamoid migration or impaction
- MR: disruption of the capsuloligamentous complex may be demonstrated.

Plantar fasciitis

- Due to repetitive microtrauma at the aponeurosis of the plantar fascia and medial process of the calcaneal tuberosity

Modalities

- Diagnosis is usually clinical, though imaging is often useful.
- *X-ray*: first line; often equivocal
- *MR*: consider if other modalities equivocal, or other soft tissue injury a concern
- *US*: adjunct
- *Bone scan*: adjunct

Additional views

- Axial (Harris–Beath) view of heels

Findings

- Thickened plantar fascia and fat pad abnormalities may be demonstrated.
- MR: thickening of plantar fascia and hyperintense T2 signal at aponeurosis
- US: thickening of plantar fascia, hypoechogenicity at aponeurosis, and ill-defined boundary of fascia and surrounding tissue
- Bone scan: increased activity at aponeurosis
- Associated with calcaneal spur

Tarsal coalition

- Fibrous or bony connection between tarsals; most often of the calcaneonavicular and/or talocalcaneal joints

Modalities

- *X-ray*: first line; often equivocal
- *CT*: used if X-ray equivocal
- *MR*: used if other modalities equivocal, or if nonosseous coalitions suspected
- *Bone scan*: useful for localization if X-ray equivocal, though usually other modalities preferred

Additional views

- Oblique foot views
- Bilateral views should be obtained.
- Axial (Harris–Beath) heel view for talocalcaneal coalition

Findings

- Irregularity, narrowing, and sclerosis of the joint space
- Talar beaking, anterior calcaneal process elongation, navicular dorsal subluxation, and subtalar convexity with distal tibial concavity
- A "C sign" made by the medial talar dome and the inferior sustentaculum tali of the calcaneus is associated with talocalcaneal coalition.
- Bone scan: increased activity at coalition
- Associated with degenerative changes in surrounding non-coalition joints

Shoulder

Plain radiographic views of the shoulder

Standard views

- *AP*: patient supine with arms at side, external rotation, elbows extended, contralateral shoulder externally rotated 40°, cassette behind shoulder; beam vertical and centered on humeral head
- *Axillary*: AP with arm abducted as close to 90° as close to as possible, cassette superior to shoulder; beam directed vertically toward femoral head
- *Transscapular* ("Y view"): anterior shoulder against cassette, contralateral shoulder externally rotated 40°; beam directed anteriorly parallel with the scapular spine

Additional views

- *Serendipity*: AP centered on the sternoclavicular joint; beam tilted 40° cephalad
- *Stryker notch*: AP with palm of hand placed on top of head with fingers pointing posteriorly; beam directed toward coracoid process and tilted 10° cephalad
- *West point*: patient prone, head turned from involved side, shoulder elevated, cassette placed superior to shoulder; beam directed toward axilla and tilted 25° down and 25° medially
- *Zanca*: AP centered on the acromioclavicular joint; beam tilted cephalad 10°

Acromioclavicular (AC) joint separation

- Classified by position of clavicle relative to acromion and coracoid

Modalities

- *X-ray*: first line; usually diagnostic
- *MR*: useful to differentiate type of separation, especially in preparation for surgery

Additional views

- Zanca acromioclavicular view
- Bilateral views should be obtained.

Findings

- Increased AC joint space and coracoclavicular distance
- MR: marrow edema indicated by hyperintense T2 signal and subchondral cyst formation

Adhesive capsulitis (frozen shoulder)

- Contraction and thickening of the glenohumeral joint capsule with adhesion formation

Modalities

- *X-ray*: first line; usually equivocal
- *MR*: consider with or without arthrography if concomitant soft tissue pathology a concern and X-ray equivocal

Findings

- Greater tuberosity osteopenia, subchondral cysts, rotator cuff tendon calcification may be demonstrated
- MR: joint capsule and synovial membrane thickening with hyperintense T2 signal. Arthrographic findings include decreased joint volume (<10 mL), loss of axial fold, and contrast within the biceps tendon sheath.

Biceps tendon rupture

- Usually occurs at the proximal head of the long tendon

Modalities

- Diagnosis usually clinical
- *X-ray*: adjunct; usually equivocal
- *MR*: adjunct; most accurate modality
- *US*: adjunct

Additional views

- AP with arm in external rotation

Findings

- Calcification within bicipital groove, hypertrophic spurring, and bony irregularities may be demonstrated.
- MR and US: tendon discontinuation within bicipital groove
- Associated with rotator cuff tear

Calcific tendonitis

- Rotator cuff tendon degeneration with calcification and inflammation

Modalities

- *X-ray*: usually diagnostic
- *MR*: used if other modalities equivocal
- *US*: preferred first line

Findings

- Calcium deposits can appear localized or diffuse, homogenous or heterogeneous, and be well or poorly demarcated.
- MR: calcium deposits have hypointense T1 signal. There may be surrounding edema with hyperintense T2 signal.

Clavicle fracture

- Classified by fracture location in middle (group I), lateral (group II), or medial (group III) third of clavicle

Modalities

- *X-ray*: first line; diagnostic

Additional views

- Serendipity sternoclavicular view

Findings

- Medial fragment usually lies superior to lateral fragment
- Associated with pneumothorax

Distal clavicle osteolysis

Modalities
- *X-ray*: first line; usually diagnostic, though may initially be equivocal
- *Bone scan*: considered if X-ray equivocal

Additional views
- Zanca acromioclavicular view

Findings
- AC joint widening, subchondral cysts, and osteopenia and tapering of the distal clavicle
- Bone scan: increased activity correlates with healing

Glenohumeral subluxation and dislocation

Modalities
- *X-ray*: often obtained before and/or after reduction
- *CT*: used if X-ray equivocal
- *MR*: used if concomitant assessment of soft tissue injury desired

Additional views
- Stryker notch view can specifically evaluate for Hill–Sachs deformity.
- West Point axillary view can specifically evaluate for anteroinferior Bankart lesion.

Findings
- Anterior dislocation: anterior, inferior, and medial displacement of humeral head.
- Posterior dislocation: internal rotation of humeral head gives it a rounded appearance (light bulb sign). Superimposition of medial humeral head and anterior glenoid (rim sign) or >6 mm space between the two structures. Two parallel lines of cortical bone of the medial humeral head indicate a reverse Hill–Sachs deformity (trough line sign).
- Inferior dislocation (luxatio erecta): inferior displacement of the humeral head below the coracoid or glenoid
- Associated findings include humeral head compression fracture (Hill–Sachs deformity), and fragmented bony glenoid labrum (bony Bankart lesion), greater tuberosity fractures, and femoral neck fractures.

Glenoid labral tear

Modalities
- *X-ray*: nondiagnostic, but usually obtained to rule out other pathology
- *CT*: used with arthrography only if MR contraindicated or unavailable
- *MR*: preferred diagnostic modality; most accurate with arthrography or with high field strength (3T)

Findings
- Fluid within the labrum or between the labrum and the bony glenoid, detachment of the labrum from the bony glenoid, and blunting truncation of the labrum
- Associated findings include paralabral cyst, humeral head compression fracture (Hill–Sachs deformity), and fragmented bony glenoid labrum (bony Bankart lesion) (Fig. 20.8).

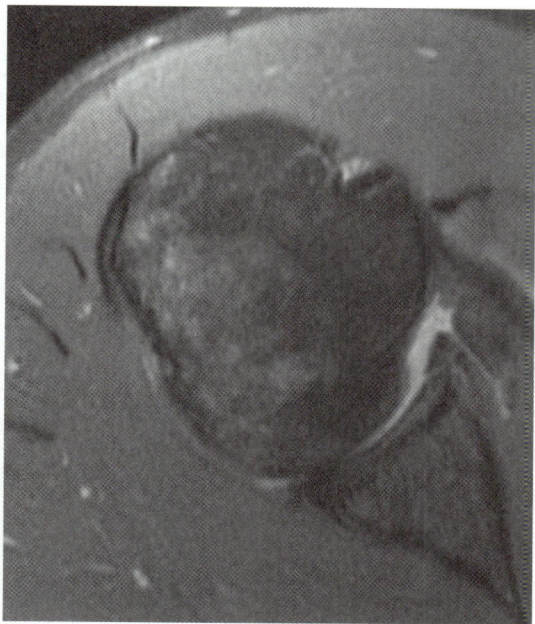

Figure 20.8 Axial MR arthrogram demonstrating extension of hyperintense contrast within and beneath the anterior glenoid labrum, characteristic of a tear. Hyperintense signal within the posterior humeral head represents a Hill–Sachs deformity associated with anterior dislocations and labral tears.

Humerus fracture

Modalities

- *X-ray*: first line; usually diagnostic
- *CT*: consider if X-ray equivocal or to further assess fractures of the humeral head, neck, articular surface, or complex fractures

Findings

- Common fractures include transverse, spiral, and oblique fractures of the shaft along with fractures of the humeral neck, head, greater tuberosity, and lesser tuberosity.

Rotator cuff tear

- Supraspinatus is most commonly involved, followed by the infraspinatus, teres minor, and, rarely, the subscapularis.

Modalities

- *X-ray*: usually equivocal
- *MR*: used if US is equivocal, or for concomitant assessment of other soft tissue injury
- *US*: often first line; can be extremely useful for diagnosis

Findings

- Sclerosis, osteophytes, and subchondral cyst formation may occur at the acromion or greater tuberosity.
- Migration of the humeral head toward the acromion may be demonstrated.
- MR: fiber discontinuity and hyperintense T1 and T2 signal at the tear site. Muscle wasting may indicate chronic injury.
- US: thickening, hypoechogenicity, and discontinuation of tendon fibers. Hypoechoic or hyperechoic foci within the tendon may be demonstrated.
- Associated with hooked (type 3) acromion

Shoulder impingement syndrome

- Rotator cuff, biceps tendon, and/or subacromial bursa compression between acromion and greater tuberosity of humerus

Modalities

- *X-ray*: reserved unless treatment is refractory; often equivocal
- *MR*: used if X-ray equivocal

Findings

- Rotator cuff tendon calcification, decreased space between superior humeral head and inferior acromion, and erosion or sclerosis of the greater tuberosity
- MR: bone spur compression of the supraspinatus tendon or subacromial bursa as well as acromioclavicular joint hypertrophy may be demonstrated.
- Associated with hooked (type 3) acromion

Sternoclavicular subluxation

Modalities

- *X-ray*: often first line; often equivocal
- *CT*: preferred modality
- *MR*: consider if concomitant soft tissue injury a concern

Additional views

- Serendipity sternoclavicular view

Findings

- Displacement of the clavicle and medial sclerosis

Thoracic outlet syndrome

- Anatomic compression or obstruction of neurovasculature serving the arm

Modalities

- *X-ray*: first line, often equivocal
- *CT*: used if cervical disk disease a concern or if MR unavailable or contraindicated
- *MR*: preferred modality if spinal cord disease or other soft tissue anomaly suspected
- *US*: Doppler flowmetry useful to assess vascular flow

Additional views

- Flexion and extension cervical spine views
- AP and lateral chest views

Findings

- Distortion or displacement of tissue surrounding the brachial plexus may be demonstrated.
- MR may demonstrate hyperintense T2 signal intensity at the site of nerve entrapment.
- US: interruption of blood flow may be demonstrated with Doppler flowmetry.
- Pancoast tumor and other mass lesions can be associated.
- Associated abnormalities include a cervical rib, clavicle deformities, elongated C7 transverse process, and degenerative changes of the cervical spine such as loss of disc space, disc herniation, and osteophytes.

Elbow

Plain radiographic views of the elbow

Standard views
- AP: arm supine resting on cassette with elbow extended and fingers in neutral flexion; beam directed perpendicularly toward elbow
- Lateral: elbow flexed 90 with ulnar side on cassette; beam directed vertically toward radial head

Additional views
- Radiocapitellar: lateral with beam tilted 45° anterior
- External oblique: lateral with arm abducted 45°

Elbow dislocation

Modalities
- *X-ray*: first line. Pre- and post-reduction views should be obtained.
- *CT*: used if enhanced assessment of concomitant fracture desired

Findings
- Displacement of the radius and/or ulna, typically posteriorly relative to the humerus
- Misalignment of radiocapitellar line through shaft of radius and center of capitellum
- Widening of joint
- Associated with concomitant fractures, especially of the radial head

Epicondylitis
- Lateral epicondylitis (tennis elbow)
- Medial epicondylitis (golfer's elbow)

Modalities
- Diagnosis is usually clinical, although imaging is usually obtained with acute, complicated, or obscure presentation.
- *X-ray*: adjunct; usually equivocal
- *MR*: especially useful with arthrography for evaluation of medial collateral ligament and for surgical assessment
- *US*: adjunct

Findings
- Chronically, tendon calcification and surface irregularity near insertion may be demonstrated.
- MR: hyperintense signal within tendon near insertion. Arthrography can reveal occult tears to the deep fibers of the medial collateral ligament, demonstrated by extension of contrast between the ligament and its ulnar attachment ("T sign") (Fig. 20.9).
- US: thickening, inhomogeneity, and hypoechogenicity of the tendon, along with local fluid collection

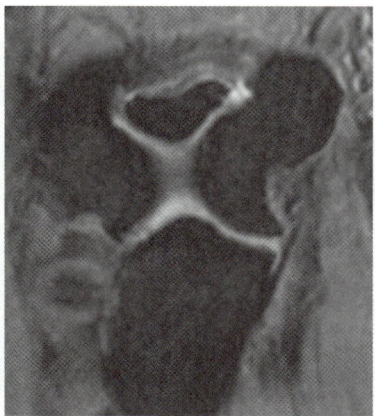

Figure 20.9 Coronal MR arthrogram demonstrating extension of hyperintense contrast between the tibia and ulnar collateral ligament (T sign), indicative of a partial tear.

Monteggia fracture

- Fracture of proximal or middle ulna with dislocation of radial head

Modalities

- *X-ray*: first line; pre and post reduction views should be obtained
- *MR*: adjunct
- *US*: adjunct

Additional views

- Orthogonal forearm views that include the elbow and wrist joints
- External oblique elbow view
- AP and lateral wrist views

Findings

- Ulna fracture typically apparent; greenstick fractures common in children, especially at site of ulnar metaphysis
- Radial head dislocation typically points in same direction as ulna apex
- Misalignment of radiocapitellar line through shaft of radius and center of capitellum
- Widening of joint
- Associated with concomitant fractures, especially of radial head

Radial head fracture

- Most common elbow fracture in adults

Modalities

- *X-ray*: first line
- *CT*: used if X-ray equivocal or enhanced visualization of fracture desired; especially for comminuted fractures of the entire radial head

Additional views

- Radiocapitellar elbow view
- Additional AP and pronated lateral wrist views for comminuted fracture of entire head

Findings

- Fractures range from occult with no displacement to comminuted fractures of the entire radial head with complete displacement of fragments.
- Occult fracture may be indicated in lateral view by fat pad triangular lucency anterior and/or posterior of the distal humerus (sail sign).
- Comminuted fractures of the entire radial head may demonstrate proximal translation of radius and dorsal subluxation of the ulna on pronated lateral wrist view.

Radial neck fracture

Modalities

- *X-ray*: first line; diagnostic

Additional views

- Radiocapitellar elbow view

Findings

- Fracture is typically through the physis with metaphyseal fragment (Salter–Harris II)
- >15° valgus rotation of radial neck
- Misalignment of radiocapitellar line through shaft of radius and center of capitellum
- Fat pad triangular lucency posterior to distal humerus on lateral view (sail sign)

Ulnar, radial, and median neuropathy

- Typically entrapment occurs near the elbow, though the entire course of the nerve is vulnerable.

Modalities

- *X-ray*: first line, often equivocal
- *CT*: used if cervical degenerative disk disease a concern or if MR unavailable or contraindicated
- *MR*: preferred modality cervical degenerative disk disease or other soft tissue anomaly suspected
- *US*: adjunct

Additional views
- AP and lateral wrist views
- Flexion and extension cervical spine views
- PA and lateral chest views

Findings
- Distortion or displacement of surrounding tissue along the course of the nerve may be demonstrated.
- MR: hyperintense T2 signal at site of nerve entrapment may be demonstrated.
- US: may reveal nerve thickening, or mass lesions such as ulnar canal cyst
- Associated abnormalities at the elbow include valgus deformity, shallow olecranon groove, bone fractures or fragments, dislocations, osteophytes, and other abnormal calcifications.
- Associated abnormalities at the wrist include fracture of the hook of the hamate and carpal dislocations.
- Other associated abnormalities include a cervical rib, clavicle deformities, elongated C7 transverse process, and degenerative changes of the cervical spine such as loss of disc space, herniation, and osteophytes.
- Pancoast tumor and other mass lesions such as ganglion cyst or lipoma can be associated.

Wrist and hand

Plain radiographic views of the wrist and hand

Standard views
- *AP*: elbow flexed 90° dorsum of hand resting on cassette; beam perpendicular to cassette
- *Lateral*: arm abducted; beam directed parallel with carpals and perpendicular to cassette

Additional views
- *Brewerton*: AP with phalanges on cassette and metacarpophalangeal joints flexed 45°; beam directed toward third metacarpal head and tilted 20° to ulnar side
- *Carpal tunnel*: hand dorsiflexed to maximum with palm on cassette; beam directed toward cup of palm and tilted 15°
- Clenched fist: PA view with fist clenched as tightly as possible
- *PA*: palm of hand resting on cassette, elbow and shoulder both flexed 90°; beam perpendicular to cassette
- *Pronated oblique*: AP with hand resting on ulnar side and tilted 45° palmarly, fingers slightly flexed; beam directed toward center of carpus
- *Robert*: true AP of thumb with maximum pronation; beam directed toward first carpometacarpal joint
- *Scaphoid*: AP with ulnar deviation; beam tilted cephalad 30°
- Supinated oblique (hook of hamate view): AP with hand resting on ulnar side and tilted 30° dorsally, thumb slightly abducted; beam directed toward center of carpus

Bennett fracture
- Intra-articular fracture and dislocation of first carpometacarpal joint

Modalities
- *X-ray*: first line
- *CT*: useful for occult or complex fractures

Additional views
- Oblique thumb view
- 30° pronated lateral thumb view
- Robert thumb view

Findings
- Radial dislocation and supination of first metacarpal
- Oblique intra-articular fracture creating triangular proximal fragment with trapezium attachment maintained
- Disruption of the "V" formed by the trapeziometacarpal joint (broken V sign)
- Widened carpometacarpal joint may indicate soft tissue interposition and irreducible dislocation.

Carpal tunnel syndrome

- Median nerve compression at the carpal tunnel

Modalities

- Diagnosis is usually clinical.
- *X-ray*: not useful unless concomitant bone trauma suspected
- *MR*: used if complicated or equivocal presentation; preferred modality for lesion detection within the canal
- *US*: adjunct

Additional views

- Carpal tunnel wrist view if bone trauma suspected

Findings

- *MR*: synovial hypertrophy, effusion, mass effect on the median nerve, and hyperintense T2 signal may be demonstrated.
- *US*: median nerve thickening and signs of synovitis such as proliferation and hypoechoic effusion

Distal radius (Colles or Smith) fracture

Modalities

- *X-ray*: first line; usually diagnostic
- *CT*: consider for complex or occult fractures and for surgical assessment
- *MR*: consider for complex or occult fractures and for surgical assessment
- Bone scan: adjunct

Additional views

- Oblique wrist view

Findings

- Fracture may demonstrate dorsal displacement and angulation (Colles) or palmar displacement and angulation (Smith), as well as decreased radial inclination and positive ulnar variance.
- Occult fracture may be indicated in lateral view by a convex dorsal subcutaneous fat line and convex or absent deep fat pad of pronator quadratus.
- Bone scan: increased activity at fracture site
- Associated with ulna and carpal fractures, ulna styloid fracture, scapholunate dislocation, and triangular fibrocartilage complex injury

Hamate fracture

Modalities

- *X-ray*: first line
- *CT*: used if X-ray equivocal
- *MR*: adjunct

Additional views

- Supinated oblique and carpal tunnel wrist views

Findings

- Fractures may occur within the body, the hook, or as an avulsion from the distal articular surface.
- Some individuals have a bipartite hamate, which demonstrates smooth margins without cortical disruption.

- *MR*: fracture is indicated by linear hypointense T1 signal surrounded by hyperintense T2 signal.
- Chronic fractures of the hook of hamate may develop avascular necrosis.

Mallet fracture and jersey finger

- Long extensor (mallet fracture) or flexor digitorum profundus (jersey finger) tendon rupture or avulsion from distal interphalangeal joint

Modalities

- *X-ray*: first line

Additional views

- AP and lateral views of injured finger

Findings

- Facture, avulsion, or subluxation of the distal phalanx

Metacarpal fractures and dislocations

Modalities

- *X-ray*: first line
- *CT*: used for occult or complex fractures, especially metacarpal head fractures and dislocations

Additional views

- Oblique hand view
- 30° pronated lateral view: second and third metacarpals, or 30° supinated lateral view for fourth and fifth metacarpals
- Robert view: first metacarpal base fracture
- Clenched fist: metacarpal base fractures
- Brewerton view: metacarpal head fractures and collateral ligament avulsion fractures.
- Traction PA and lateral views may be considered for comminuted fractures and carpometacarpal or metacarpophalangeal dislocations only after avulsion fracture is ruled out with standard views.

Findings

- Shaft fractures may be transverse, oblique, or spiral.
- Shaft fractures typically demonstrate dorsal angulation of the proximal fragment and volar angulation of the distal fragment.
- Oblique and spiral fractures tend to rotate and shorten.
- Metacarpal head fractures tend to be comminuted.
- In carpometacarpal dislocation, the metacarpal usually migrates dorsally with loss of joint space on the AP view; associated with dislocation and fracture of surrounding joints.
- In metacarpophalangeal dislocation, the phalanx usually migrates dorsally with overlap of metacarpal head on AP view.
- Base fractures are particularly associated with carpometacarpal dislocations and avulsions.

Scaphoid fracture

- Most common hand fracture

Modalities

- *X-ray*: first line, usually diagnostic
- *CT*: used if X-ray equivocal and unnecessary splinting contraindicated for athletic or professional reasons, for complex injury, or if 7- to 10-day follow-up X-ray equivocal; more accurate than bone scan
- *MR*: adjunct; high accuracy
- *Bone scan*: adjunct; very high sensitivity, low specificity

Additional views

- Bilateral PA in ulnar deviation, semipronated oblique, and scaphoid wrist views

Findings

- Fracture may appear as a lucent line disrupting cortex or as an opaque line due to overriding fragments.
- Scapholunate angle >70°
- Capitolunate angle >20°
- Intrascaphoid angulation at fracture (humpback deformity)
- Disruption of longitudinal radius, lunate, capitate, and third metacarpal axis
- Displacement or absence of scaphoid fat stripe may indicate occult fracture.
- MR: fracture indicated by linear hypointense T1 signal surrounded by hyperintense T2 signal (Fig. 20.10)
- Bone scan: increased activity

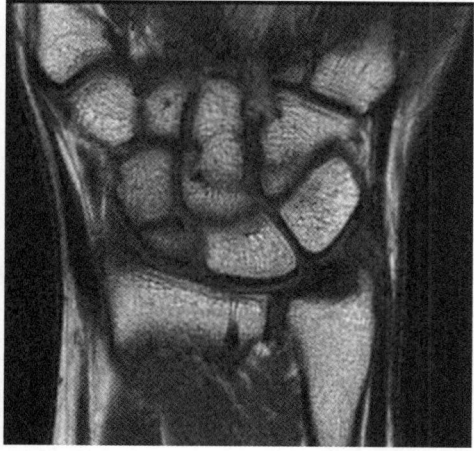

Figure 20.10 Coronal MR demonstrating scaphoid fracture with hypointense signal across the proximal pole.

- Associated with distal radius fractures and carpal instability
- Chronically, avascular necrosis may develop, especially with fractures of the proximal one-third.

Scapholunate instability or dislocation

- Most common wrist injury

Modalities

- *X-ray*: first line, usually diagnostic
- *CT*: used if X-ray equivocal, or with complex injury

Additional views

- Clenched fist view AP in ulnar deviation
- Oblique wrist view

Findings

- Increased scapholunate gap on clenched fist AP view compared to uninjured side or compared to lunotriquetral gap (Terry Thomas sign)
- Scapholunate angle >70°
- Capitolunate angle >20°
- Scaphoid rotation with proximal pole becoming posterior and distal pole becoming anterior
- Disruption of the smooth arc created by the proximal borders of the scaphoid, lunate, and triquetrum
- Disruption of longitudinal radius, lunate, capitate, and third metacarpal axis
- Associated with negative ulnar variance
- Chronically, may see proximal migration of capitate and degenerative changes of the radioscaphoid, capitolunate, and scaphotrapezotrapezoidal (STT) joints

Triangular fibrocartilage complex (TFCC) injury

Modalities

- *X-ray*: first line, usually equivocal
- *MR*: most accurate modality

Findings

- MR: discontinuity of the TFCC with hyperintense T2 signal
- Associated findings include positive ulnar variance, ulnar styloid avulsion, and flattening and subchondral sclerosis of the lunate, triquetrum, and distal ulna.

Ulnar collateral ligament injury (gamekeeper's thumb or skier's thumb)

- Instability of first metacarpophalangeal joint due to ulnar collateral ligament disruption

Modalities

- *X-ray*: first line
- *MR*: considered for surgical assessment

Views
- PA and lateral thumb views
- Bilateral extension and flexion thumb views with valgus stress only after avulsion fracture ruled out with standard views

Findings
- Avulsion of ulnar collateral ligament from base of phalanx (gamekeeper's fracture)
- Volar subluxation of proximal phalanx, >3 mm indicates significant instability.
- 15° difference in laxity on stress views compared to uninjured thumb indicates instability.
- >30° of total laxity on stress views likely indicates complete ligament tear.
- Chronically, degenerative joint changes may be demonstrated

Head and spine

Cervical radiculopathy

- Neck and upper extremity pain, parasthesia, and numbness due to cervical nerve root pathology; typically C6 or C7

Modalities

- *X-ray*: first line; often equivocal
- *CT*: consider with myelography if X-ray equivocal and MRI contraindicated or unavailable
- *MR*: preferred modality if X-ray equivocal

Views

- AP, lateral, and oblique cervical spine views
- Swimmer's view if enhanced visualization of C7 desired

Findings

- Cervical spine degenerative changes such as narrowed disc space, herniation, osteophytes, and fracture
- MR: soft tissue abnormalities of the ligaments or intervertebral discs may be demonstrated.

Cervical spine trauma

Modalities

- *X-ray*: often first line
- *CT*: preferred first line if fracture suspected
- *MR*: used if other modalities equivocal for soft tissue injury or especially for ligamentous, intervertebral disc, or spinal pathology suspected

Views

- AP, cross-table lateral (Fig. 20.11), and open-mouth odontoid cervical spine views
- Standard cervical spine trauma series: AP, cross-table lateral, open-mouth odontoid, left and right oblique, and swimmer's views.
- Cross-table lateral: demonstrates all cervical vertebral bodies and cervicothoracic junction; excellent for evaluation of spondylosis
- Odontoid: enhanced view of C1 and C2, including dens
- Oblique: demonstrates pedicles, lamina, and neural foramen
- Swimmer's: enhanced view of cervicothoracic junction
- Flexion and extension lateral: evaluate cervical stability and compression fractures; contraindicated in traumatic injury that has not been radiographically cleared

Findings

- Disruption of the anterior, posterior, or spinolaminar contour lines indicates bony or ligamentous injury.
- Loss of intervertebral space may indicate disc herniation or fracture.
- Widening of the prevertebral space is indicative of occult fracture.
- Spinous process fracture may be demonstrated as avulsion on lateral view.

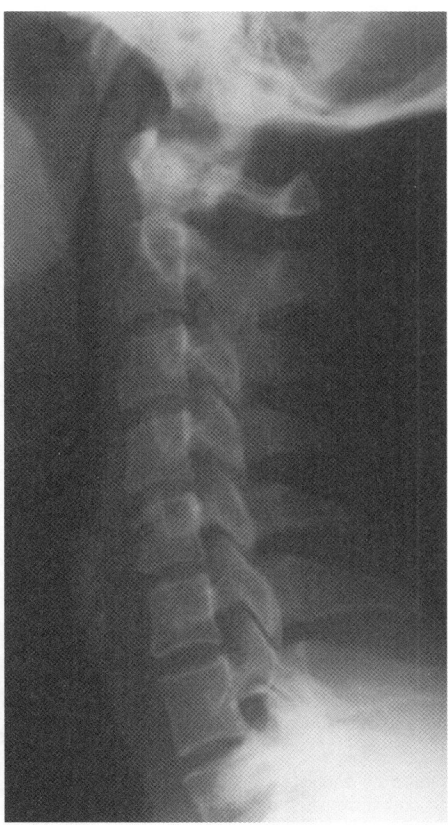

Figure 20.11 Lateral X-ray of normal cervical spine.

- Odontoid process fractures at the base (type II) or within the body of the axis (type III) may be displaced, with posterior displacement most concerning for spinal cord injury. Tip avulsion fractures (type I) are associated with atlanto-occipital dislocation, which is demonstrated by dissociation of the occiput and C1. Instability is indicated by an atlantodental interval of >3 mm (from dens to posterior of C1 anterior arch).
- Anteriorly shortened and sclerotic vertebral body is indicative of compression fracture.

- Flexion teardrop fracture is demonstrated by a triangular fragment at the anteroinferior portion of the vertebral body with anterior intervertebral space narrowing.
- Burst fracture is demonstrated by comminuted vertebral body with displacement of fragments into spinal canal. Instability is indicated by loss of over half the vertebral height or displacement into >30% of the canal diameter.
- Increased interlaminar space may indicate vertebral subluxation.
- Unilateral facet dislocation is indicated by malalignment of the spinous processes and anterior displacement of the vertebral body by less than half of its diameter. Instability is indicated by >3.5 mm of translational displacement.
- Bilateral facet dislocation is indicated by anterior displacement of a vertebral body by over half its diameter.
- Diminished cross-sectional area of the spinal canal with displacement of spinal fluid and cord compression is indicative of spinal stenosis.
- Cervical spine instability can be demonstrated by >20° of sagittal plane rotation of a vertebrae in subsequent flexion and extension films, or >11° of angulation between adjacent vertebrae in one view.

Degenerative disc disease
- Disorders include herniation, fissuring, and degeneration.

Modalities
- *X-ray*: often first line; often equivocal
- *CT*: most accurate modality when combined with myelography; consider for surgical assessment if other modalities equivocal
- *MR*: preferred first line

Views
- Standing AP and lateral spine views
- Flexion and extension lateral cervical spine views if instability suspected
- Oblique view if enhanced evaluation of neural foramen desired

Findings
- Loss of intervertebral space, endplate irregularity, osteophyte formation, and subchondral sclerosis and cyst formation
- Hypertrophy, irregularity, and misalignment of the facets may lead to neural foramen stenosis and radiculopathy.
- CT may demonstrate peripheral bulging of disc material beyond margins of vertebral bodies and decreased attenuation within the disc.
- With myelography, the spinal cord can be visualized within the canal; nerve root impingement from disc, bone spur, or foraminal encroachment may be evident.
- Diminished cross-sectional area of the spinal canal with displacement of spinal fluid and cord compression is indicative of spinal stenosis; a diameter of <10 mm is suggestive.
- MR: hypointense T1 and T2 signals within the disc. Cartilaginous endplate may demonstrate hyperintense T1 and T2 signal. Nerve compression may demonstrate hyperintense T2 signal.
- Associated with spondylosis, spondylolysis, and spondylolisthesis

Head trauma

Modalities

- *X-ray*: adjunct
- *CT*: preferred modality for acute head trauma
- *MR*: consider if CT equivocal; especially useful for evaluation of parenchymal contusion or if follow-up imaging desired
- Bone scan: consider for children with suspected nonaccidental injury

Views

- AP, lateral, and open-mouth odontoid cervical spine views
- AP and lateral chest views may be considered with traumatic injury.

Findings

- Skull fractures can be distinguished from skull sutures by their depth, variable width, sharp margins, and linear course with angular turns.
- Air collection in the paranasal sinuses or pneumocephaly may indicate occult skull fracture.
- Cerebral contusion is often initially isoattenuating, but later demonstrates hyperattenuating foci surrounded by a large zone of hypoattenuation; coup and countercoup lesions may be present.
- Intracranial hematoma, hemorrhage, or edema often demonstrates parenchymal mass effect with midline shift, ventricular compression, and sulci obliteration.
- Intracranial hematomas are initially hyperattenuating. Chronically, attenuation will decrease, becoming heterogeneous at approximately 2 weeks, and hypoattenuating; focal area of low or heterogeneous attenuation (swirl sign) indicates active bleeding.
- Epidural hematomas stereotypically present as a lenticular-shaped mass with smooth margins between the brain and skull and rarely cross suture lines.
- Subdural hematomas stereotypically present as a unilateral crescent-shaped lesion adjacent to the inner skull with smooth margins.
- MR: Cerebral contusions acutely demonstrate hyperintense T2 signal and chronically appear as areas of irregular brain contour with loss of gray and white matter discrimination. Intracranial hematomas initially demonstrate hypointense T2 signal followed over weeks by hyperintense T1 and T2 signal and afterward may last for many months as hypointense T1 signal.
- Bone scan: fractures demonstrate increased activity.

Maxillofacial and orbital fractures

Modalities

- *X-ray*: consider if low suspicion for complex fracture and no ocular symptoms
- *CT*: preferred modality, especially if intracranial injury suspected; 3D construction helpful for surgical assessment
- *MR*: consider with soft tissue or nervous injury and equivocal CT; contraindicated if ferromagnetic foreign body may have been introduced with trauma

Views
- *Standard skull series*: Waters, Caldwell, submental vertex (jug-handle), and cross-table lateral views
- *Waters*: for evaluation of inferior orbital rim and orbital floor (maxillary sinus); can also evaluate zygomatic arch and tripod fractures
- *Caldwell*: for evaluation of lateral orbital rim and ethmoid fractures; can also evaluate zygomatic arch and tripod fractures
- *Submental vertex* (jug-handle): for evaluation of zygomatic arch and tripod fractures; contraindicated if cervical spine injury suspected
- PA chest film if teeth are missing
- AP, lateral, and open-mouth odontoid cervical views and AP and lateral chest views may be obtained as part of a trauma series.

Findings
- Zygomatic arch fractures typically have a break on each end and a third in the middle.
- Concomitant fractures of the lateral orbital wall, inferior orbital floor, and the zygomatic arch indicate a tripod fracture.
- Increased opacity or air–fluid level in the maxillary or ethmoid sinuses may indicate presence of a Le Fort, orbital floor (maxillary sinus), or ethmoid fracture.
- With orbital fractures, CT may identify extraocular muscle entrapment, involvement of the optic nerve by bone fragments, and optic nerve stretching due to retro-ocular edema or hematoma.

Mandible fracture
Modalities
- *X-ray*: first line
- *CT*: preferred modality if complex maxillofacial fracture or intracranial injury suspected; 3D construction helpful for surgical assessment

Views
- *Panorex*: preferred view that creates a 2D panoramic projection of the entire mandible
- *Mandible series*: diagnostically equivalent to Panorex view; includes PA, bilateral lateral oblique, Towne, and occlusal views of the mandible.
- *Lateral oblique*: excellent visualization of mandible angle and ramus
- *Towne view*: excellent condyle visualization.
- *Occlusal*: for evaluation of body fracture displacement
- *Periapical*: for evaluation of teeth and roots
- PA and lateral chest views if teeth are missing.
- AP, lateral, and open-mouth odontoid cervical views and AP and lateral chest views may be obtained as part of a trauma series.

Spondylolysis

- Stress fracture of the pars interarticularis

Modalities

- *X-ray*: first line
- *CT*: more specific than single-photon emission computed tomography (SPECT), consider if SPECT equivocal
- *MR*: adjunct, used if concomitant soft tissue injury a concern
- *Bone scan*: SPECT has higher sensitivity than X-rays and correlates well with symptomatic etiology. It is often used if fracture is discovered on X-ray or X-ray equivocal.

Views

- AP, lateral, and lateral oblique lumbosacral spine views
- Lateral spot view of the lumbosacral junction may be considered.
- Flexion and extension lateral views if instability suspected

Findings

- The pars interarticularis has a "Scottie dog" appearance in lateral oblique view; a linear lucency through the "collar" of the Scottie dog is pathognomonic for spondylolysis (Fig. 20.12).
- In unilateral spondylolysis, sclerosis of the contralateral pars interarticularis may be demonstrated.
- Anterior displacement of the vertebral body (spondylolisthesis) may accompany bilateral spondylolysis (Fig. 20.13).
- Spondylolysis most commonly occurs at L5, allowing displacement over the sacrum.
- MR: acutely, the fracture is seen as linear hypointense T1 signal surrounded by hyperintense T2 signal. Nerve compression may demonstrate hyperintense T2 signal.
- Bone scan: SPECT demonstrates increased activity at the fracture site; activity correlates well with the degree of symptoms.
- Associated with spina bifida occulta

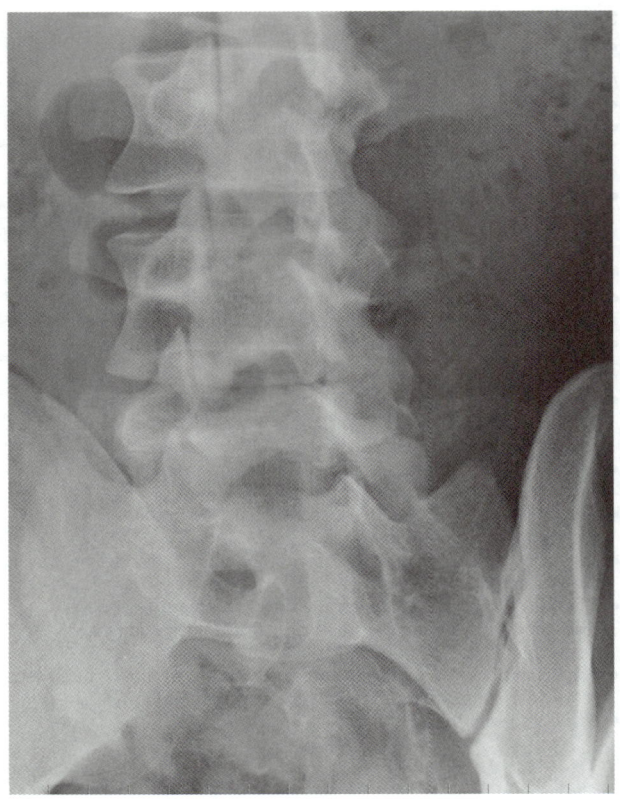

Figure 20.12 Lateral oblique X-ray of the lumbosacral spine demonstrating L5 spondylolysis with the characteristic lucency through the collar of the "Scottie dog."

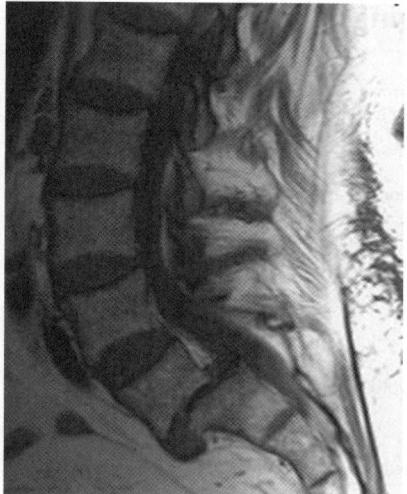

Figure 20.13 Sagittal MR demonstrating severe spondylolisthesis of the L5–S1 junction.

Pediatric imaging

Ewing sarcoma
- Malignant neuroectodermal tumor
- Most often occurs in the femur, tibia, fibula, humerus, pelvis, or ribs

Modalities
- *X-ray*: first line
- *CT*: preferred modality for metastatic evaluation of thorax, and for focal lesions if MR unavailable or contraindicated
- *MR*: preferred modality for focal lesions, and surgical assessment
- *Bone scan*: preferred modality for metastatic evaluation of entire skeleton

Views
- These vary with anatomic location, but at least two orthogonal views should be obtained.
- The entire extent of involved bone and adjacent joints should be imaged.

Findings
- Lytic lesions with permeative "moth-eaten" appearance and wide zone of transition
- Aggressive periosteal reaction characteristically has lamellated "onion-skin" appearance but may demonstrate Codman's triangle or sunburst appearance.
- *MR*: lesions demonstrate hypointense T1 and hyperintense T2 signal.
- *Bone scan*: increased activity

Lateral condyle fracture
Modalities
- *X-ray*: first line; can be equivocal, especially initially
- *MR*: used if X-ray equivocal and for surgical assessment

Views
- Bilateral AP, lateral, and internal oblique elbow views
- Consider full elbow extension to accentuate fragment displacement.

Findings
- Identification of fracture line may be difficult before ossification of capitellum occurs.
- Lateral soft tissue swelling in the AP view and fat pad triangular lucency anterior and/or posterior of distal humerus in the lateral view (sail sign)

Osteochondroma
- Benign bony tumor with cartilaginous cap
- Most often occurs in the distal femur, proximal tibia, or proximal humerus

Modalities

- *X-ray*: first line, often diagnostic
- *CT*: used if X-ray equivocal or for surgical planning
- *MR*: used if other modalities equivocal
- *US*: can be used to visualize the cartilaginous cap

Views

- These vary with anatomic location, but at least two orthogonal views should be obtained.

Findings

- Well-defined bony projection with mottled density, most often located at the metaphysis of long bones
- Cartilaginous cap may contain flakes of calcification.
- MR: cartilaginous cap demonstrates hyperintense T2 signal intensity. Hyperintense T2 signal in adjacent muscle may indicate impingement.
- US: hypoechoic cartilaginous cap covering hyperechoic bony projection

Osteochondrosis, pediatric

- Degenerative changes of epiphyses that occur in rapidly growing children; usually idiopathic
- Classified by anatomic location

Modalities

- *X-ray*: first line, usually diagnostic
- *CT*: used if X-ray equivocal and MR unavailable or contraindicated
- *MR*: most accurate modality; preferred if X-ray equivocal
- *Bone scan*: initially more sensitive than X-ray, but less specific

Views

- Vary with anatomic location
- Bilateral comparison views are often helpful.
- Capitellum (Panner disease): AP, lateral, and oblique elbow views.
- Femoral head epiphysis (Legg–Calvé–Perthes disease): AP and frog-leg lateral hip views
- Metatarsal (Freiberg infarction): AP, lateral, and oblique foot views
- Navicular (Köhler disease): lateral and oblique foot views, and coned-down AP view of the navicular
- Tibial tuberosity (Osgood–Schlatter disease): AP and lateral knee views with slight internal rotation
- Vertebral bodies (Scheuermann disease): standing AP and lateral spine views

Findings

- Joint effusion, progressing to patchy sclerosis, subchondral lucency and collapse, and finally articular surface fragmentation with variable displacement of fragments
- Metatarsal (Freiberg infarction): cortical hypertrophy of affected metatarsal; associated with second metatarsal longer than first

- Tibial tuberosity (Osgood–Schlatter disease): thickening and calcification of the patellar tendon and fragmentation at the tibial tubercle may be demonstrated; this is associated with high-riding patella.
- Vertebral bodies (Scheuermann disease): 5° or more of anterior wedging in at least three adjacent thoracic vertebrae in lateral view is diagnostic; irregularities of the cartilage endplate (Schmorl's nodes) may be demonstrated.
- MR: unilateral decreased T1 signal intensity
- Bone scan: initially decreased activity followed by increased activity during reossification

Osteosarcoma

- Malignant bony tumor
- Usually occurs in distal femur, proximal tibia, or proximal humerus

Modalities

- *X-ray*: first line; may be equivocal
- *CT*: preferred for metastatic evaluation of thorax and for focal lesions if MR unavailable or contraindicated
- *MR*: preferred for focal lesions and surgical assessment
- Bone scan: preferred for metastatic evaluation of entire skeleton

Views

- These vary with anatomic location, but at least two orthogonal views should be obtained.
- The entire extent of involved bone and adjacent joints should be imaged.

Findings

- Skip lesions that are osteolytic, osteoblastic, or a mixture of both
- Wide zone of transition, sclerosis, and aggressive periosteal reaction with Codman's triangle or sunburst appearance may be demonstrated.
- MR: lesions have heterogeneously hyperintense and hypointense T1 and T2 signal. Invasion of marrow, joints, and soft tissue may be demonstrated.
- Bone scan: increased activity

Physeal (growth plate) fractures

Modalities

- *X-ray*: first line; often initially equivocal (especially for type I and type V)
- *CT*: used for severely comminuted fractures
- *MR*: most accurate modality, especially within 10 days post-injury

Views

- Vary with anatomic location
- Stress views may reveal occult fracture (especially of knee and elbow), though contraindicated if further physeal damage may occur

Findings

- *Salter–Harris type I*: physeal widening that may not be apparent initially, soft tissue swelling over the physis. After 1 week, adjacent sclerosis and periosteal reaction occur (Fig. 20.14).
- *Type II*: fracture through physis and includes fragment of metaphysis (Fig. 20.15)
- *Type III*: fracture through physis and epiphysis to the articular surface (Fig. 20.16)
- *Type IV*: fracture through the metaphysis, physis, and epiphysis to the articular surface (Fig. 20.17)
- *Type V*: crushing of the physis usually not initially apparent, soft tissue swelling over the physis

Slipped capital femoral epiphysis (SCFE)

- Displacement of the epiphysis from the physis

Modalities

- *X-ray*: first line; usually diagnostic
- *CT*: adjunct
- *MR*: used if X-ray equivocal

Views

- AP and bilateral frog-leg lateral hip views of pelvis (Care should be taken with abduction during the frog-leg lateral view to avoid exacerbating the condition; when in doubt a true lateral view may be substituted.)

Findings

- Blurring and displacement of the metaphysis–physis junction
- Widening of the physis with epiphysis displacement
- Epiphysis appears reduced in size in AP view from posterior rotation. This also leads to the appearance of "blanching" increased density of the metaphysis
- MR: surrounding edema demonstrates hyperintense T2 signal.

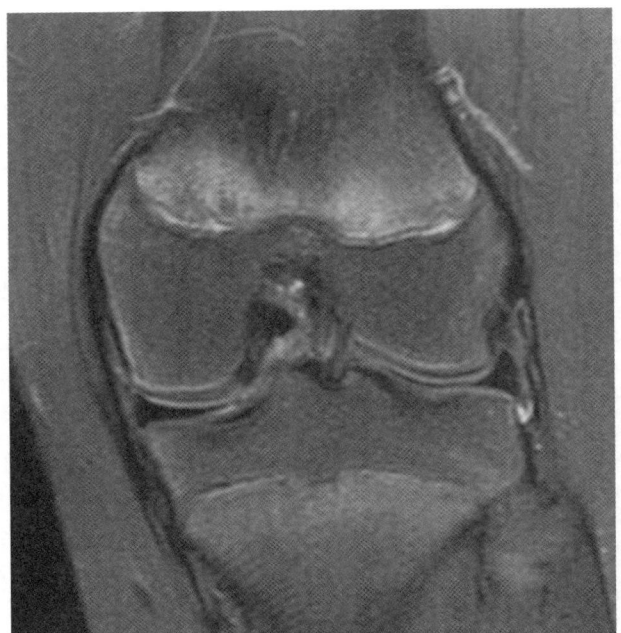

Figure 20.14 Coronal MR demonstrating Salter–Harris type I fracture with widening and hyperintense signal within the distal femoral physis.

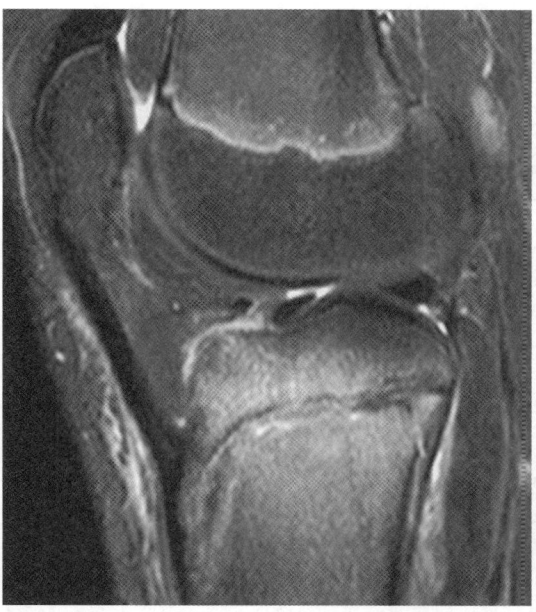

Figure 20.15 Sagittal MR demonstrating Salter–Harris type II fracture with widening of the proximal tibial physis and fracture extending through the posterior metaphysis.

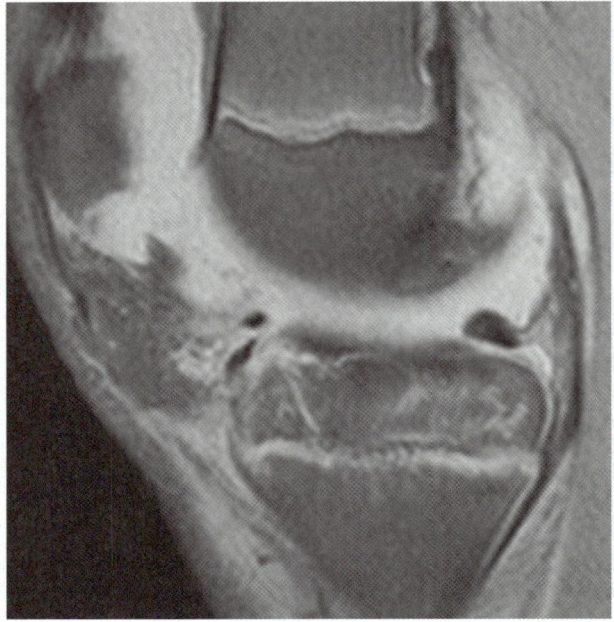

Figure 20.16 Sagittal MR demonstrating Salter–Harris type III fracture with widening of the proximal tibial physis and fracture extending through the anterior epiphysis to the articular surface.

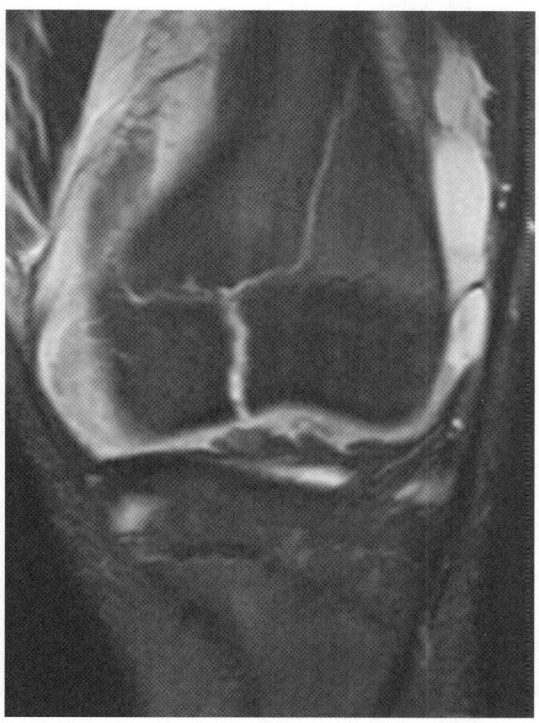

Figure 20.17 Coronal MR demonstrating Salter–Harris type IV fracture with fracture extending through the distal femoral metaphysis, physis, and epiphysis to the articular surface.

Sports psychology

Introduction

Sports psychology is the study of the psychologica. variables that impact sports performance. Most would agree that there is a mental side of sports. Athletic commentators are constantly discussing the confidence, focus, and attitude of athletes on the fields and courts. The percentage contribution of psychological skills on athletic performance may not be measurable, but the relative impact on performance outcome cannot be ignored.

This chapter will cover major internal and external factors impacting athletic performance and psychological skills that can be practiced and used to enhance performance success.

There are numerous factors that influence sports performance. In this chapter we cover the following (a) motivation; (b) emotional control; (c) anxiety, arousal, and stress; (d) self-confidence; (e) commitment; (f) attention; and (g) injury. These seven subjects were chosen because of their significance with regard to performance outcome and general patterns of participation.

Motivation and sports performance

The ability to be the best or merely to excel in any performance arena requires the "want to." Many individuals possess a certain degree of talent early on, but few ever achieve the prominence and success of a Tiger Woods, Roger Federer, or Laila Ali. People often claim that they would do anything to be an NBA, NFL, or Olympic star, yet few have the drive to work through the obstacles and keep pushing through failures. Few individuals are motivated enough to truly be great.

In sports, *motivation* can be described as one's desire to move toward a goal and the intensity of energy one is willing to produce in order to execute the required behaviors. People may be motivated by a variety of factors, including an intrinsic desire to perform, extrinsic rewards or glory, a desire to succeed, or a fear of failure.

General categories of motivation and orientation impacting motivation

- *Intrinsic motivation:* People who are driven to action on the basis of their personality, needs, interests, and goals.[1] These people will likely continue toward their goal regardless of the environment.
- *Extrinsic motivation:* People who are driven to action because of factors outside their control, including family, coaches, money, and prizes.[1] These individuals will require a variety of tangible or intangible rewards (i.e., praise, play time, trophy) in order to maintain their motivational level.
- *Desire to approach success:* People approach competitive situations because of a desire to compete and progress in skill level. They generally accept challenges.
- *Desire to avoid failure:* People compete in order not to lose. Often they avoid situations in which their competitive advantage is minimal or closely parallels that of a competitor, for fear of losing. They avoid risky situations or challenges and often perform below capabilities.
- *Outcome orientation:* People may be motivated to complete a task only because they want to finish, win, or receive the accolades for finishing.
- *Task orientation:* Others are motivated to perform tasks because they enjoy the process, learning, and ups and downs associated with trials.
- *Social orientation:* Some people engage in activities merely to be a part of the group and to enhance their socialization experiences.

Although an individual may be more personally motivated by the task, outcome, or social situation, there is evidence that others may influence motivational tendencies. Parents, coaches, or other socializing agents can influence goal orientation by influencing the motivational climate.[2] The motivational climate is determined by a variety of factors surrounding the task, competition level, feedback provided, and groupings of athletes in a given achievement setting.[1]

A positive motivational climate can be established by the following:
- Setting task-specific goals
- Providing instructional feedback about behaviors and skills that encourage corrections (e.g., "Your footwork was better, but next time stay on your toes.") instead of results (e.g., "You missed again.')
- Identifying athletes' goal orientation in order to match the needs of the athlete and the setting

1 Weinberg RS, Gould D (2007). *Foundations of Sport and Exercise Psychology*. Champaign, IL: Human Kinetics.
2 Nicholls JG (1984). Conceptions of ability and achievement motivation. In Ames R, Ames C (eds.), *Research on Motivation in Education: Student Motivation* (Vol. I). New York: Academic Press.

Emotional control and sports performance

Once athletes are motivated to achieve success, they must learn to recognize and control their emotions in both positive and negative situations. According to Deci,[1] *emotions* are defined as reactions to real or imagined stimulus that lead to physical changes, facial manipulations, and behavior changes.

Additional theories concerning the impact of emotions on performance include the following:

According to Lazarus's[2] cognitive–motivational–relational theory (CMRT), appraisal of the situation and coping abilities influences emotions and performance. If the athlete interprets the situation as dangerous, positive, negative, or inconsequential, different respective emotions will emerge. These emotions may be positive or negative, depending on whether athletes feel future success or failure is likely.[3]

Different emotions will emerge on the basis of athletes' feelings concerning their coping abilities. Feelings of anger and frustration may emerge if an athlete feels incapable of handling the demand, whereas athletes may respond more positively if they feel strong and in control over the situation.

According to Hackfort's[4,5] action theory, emotions and actions influence each other in a reciprocal fashion. Actions can invoke certain emotions or cause a change to emotions experienced.

Emotions can be categorized as either beneficial or costly[4] depending on the action or behavior that follows. Fear may benefit an athlete in a high-risk sport by influencing the athlete to modify a behavior, be more aware of surroundings, or recognize danger. However, fear also could be costly to performance outcome if it leads to tightness in muscles, narrowing of attention, and focus on irrelevant cues.

Emotions consist of the following[6,7]:

- *Physiological changes:* changes in heart rate, blood pressure, skin response, and facial expression
  - Ex. A person who is embarrassed may turn red; happy people smile; angry people frown.
  - Ex. Excitement and anger both lead to increased heart rate
- *Action tendencies:* compulsions to move or respond in a certain manner (though not always acted upon) are based on certain emotions.
  - Ex. Feelings of anger involve the action tendency to punch (clearly, societal rules do not allow this in most situations).
- *Subjective experiences:* athlete's interpretation of the experience
  - Ex. An athlete may see a large crowd at an event and perceive it to be scary, whereas a different athlete views that same experience as exciting.

The impact of emotions on sport performance includes the following:

- Emotions can affect the amount of energy athletes possess and lose prior to competition by influencing arousal level.[5]
- Emotions can affect cognition and focus.

Suggestions for enhancing emotional control include the following[6]:

- *Self-talk:* Use positive statements to replace maladaptive self-talk and use self-talk to trigger beneficial emotions for performance.
- *Imagery:* Fostering images of calm and relaxing scenarios can stimulate more positive emotions. Fostering images of previous success may increase feelings of pride and happiness. Creating images of recent failings or mistakes make increase feelings of frustration or anger. By practicing imagery, athletes can learn to stimulate the most ideal emotion for a given situation.
- *Modeling others:* One can learn which emotions are effective and ineffective in certain situations by watching the behaviors of others and the ramifications of their emotional responses.
- *Self-analysis:* Keeping a journal of emotional responses and situations may help athletes identify patterns of responses and encourage positive changes.

1 Deci EL (1980). *The Psychology of Self-Determination*. Lexington, MA: Heath.

2 Lazarus RS (1991). *Emotion and Adaptation*. Oxford, UK: Oxford University Press.

3 Weiner B. (1985). *An Attributional Theory of Motivation and Emotion*. New York: Springer-Verlag.

4 Hackfort D (1989). Emotion and emotion control in sports: benefits and costs. First IOC World Congress on Sport Sciences, Oct. 28–Nov. 3.

5 Hackfort D (1991). Emotion in sports: an action theoretical analysis. In Spielberger CD, Sarason JG, Van Heck WL (eds.) *Stress and Emotions*, Vol. 14 (pp. 56–73). New York: Hemisphere.

6 Jones MV (2003). Controlling emotions in sport. Sport Psychologist **17**(4):471–486.

7 Vallerand RJ, Blanchard CM (2000). The study of emotion in sport and exercise: historical, definitional, and conceptual perspectives. In Hanin YL (ed.). *Emotions in Sport*. Champaign IL: Human Kinetics, pp. 3–37.

Anxiety, arousal, and stress and sports performance

Anxiety, arousal, and stress have been found to detract from performance outcomes. Fans, parents, coaches, teammates, and athletes themselves increase the stressfulness of a situation, leading to increased arousal, a perceived inability to cope with the situation, anxious feelings, and, ultimately, a negative performance outcome.

It is important to note that although the terms *anxiety, arousal,* and *stress* are often used interchangeably, these are distinctly different concepts. Basically, the differences between these three concepts concern a focus on the body (arousal), the mind (anxiety), or the interpretation (stress).

- *Anxiety* refers to a negative cognitive or emotional state resulting in nervousness, worry, and physical arousal.[1]
- *Arousal* concerns the body and mind's activation from deep sleep to intense excitement.[1]
- *Stress* is defined as a state of anxiety resulting from one's interpretation that demands and responsibilities exceed coping ability.[2]

Detrimental effects of anxiety

Physical implications that may lead to early fatigue or exhaustion:

- Increased muscle tension
- Increased heart rate
- Increased sweating

Psychological implications that can lead to poor decision-making or errors in performance or that can decrease self-confidence:

- Negative thinking
- Irrational thoughts
- Unfocused thinking

Suggestions for minimizing stress and anxiety and identifying an ideal arousal level

Identification

Athletes must identify what is leading to this physical or psychological response. It is easier to prepare for and modify responses when the trigger is known. Also, athletes must identify the level of arousal that leads to their optimal physical performance. This will help them identify the need to "psych up" or "calm down" prior to competition.

Reduce uncertainty

Much stress and anxiety results from not knowing what is to come. Athletes must prepare for as many scenarios, under various conditions, as possible to better be prepared for the unexpected. In addition, it's important for athletes to realize in advance that surprises do happen and to feel confident enough in their skills to know that they can cope, adjust, and be successful regardless of the situation.

Appraisal of physical reaction

The physical responses to intense excitement or severe nervousness are essentially the same. If athletes can train their brains to define "butterflies in the stomach" as a sign of readiness instead of fear, they will soon realize that it is possible to play through the physiological arousal. Once the performance begins and thoughts are redirected toward the game, match, or event, increased heart rate, butterflies, and muscle tension disappear.

There always will be stressors in sports, but they only lead to performance detriments if they are interpreted as being beyond one's control. Self-doubt resides in athletes' minds. If they hope to erase the stress, first they must believe in their capabilities to cope with the situation. Thus, building self-confidence can lead to decreases in stress and anxiety.

1 Weinberg RS, Gould D (2007). *Foundations of Sport and Exercise Psychology*. Champaign, IL: Human Kinetics.
2 Seaward BL (2006). *Essentials of Managing Stress*. Sudbury, MA: Jones and Bartlett.

Self-confidence and sports performance

The most commonly cited definition of self-confidence is the belief that you can accomplish a desired behavior. Interestingly, self-confidence, as measured by the Competitive State Anxiety Inventory (CSAI-2), is the absence of cognitive anxiety. Thus, *confidence* is defined basically as believing in your ability to accomplish a task without any accompanying anxious thoughts.

This does not mean that the person will always accomplish the task, but rather that the person possesses the mindset necessary to keep working toward a desired goal without fear or nervousness over the outcome.

Characteristics of confident athletes

Confident athletes are more likely to

- Stay calm and relaxed under pressure because of a more positive appraisal and lack of anxiety.
- Focus on important cues and be able to play in the moment as a result of fewer distracting thoughts.
- Persist in a task or game even when they are losing or behind because they believe they have the ability to turn it around.
- Perform to the best of their abilities.

Influences on athletes' level of confidence

- The athletes (personality, goal orientation, optimism, gender, etc.)
- The culture or social climate (competitive level, motivational climate, coach behavior, program expectations, etc.)
- Achievements (previous successes and failures in similar ventures)

Suggestions for increasing confidence

- *Identify strengths and weaknesses:* Assess current capabilities, focusing on both strengths and weaknesses, acknowledging that everyone possesses both.
- *Goal setting:* Set realistic yet challenging goals that allow for small successes along the way.
- *Self-talk:* Use positive self-talk. Avoid personal attacks, such as "You suck," "Are you ever going to get that right?," or "You should not even be on the team."
- *Restructuring extrinsic negatives:* Individuals who hear negative comments from coaches, teammates, fans, or parents must learn how to accept the message while ignoring the tone or negativity. This is most easily done by rephrasing the comment into a useful, behavior-focused statement.
- *Accept mistakes:* Know that the more risks athletes take and the more mistakes they make, the better they will become.
- *Take pride in small accomplishments:* A confident athlete can find the one good play in a bad game.

When confident athletes take the field or court or step up to the plate, others can see it in their eyes and read it in their body language. This posturing affects the athletes themselves and those around them.

Sometimes confidence is easy, but sometimes it takes work. All athletes can work on the external demonstration of confidence while simultaneously working on changing their thoughts. It is important to make clear that although confidence is critical, it will not improve play without accompanying talent and skill.

Commitment and sports performance

An athlete may have all the talent and confidence in the world, but if they are unwilling to put in the time and effort, the athlete will never reach their peak. Commitment is an essential quality in top-level athletes. Great athletes can maintain an incredible focus, keep their bodies fit, and work on their skills and mental game while preserving a perspective that allows life to go on, regardless of whether they win or lose.

Those who lack balance tend to overcommit to their sport, which leads to dysfunctional behaviors and thoughts. Athletes in this category may overtrain, become anxious when not training, and use performance-enhancing drugs.[1,2]

Defining commitment

- A desire and resolve to stay with a sport over time [3]
- Persistence when others want to quit
- The willingness to give a little extra, keep going when tired, placing sports on top of the priority list, and continually try to improve [4]
- The willingness to sacrifice for your sport

Internal factors and barriers impacting sport commitment

- *Vision:* the ability to see yourself attaining the "dream" [4]
- *Motivation:* the desire and willingness to push through obstacles to achieve success.
- *Athletic identity:* the amount to which you identify yourself by your athletic endeavors [5]

External factors and barrier that impact sport commitment

- *Coaches:* Words of motivation, amount and type of reinforcement, and conflicts between athletes and coaches have been found to positively or negatively affect an athlete's commitment.[6]
- *Teams:* More task-cohesive teams demand commitment of all members.[7] Therefore, committed athletes breed further commitment from their teammates.

1 Coen SP, Ogles BM (1993). Psychological characteristics of the obligatory runner: a critical examination of the anorexia analogue hypothesis. *J Sport Exercise Psychol* **15**:338–354.

2 Hughes R, Coakley J (1991). Positive deviance among athletes: the implications of overconformity to the sport ethic. *Social Sport J* **8**:307–325.

3 Scanlan TK, Simons JP, Carpenter PJ, Schmidt GW, Keeler B (1993). The sport commitment model: measurement development for the youth-sport domain. *J Sport Exercise Psychol* **15**:16–38.

4 Orlick T (2000). *In Pursuit of Excellence: How to Win in Sport and Life Through Mental Training* (3rd ed.). Champaign, IL: Human Kinetics.

5 Horton RS, Mack DE (2000). Athletic identity in marathon runners: functional focus or dysfunctional commitment? *J Sport Behav* **23**(2):101–119.

6 Whisenant W (2005). Organizational justice and commitment in interscholastic sports. *Sport Education, and Society* **11**(3):343–357.

7 Carron AV, Hausenblas HA (1998). *Group Dynamics in Sport* (2nd ed). Morgantown, WV: Fitness Information Technology.

Attentional focus and sports performance

Attentional focus varies from player to player and often from situation to situation. However, it is clear that in order to be successful in sports, there is an ideal focus, and one must learn to control the mind and direct attention to what is important.

There are four main areas of attention athletes must work on.[1]

Maintain focus on relevant cues
- Ignore distractions both before and during competitions.
- Focus on the play, teammates, and the skill you are performing.

Staying focused over time
- The ease of focusing depends on the time of year, point in a competition, or internal and external distractions.
- Athletes must learn to "turn on" and "turn off" focus—this teaches control of the mind at critical times.

Being aware of the situation
- Lack of awareness can lead to mistakes in judgment, errors in performance, and injuries.
- Awareness on and off the field of play is critical for athletes and coaches.

Shifting attention when necessary
Understanding and using different attentional styles to suit the situation improves play. One style may be more or less useful depending on the sport. However, most sports require the ability to shift between these styles.

There are basically four types of attentional styles[2]
- *Broad-external*: ability to see the entire field
- *Broad-internal*: ability to identify each muscle tightening and each feeling and thought
- *Narrow-external*: ability to focus on a single external target and block out the remaining visual field
- *Narrow-internal*: ability to focus on a single thought or feeling from within

Common errors in attentional focus

Too much focus on single item, situation, or factor
Too much attention internally has been said to lead to a "paralysis by analysis," otherwise known as overthinking.[3]

Lack of focus
Too little focus on any single aspect of the game may lead to a failure to plan or see what is right in front of you.
- Ex. If an athlete is so narrowly focused on a teammate, the athlete may miss seeing the defender waiting on the side to pick off the pass.

Incorrect focus

Sometimes athletes are focused on the wrong cues.

- Ex. An athlete who is focused on winning the game cannot possibly be thinking about the important cues needed to execute the skill. Our mind is able to switch between thoughts quickly, but we are not so capable of thinking two thoughts simultaneously.

Focused on distractors

Sometimes athletes focus on other people, events, and thoughts.

- Ex. Individuals focused on the fans, school work, or a fight they had earlier with a friend will not be focused on the ball, the teammate, the opponent, or the game.

Suggestions for improving attentional focus and shifting attention

- *Awareness:* Recognize thoughts to be better able to control and change them.
- *Practice:* Just as athletes must practice hitting, throwing, and shooting, they must also practice attentional shifting.
- *Cue words:* Create cue words that focus you on the proper technique for certain skills. Link the cue words with skill execution.
- *Goal setting:* Write a goal every day before practice and competition on your hand, a piece of equipment, or a piece of paper. When attention begins to shift to irrelevant cues, look at the paper or reminder and refocus on the moment.
- *Avoiding off-field distractors:* Prior to practice or competition, write down all possible distractors for that day. Place that list in your bag or locker with a note saying, "I will deal with these later."
- *Avoiding on-field distractors:* Be aware of your thoughts. Use cue words. And, remind yourself of your goal.

1 Weinberg RS, Gould D (2007). *Foundations of Sport and Exercise Psychology.* Champaign, IL: Human Kinetics.

2 Nideffer RM, Sagal M (2001). Concentration and attention control training. In Williams JM (ed.), *Applied Sport Psychology* (4th ed). Mountain View, CA: Mayfield, pp. 312–332.

3 Nideffer and Sagal (2001), p. 315.

Injury and sports

Research in the area of sports injury has addressed psychological factors that may increase the likelihood of getting injured and psychological reactions post-injury. There are inconsistencies in the literature attempting to predict a predisposition to injury.[1,2] The main findings, however, point to the impact of certain personality traits on the stress response.[3]

According to Williams and Anderson,[4] stress is a mediating variable between personality and injury. Results have identified that athletes low in optimism, low in hardiness, and low in perceived control may be more likely to incur injuries than their counterparts because of increased stress.[3] Stress leads to disruptions in attention and muscle tension.[5] Distracted thoughts and tight muscles lead to errors in judgment, errors in technique, and thus the greater likelihood of injury.

Aside from reducing stress, using appropriate equipment, teaching proper techniques, and using safe venues, there is little else athletes can do to prevent injury. Therefore, it is important to understand athletes' responses to injury.

It was originally suggested that athletes experience a response to injury similar to the grief response.[6] This is characterized by the following stages:
- Denial
- Anger
- Bargaining
- Depression
- Acceptance

More recent evidence has identified the response as being less orderly; athletes go back and forth between stages.[5] Regardless of the exact progression of responses, researchers[6–8] have found that injured athletes experience the following:
- Pain
- Anger
- Irritability
- A lack of control
- Loss of identity
- Fear
- Loss of confidence

Additional issues faced by injured athletes are as follows:
- Distrust in the medical staff
- Playing through injury, masking pain
- Frustration over missing games
- Fear of losing starting position
- Lack of communication with coaches
- Negative response on school and other areas of life

Sports are all about pushing limits and doing more than you did before. According to Coakley's[9] sport ethic, athletes are expected to (a) make sacrifices for the game, (b) strive for distinction, (c) accept risks and play through pain, and (d) accept no limits while pursuing the possibilities of sport. This message, though engrained in the minds of many tcp athletes and coaches, can be very detrimental to the health and well-being of many athletes.

In order to improve athletes' responses to injury and ultimate recovery, it is important to do the following:

- Ensure that all athletes know to listen to their bodies, as a small pain now may lead to a bigger pain later. This is necessary for preventing injuries and intensifying injuries.
- Create open communication between athletes, medical staff, and coaches.
- Provide social support to injured athletes to help them through the recovery process.
- Do not allow injured athletes to isolate themselves or be isolated by the team.
- Teach athletes to use imagery during their recovery. Although they may not be able to physically partake in practice, visualizing the plays on the sideline may increase their preparedness once they are ready to return to play.
- Recognize that recover from injury may not be quick or linear, thus prepare for setback and practice patience.

1 Passer MW, Seese MD (1983). Life stress and athletic injury: examination of positive versus negative life events and three moderator variables. *J Hum Stress* 9:11–16.

2 Petrie TA (1993). Coping skills, competitive trait anxiety, and playing status: moderating effects on the life stress-injury relationship. *J Sport Exercise Psychol* 15:261–274.

3 Ford IW, Eklund RC, Gordon S (2000). An examination of psychosocial variables moderating the relationship between life stress and injury time-loss among athletes of a high standard. *J Sports Sci* 18.5:301–312.

4 Anderson, M., Williams, J. (1988). A model of stress and athletic injury: prediction and prevention. *J Sport Exercise Psychol* 10(3):294–306.

5 Weinberg RS, Gould D (2007). *Foundations of Sport and Exercise Psychology.* Champaign, IL: Human Kinetics.

6 Hardy CJ, Crace RK (1993. The dimensions of social support when dealing with sport injuries. In Pargman D (ed.), *Psychological Bases of Sport Injuries.* Morgantown, WV: Fitness Information Technology, pp. 121–144.

7 Petitpas A, Danish S (1995). Caring for injured athletes. In Murphy S (ed.), *Sport Psychology Interventions.* Champaign, IL: Human Kinetics, pp. 255–281.

8 Silva JM, Hardy CJ (1991). The sport psychologist: psychological aspects of injury in sport. In Mueller FO, Ryan A (eds.). *The Sports Medicine Team and Athlete Injury Prevention.* Philadelphia: FA Davis, pp. 114–132.

9 Coakley J (2001). *Sport in Society: Issues and Controversies,* 7th edition. McGraw-Hill.

Further reading

Carron AV, Hausenblas HA (1998). *Group Dynamics in Sport*, 2nd ed. Morgantown, WV: Fitness Information Technology.

Coen SP, Ogles BM (1993). Psychological characteristics of the obligatory runner: a critical examination of the anorexia analogue hypothesis. *J Sport Exercise Psychol* **15**:338–354.

Deci EL (1980). *The Psychology of Self-Determination*. Lexington, MA: Heath.

Ford IW, Eklund RC, Gordon S (2000). An examination of psychosocial variables moderating the relationship between life stress and injury time-loss among athletes of a high standard. *J Sports Sci* **18.5**:301–312.

Hackfort D (1989). Emotion and emotion control in sports: benefits and costs. First IOC World Congress on Sport Sciences, Oct. 28–Nov. 3.

Hackfort D (1991). Emotion in sports: an action theoretical analysis. In Spielberger CD, Sarason JG, Van Heck WL (eds.) *Stress and Emotions*, Vol. 14. New York: Hemisphere, pp. 56–73.

Hardy CJ, Crace RK (1993). The dimensions of social support when dealing with sport injuries. In Pargman D (ed.), *Psychological Bases of Sport Injuries*. Morgantown, WV: Fitness Information Technology, pp. 121–144.

Horton RS, Mack DE (2000). Athletic identity in marathon runners: functional focus or dysfunctional commitment? *J Sport Behav* **23**(2):101–119.

Hughes R, Coakley J (1991). Positive deviance among athletes: the implications of overconformity to the sport ethic. *Sociol Sport J* **8**:307–325.

Jones MV (2003). Controlling emotions in sport. *Sport Psychologist* **17**(4):471–486.

Lazarus RS (1991). *Emotion and Adaptation*. Oxford, UK: Oxford University Press.

Nicholls JG (1984). Conceptions of ability and achievement motivation. In Ames R, Ames C (eds.), *Research on Motivation in Education: Student Motivation* (Vol. I). New York: Academic Press.

Nideffer RM, Sagal M (2001). Concentration and attention control training. In Williams JM (ed.), *Applied Sport Psychology*, 4th ed. Mountain View, CA: Mayfield, pp. 312–332.

Orlick T (2000). *In Pursuit of Excellence: How to Win in Sport and Life Through Mental Training*, 3rd ed. Champaign, IL: Human Kinetics.

Passer MW, Seese MD (1983). Life stress and athletic injury: examination of positive versus negative life events and three moderator variables. *J Hum Stress* **9**:11–16.

Petrie TA (1993). Coping skills, competitive trait anxiety, and playing status: moderating effects on the life stress-injury relationship. *J Sport Exercise Psychol* **15**:261–274.

Petitpas A, Danish S (1995). Caring for injured athletes. In Murphy S (ed.), *Sport Psychology Interventions*. Champaign, IL: Human Kinetics, pp. 255–281.

Scanlan TK, Simons JP, Carpenter PJ, Schmidt GW, Keeler B (1993). The sport commitment model: measurement development for the youth-sport domain. *J Sport Exercise Psychol* **15**:16–38.

Seaward BL (2006). *Essentials of Managing Stress*. Sudbury, MA: Jones and Bartlett.

Silva JM, Hardy CJ (1991). The sport psychologist: psychological aspects of injury in sport. In Mueller FO, Ryan A (eds.). *The Sports Medicine Team and Athlete Injury Prevention*. Philadelphia: FA Davis, pp. 114–132.

Vallerand RJ, Blanchard CM (2000). The study of emotion in sport and exercise: historical, definitional, and conceptual perspectives. In Hanin YL (ed.), *Emotions in Sport*. Champaign IL: Human Kinetics, pp. 3–37.

Weiner B. (1985). *An Attributional Theory of Motivation and Emotion*. New York: Springer-Verlag.

Weinberg RS, Gould D (2007). *Foundations of Sport and Exercise Psychology*. Champaign, IL: Human Kinetics.

Whisenant W (2005). Organizational justice and commitment in interscholastic sports. *Sport Education, and Society* **11**(3):343–357.

The team physician

The medical care of a team or squad of athletes is an integral part of the role of the sports medicine specialist and potentially one of the most rewarding aspects of sports medicine practice.

The specifics of the team physician role will depend on a variety of issues including the sport involved, the nature of the event, e.g., single sport or multi-sport, and the level of competition or ability of the athletes. There are, however, a number of general principles that are relevant to team medical support in general and some special circumstances.

Team physician definition

The team physician must have an unrestricted medical license and be an M.D. or D.O. who is responsible for treating and coordinating the medical care of athletic team members. The principal responsibility of the team physician is to provide for the well-being of individual athletes, enabling each to realize his or her full potential.

The team physician should possess special proficiency in the care of musculoskeletal injuries and medical conditions encountered in sports. The team physician also must actively integrate medical expertise with other health-care providers, including medical specialists, athletic trainers, and allied health professionals.

The team physician must ultimately assume responsibility within the team structure for making medical decisions that affect the athlete's safe participation. Such responsibility includes the following:

- Provide for proper preparation for safe return to participation after an illness or injury
- Integrate medical expertise with that of other health-care providers, including medical specialists, athletic trainers, and allied health professionals
- Provide for appropriate education and counseling regarding nutrition, strength and conditioning, ergogenic aids, substance abuse, and other medical problems that could affect the athlete
- Provide for proper documentation and medical-record keeping

The bottom line of the team physician is the health and welfare of the athlete.

The qualifications of a team physician

The primary concern of the team physician is to provide the best medical care for athletes at all levels of participation. To this end, the following qualifications are necessary for all team physicians:

- Have an M.D. or D.O. in good standing, with an unrestricted license to practice medicine
- Possess a fundamental knowledge of emergency care regarding sporting events
- Be trained in CPR
- Have a working knowledge of trauma, musculoskeletal injuries, and medical conditions affecting the athlete

In addition, it is desirable for team physicians to have clinical training and experience and administrative skills in some or all of the following:

- Specialty board certification
- Continuing medical education in sports medicine
- Formal training in sports medicine (fellowship training, board-recognized subspecialty in sports medicine, known as a certificate of added qualification [CAQ] in sports medicine)
- Additional training in sports medicine
- 50% or more of practice involving sports medicine
- Membership and participation in a sports medicine society
- Involvement in teaching, research, and publications relating to sports medicine
- Training in advanced cardiac life support
- Knowledge of medicolegal, disability, and workers' compensation issues
- Training in media skills

The medical kit

The equipment that the team physician takes to an event will depend on a number of factors and can be as basic or extensive as one desires. However, there should always be a standard amount of equipment in any one kit.

Experience of practitioner

Carry equipment that you are competent to use. If covering a sport that might require a particular piece of equipment, seek appropriate training before agreeing to cover that event. If your level of knowledge and experience does not commensurate with that required to provide a duty of care for those you are looking after, you should not be there, no matter how attractive the opportunity.

Medical risk assessment

A vital part of team coverage is medical risk assessment. This means identifying what problems you are likely to encounter, what facilities will be at your disposal to deal with such events, and what additional equipment you need to provide or arrange to have provided. A number of issues will govern the medical risk associated with a particular event.

Sport

Different sports clearly carry different injury profiles, e.g., the high risk of contact trauma associated with football or rugby compared with the low risk associated with tennis or cross-country. You must have an appreciation of the injury profile of the sport to be able to adequately plan.

For example, it would be indefensible if you could not adequately immobilize the cervical spine when covering a football game, whereas serious cervical injury would be highly unlikely on a tennis court. However, knowledge of adequate cervical spine immobilization is needed in any sport or event covered.

Venue or event

The venue will influence the equipment that you carry. The equipment you will need, for example, to provide medical coverage at a high school football game will be very different from that required to cover a Division I college football game. Similarly, consider the role of the medical staff for the Boston Marathon, run over the same distance as another on the foothills of Mount Everest.

The following list, although not exhaustive, covers many of the important factors:

- Will you be a solo practitioner or part of a team of clinicians? If part of a team, what is their experience and what equipment are they likely to bring?
- What medical equipment will be provided by the venue (e.g., is there a fully equipped medical tent or training room)?
- Will emergency medical support be present (will there be a paramedic ambulance on site)? If not, what is the time frame for arrival to the event if called?

- Where will you be situated in relation to the field of play and what access to the field of play do you have?
- Where are the nearest emergency care and hospital facilities?
- What is the transfer time to these facilities and how might that change on the day of competition?
- Environment and climate considerations

The team you are covering

Most athletes are by definition healthy; however, they may have medical conditions, e.g., diabetes, asthma, or disabilities, that will influence the type of equipment you require. Furthermore, you will almost certainly be responsible for the health of those individuals supporting the athletes, e.g., performance directors, coaches, and medical and paramedical staff.

Support staff may have a variety of chronic illnesses and medical requirements and you should be prepared for these. If you are traveling with a team with whom you don't usually work, it is useful to send out a questionnaire prior to departure requesting key current and past medical history, medications, and allergies.

Basic medical equipment

- Soft water bottle—this allows pressure to be exerted when irrigating wounds
- Device to remove helmet (Trainer's Angel, etc.)
- Tape
- Assorted plasters, sterile wound dressings, and bandages
- Stethoscope
- Portable sphygmomanometer
- Oto- and opthalmoscope, spare batteries
- Penlight
- Scissors
- Tongue depressors
- Thermometer
- Oropharyngeal airways (multiple sizes)
- Nasopharyngeal airways (6–8 mm)
- Petroleum gel
- Pocket mask with mouthpiece and O_2 inlet
- Alcohol wipes
- Antimicrobial soap and hand sanitizer
- Cleaning fluid (e.g., chlorhexidine, Betadine)
- Semipermeable dressing (e.g., Tegaderm) of various sizes
- Low-adherence dressing (various sizes)
- Sterile gauze swabs and cotton balls
- Tubular bandage (e.g., Tubigrip)
- Supportive bandage
- Cohesive bandage (e.g., Coban)
- Permeable adhesive tape
- Blister pack
- Sterile and nonsterile gloves
- Adhesive strips (e.g., Steri-strip) with mastisol
- Tissue adhesive (e.g., Dermabond)
- Suture kit and staples
- Suture removal kit and staple remover
- Scalpel and blades (preferably disposable)
- Razor
- Sharps container
- Assorted needles and syringes
- Tourniquet
- Blood and specimen bottles and culturettes
- Peak flow meter and disposable mouthpieces
- Assorted cannulae
- 1000 mL bag of normal saline or lactated Ringer's solution
- IV set up with 16,18, and 22 g catheters
- Adjustable hard collar
- Safety pins

- Tape measure
- Urinalysis testing strips (e.g., Clinitest)
- Glucose testing meter and test strips
- Save-a-tooth kit
- Contact saline solution and contact lens container

Don't forget the obvious nonmedical items—e.g., pen, paper, incident report form, standardized concussion testing form, cell phone or walkie-talkie, and useful contact numbers.

A driver's license and medical license are often helpful. Carrying a prescription pad is also useful.

Essential drugs and medications

If providing medical support to a large team or squad competing nationally or internationally, you will need an extensive drug list to cover most medical situations. Irrespective of the drugs you have available, at base there are essential drugs and medications that you should carry with you. This list is a guide to essentials; it will also be influenced by the medical history of your team members.

- Epinephrine (adrenaline) (1/10,000) 1 mg in 10 mL prefilled syringe
- Epinephrine (adrenaline) (1/1000) 1 mg in 1 mL prefilled syringe
- Parenteral antihistamine, e.g., chlorpheniramine (10 mg/mL)
- Hydrocortisone IV 100 mg vial
- Glucogel (3 ampoule pack)
- Frusemide (IV and oral)
- Midazolam 1 mg/mL as 50 mL vial (optional)
- Parenteral opiate analgesia (e.g., meperidine 25 mg/1 mL amp or morphine)—depends on the circumstances
- Naloxone (optional; if carrying opiate analgesia, essential)
- Anesthetic (e.g., topical [EMLA], lidocaine, bupivicaine)
- Intra-articular steroid (e.g., triamcinolone, methylprednisolone)
- Sterile water ampoules for injections
- Antihistamine (oral and topical)
- Acetaminophen
- Compound analgesic (e.g., co-codamol)
- Parenteral analgesia (e.g., IM ketorolac 30–60 mg)
- Nonsteroidal anti-inflammatory drug (NSAID) (e.g., ibuprofen)
- Penicillin (IV and oral)
- Alternative broad-spectrum antibiotics, including those for penicillin-sensitive individuals, e.g., erythromycin, bactrim, etc.
- Aspirin
- Nitrolingual spray
- Antacids
- Antidiarrheal agent (e.g., loperamide)
- Laxative (e.g., biscadoyl 5 mg)
- Rehydration (Gatorade, Pedialyte)
- Antiemetic (e.g., prochlorperazine, oral and IV/IM)
- Beta-2 agonist inhaler (e.g., albuterol)
- Anesthetic throat lozenges
- Oral steroid (e.g., prednisolone)
- Silvadene
- Topical steroid (e.g., hydrocortisone)
- Antifungal cream or powder
- Antibiotic and steroid drops suitable for ocular and ear use
- Fluorescein/tetracaine eye drops

- Migraine treatment (e.g., sumatriptan or equivalent)
- Oral decongestant (if not banned by your team's governing body)
- Motion sickness medication (e.g., meclizine 25 mg)
- Anti-cough medication (benzatoate, dextromorphan, etc.)

Know the current doping regulations and which ones apply to the athletes under your care, e.g., in/out competition, IOC, NCAA, etc. It is good policy to not have any banned substance in your medical bag, even if staff members may use them.

Also, regularly check for expired medications.

Security and insurance issues

Increased security has restricted the ease with which a doctor can transport medical equipment and medication. Consider taking practical steps to preempt or avoid any related difficulties.

- Itemize, in full, the contents of your medical bag.
- Write to the embassy of the country of destination detailing your travel arrangements and seek approval for the carriage of your medical equipment; be sure to include your list.
- Do not take with you strong opiate-based analgesia, e.g., morphine, unless absolutely necessary. Seek prior agreement if you do bring it. Many countries restrict even moderate or weak opiates not intended for personal medical use.
- Where possible, obtain medications in the state or country of destination.
- Consider writing to the airline you will use, detailing your medical luggage.
- Carry a copy of your itemized medical bag and a letter confirming your medical role.
- Ensure that any prohibited "dangerous" (or potential prohibited) items are stored in the hold.
- Do not take pressurized containers, e.g., oxygen
- Ensure that you have appropriate travel insurance.
- Ensure that you have appropriate medical insurance and indemnity to practice in the state or country of destination.
- Carry separately a photocopy of your passport.

Team travel

Providing medical support to a traveling team presents the sports physician with additional challenges, and adequate and timely preparation is essential. The following considerations should help you prepare for your team travel experience.

Selecting a medical team

You may be responsible for a team of medical officers. In these circumstances, you should be involved in the appointment of your medical team. It is vitally important to get your team right from the start. This process should be just as any other professional appointment, with a job description (including essential and desired criteria), application process with open job advert, short-listing, and interview.

Your interview panel should be multidisciplinary and should include the athletic trainer, strength and conditioning staff member, etc. The appointments panel should meet prior to the interview to identify key questions that will allow the interviewee to demonstrate that they possess the necessary essential and desired qualities. In particular, the ability to work effectively within a multidisciplinary team should be assessed.

It may be useful to have, within a team, doctors of differing sports medicine backgrounds, e.g., primary care, musculoskeletal, emergency care, orthopedics, etc. These physicians should be board certified or have a certificate of added qualification (CAQ) in sports medicine.

Medical preparation

Adequate preparation is essential, whether you are the chief medical officer to an Olympic team or the team physician to a local high school team. The preparation will reflect the particular circumstances but should follow good medical practice and applies irrespective of the stature of your athletes.

Team building

Get to know your team before departure. In many circumstances, you will already be part of a well-established team or squad. For major events, however, the headquarters staff may be from different backgrounds and you will almost certainly be working with a number of strangers.

For this reason, most organizations arrange team-building sessions, usually residential and often at weekends, that you should attend, whether you are a medical team leader or another covering team member. These sessions are invaluable opportunities to get to know other team members and facilitate preparation and planning.

You should be prepared to advise your team on relevant medical issues including the ubiquitous "what-if" scenarios, e.g., what do we do if one of the team members brings into camp a highly contagious form of gastroenteritis?

You may attend training or preparation camps. These will serve a number of purposes, not least is the opportunity to ensure effective team working and meet any athletes or support staff who are new to a squad. Training, preparation, or holding camps may provide an opportunity to get to know some individual squads.

Pretravel medical assessment

Providing medical support during competition can be challenging, in addition to the complications of being in another state or foreign country with various cultural, environmental, and linguistic differences. It helps to have as much information about your destination and team members as possible.

You may have had the luxury of a pregames visit or training camp, in which case you should perform a medical risk assessment as described previously. If not, contact nonmedical colleagues who are going on a pregames visit and other medical colleagues who may have been to your destination previously, and try to make contact with local medical services. The Internet and e-mail can facilitate communication.

Team education

Invest time in educating your team prior to competition. You should have had the opportunity to meet your team at team-building sessions or at the preparticipation exam (PPE). These will usually be arranged to replicate some of the environmental challenges that may be encountered and thus provide an ideal learning opportunity for athletes and support staff.

You may wish to consider writing up a medical fact sheet, which can be sent to those on your team whom you are not able to meet.

Following are some of the issues that you might wish to cover:
- Your contact details (and those on the medical team)
- Jet lag and travel sickness
- Environmental advice (dealing with heat, humidity, cold, altitude, insects)
- Hygiene (in particular the prevention of travel-related illness)
- Fluid and nutrition
- Immunization advice
- Locality advice, e.g., details of how to access the local pharmacy opticians, hospital services, and dentist, with relevant names and contact information
- Emergency advice, e.g., what to do if you are involved in a car crash
- Medical insurance coverage (the coverage provided as a member of a team and what additional coverage individuals will have to arrange for)
- General travel advice

Immunization and vaccination

Exact immunization requirements depend on your destination. You must ensure that you are aware of the latest advice. The Centers for Disease Control and Prevention (CDC: www.cdc.gov) has the most up-to-date recommendations for immunizations and vaccinations.

Assuming that the normal vaccination program against TB, measles, mumps, rubella, pertussis, Hib, meningococcus, and polio has been completed, you may update immunization against hepatitis A and B and tetanus. Vaccination should take place as early as possible to allow sufficient time to get over any reactions.

The journey

Your role as a team doctor goes far beyond normal medical practice. You are very much a member of a team and may be able to help with other tasks, including travel logistics, e.g., helping with luggage and assisting with check in.

Ensure that you have a small medical bag in your hand luggage. It may be useful to include the following items:

- Letter of authority confirming your medical role and requirement to carry medical equipment (and a list of that equipment)
- Acetominophen
- Ibuprofen
- Prochlorperazine (buccal)
- Loperamide
- Antihistamine
- Merocaine throat lozenges
- Imitrex (50 mg tablets)
- Epinephrine (Epipen)
- Laerdal pocket mask
- Stethoscope
- Albuterol inhaler
- Aspirin
- Any specific medications, depending on the regular prescriptions of team members

Jet lag

Most of us have experienced jet lag, an almost indescribable feeling of utter uselessness. It is characterized by the following symptoms:

- Altered sleep pattern with daytime sleepiness and nighttime insomnia
- Poor concentration
- Fatigue and malaise
- Gastrointestinal disturbance

In addition to these generic symptoms, it will impair athletic performance for several days.

Jet lag is thought to be caused by disrupted circadian rhythms in those flying across three or more time zones. (A time zone is defined by a 1-hour time change for every 15° traveled in either direction from the Greenwich meridian; there are, of course, 24.) Although jet lag cannot be prevented, it can be modified and its impact reduced by taking fairly simple measures:

- Ensure adequate rest and sleep prior to departure. You may want to start adjusting your time zone prior to departure, e.g., going to bed and getting up an hour earlier or later.
- Aim to arrive late afternoon.
- Maintain good hydration.
- Synchronize your watch to the destination time zone upon departure.
- Ensure adequate relaxation during the flight. Try to eat and sleep in concordance with your new time zone.

- Upon arrival, try to remain active during any remaining daylight hours and adjust meal and bedtimes to new time zone.
- Avoid stimulants (e.g., caffeine) at times when you should be resting.
- Try to adopt a flexible routine upon arrival; a rigid routine will prolong the effects of jet lag.
- Be prepared to allow 1 day of recovery for each time zone crossed (e.g., if traveling from London to Sydney, you should expect to modify your normal training and expect altered performance for up to 10 days).

Melatonin is a hormone secreted in the evening by the pineal gland. It has been used in experiments to modify the symptoms of jet lag. Current evidence to support its use in reducing the symptoms of jet lag is inconclusive and there is a lack of data on its long-term safety.

Arrival—getting started

Upon arrival check that your team and their medical equipment have arrived complete and undamaged. Once appropriately refreshed and rested (if time permits), establish a well-organized base from which to operate from, be if the hotel room, medical room, or medical suite. You should have considered the location of your medical room prior to arrival; however, be flexible if the situation requires it.

Issues to consider when planning the location of your medical room are the following:

- Confidentiality and privacy
- Accessibility
- Security
- Space
  - An examination table should be accessible from all sides.
  - In an ideal world you will need a desk, two chairs, storage space including secure storage, and a fridge.
- Proximity to colleagues, e.g., physical therapy, emergency departments
- Environment, e.g., air conditioning, natural light
- Power, communication, computer, and IT connections
- Mobile telephone with appropriate network coverage
- Access to washing and toilet facilities
- Drug testing facility
- Isolation room

Ideally, avoid your own room becoming the medical room, to protect your privacy, although all too frequently this is what happens.

In addition, the medical team should have access to a designated car.

Managing your medical service

Organization is essential for a successful medical service. Despite the best made plans, medical support in a competitive environment will constantly be faced with new problems, requiring changes in plan and flexibility, and with unreasonable deadlines that have to be met. If you are organized, then managing change becomes more achievable.

Medical consultations

Athletes train and compete, eat and rest, at varying times, and your accessibility should reflect this. A flexible drop-in approach to appointments suits most athletes. This usually means being available from early morning to late evening.

But you also need some rest to remain fresh and enthusiastic (and don't feel guilty about it). If you are a solo physician, make everyone aware of your availability for that day, structure any down time around the likely quiet periods—e.g., athletes will frequently want to see you before and after training and competition, they are less likely to need your services during their rest time. You will need to provide 24-hour contact details in the case of an emergency.

You will almost certainly be required to provide coverage at training and competition. This is challenging in a multi-games environment. If you are part of a team, arrange a rotation.

In medical consultations, remember the following:
- Your ethical code of practice
- An athlete's right to confidentiality
- Do not practice beyond your scope of practice. If you have prepared properly, you will have made arrangements to seek specialist advice when appropriate.
- The ability to ask for a second opinion. Even if you are a solo physician, there is always someone somewhere available for advice.
- You must have professional indemnity and insurance to allow you to practice medicine in the country you are working in.
- Accurate medical-record keeping is essential. The development of a Web-based electronic record has made an important contribution to our ability to maintain an accurate medical record for athletes as patients who are constantly on the move. If it isn't documented, it didn't happen.
- You must have contingency plans in the event of contagious illness.
- Any prescribing must be within the IOC, NCAA, games organizing body, or international federation out/in competition doping regulations, and you must be aware of which rules apply. If you prescribe or use a regulated substance, you must complete and submit the relevant therapeutic use exceptions (TUE) form (or any equivalent documentation) and ensure that copies are retained by you and the athlete and scanned into any electronic record.
- Good team work and communication

You are part of a medical team, and all members of that team, acknowledging any limitations imposed by respecting an athlete's confidentiality, should be included in a multidisciplinary approach to management. You are also part of a wider athletic team. In many circumstances, the coach and performance director should also be kept informed of any athlete's medical issues, although this must be with the athlete's full consent.

Preparticipation exam (PPE)

Your appreciation of the team's previous medical history may vary from having a detailed knowledge of a team through years of working with the same individuals to having virtually no prior knowledge. That is why the PPE is vital to the sports medicine physician. This exam determines if the athlete is able to participate in a safe manner or if other testing is needed before the athlete can compete.

PPE primary goals
- Detect conditions that may predispose to injury or illness
- Detect conditions that may be life threatening or disabling
- Meet legal and insurance requirements

PPE secondary goals
- Determine general health
- Counsel on health-related issues
- Assess fitness level for certain sports

Goals and objectives

The overall goal of the PPE is to help maintain the health and safety of the athlete in training and competition. It provides a practical means for the physician to educate the young athlete on a variety of health topics.

Health education is an important aspect of the PPE with young athletes because this may be the only health maintenance exam they seek out all year. Athletes may also use this time to discuss overall health goals as they relate to their own athletic performance. A strengthening or rehabilitation program may then be developed by coaches and trainers.

The purpose of the PPE is not to disqualify athletes from competition but to promote safety, identify ongoing injuries, and prevent future injuries. Only 0.3%–1.3% of athletes are denied clearance during the PPE.

The specific objectives of the PPE may vary slightly from physician to physician, but should always include 1) detection of conditions that limit participation or may predispose to injury, 2) detection of conditions that may be life threatening or disabling, and 3) meeting of legal requirements as set forth by the state or sponsoring school or club.

Other common objectives include determining the general health of the athlete, evaluating the athlete's fitness level, and optionally assessing the athlete's level of maturity.

Timing and setting

Health-care professionals who wish to perform PPEs must be qualified on the basis of specialty, training, and clinical expertise. Each state certifies health-care practitioners qualified to perform PPEs at the secondary school level. College, professional, and international competitors are governed by their own athletic boards as to who may perform their PPE.

The primary care physician is a well-qualified candidate for performing the PPE because of their training in a broad range of problems. The primary care physician is also knowledgeable in consulting with specialty physicians when problems are detected that require further clinical expertise.

Timing

The PPE should be scheduled 6 weeks prior to the preseason. This allows adequate time for correction and rehabilitation of any problems detected. Timing for a collegiate athlete is often based on availability.

Some athletes may return to school just days before preseason begins. In this case physicians may prefer to perform outgoing physicals at the end of the season with a follow-up review of the medical history just prior to the season beginning. This would allow the physician to detect any conditions and the athlete to rehabilitate any injuries during the off-season.

Many schools will require one PPE for fall and winter sports and another for spring and summer sports. In general, however, an annual PPE is all that is required for high school athletes. Athletes who are minors are required to provide written permission from their legal guardian for the examination.

Settings

The two most common settings for performing PPEs are in a station-based environment or in the physician's office. Each setting has its own advantages and disadvantages in providing the best overall health screening of the athlete.

Station-based setting

Advantages

Station-based evaluations offer the athlete a group of clinical experts that can provide an extremely time-efficient and cost-effective examination. Hundreds of PPEs can be performed in one day with a well-trained staff.

Effective station-based setups will include the expertise of nurses, physical therapists, exercise physiologists, athletic trainers, and possibly dentists and nutritionists. Other assistants can be guided by physicians to efficiently administer sign-in, vision checks, and weights and measurements.

An athlete who receives care from a "team" setting may improve his or her communication with the medical personnel. Additionally, all members of the medical team and coaches will become more knowledgeable about each individual athlete.

Disadvantages

The disadvantages of a station-based format lie simply in its requirements—precise training and coordination of staff members and a large physical space to set up the stations. The setting itself can become confusing and noisy.

This lack of privacy may inhibit athletes from discussing personal health matters. A feeling of being rushed may also decrease the health education and counseling offered by the physician. If a disqualifying condition is detected, an athlete and his or her parents may not fully understand the need for further evaluation or disqualification from play, given the lack of time and privacy.

Finally, the continuity of care may be compromised with a station-based evaluation. Coordinating personnel and schedules can become difficult for the physician who is previously unknown to the athlete.

Station-based format

The station-based PPE can be divided into required and optional stations. Personnel best suited for each of the stations should be assigned by the physician. If more then one physician is present, divide the physical exam into two parts, medical and musculoskeletal. Female and male examining sites should be separated into two distinct areas.

A suggested format of the stations is given below:

- Station 1: check-In
- Station 2: vital signs including blood pressure, pulse, visual acuity, respiration rate, temperature, and height and weight
- Station 3: medical exam
- Station 4: orthopedic exam
- Station 5: final check and clearance
- Optional stations: concussion baseline testing (computer or balance), nutrition, flexibility and strength assessments, body composition (fat percentage), and dental exams

Office-based settings

Advantages

An office-based PPE performed by the athlete's own primary care physician offers the major advantage of familiarity. If the physician has treated the athlete throughout childhood, a complete medical history including previous physical examinations and medical records will provide a thorough review in comparison with the PPE screening evaluation form.

The previously established working relationship may make it easier for the physician to educate and counsel the athlete on sensitive health issues such as drugs, alcohol, birth control, and sexually transmitted diseases. The continuity of care provided by the athlete's own physician can be crucial in detecting, evaluating, and treating any conditions discovered during the PPE.

Disadvantages

A physician's busy office schedule often only allows for a short general health screen. This is not an adequate amount of time to detect conditions that may predispose the athlete to injury or illness. Furthermore, many primary care physicians lack the interest in or knowledge of sports-related medical problems. The physician may not be comfortable or qualified in determining clearance for an athlete.

We should not assume that all athletes have an established primary care physician. In general, athletes represent a healthy population that may not seek medical attention unless required. Additionally, not all athletes can afford the cost of a private office-based PPE.

Office-based format

The office-based PPE follows the same examination procedure as any other primary care examination. The major difference between routine office-based examinations and the PPE is allowance of extra time for the PPE.

Routine screening testing

Although issues concerning routine laboratory screening tests are frequently discussed and often controversial, some sports societies maintain that routine laboratory screening tests in asymptomatic athletes should not be required for the PPE.[1,6]

Screening tests in the young athlete must be cost-effective. Studies evaluating the use of such tests as urinalysis, CBC, chemistry profile, lipid profile sickle cell trait, and ferritin level in the PPE have not shown any cost-effectiveness.

Extensive cardiopulmonary testing for routine screening in the PPE is also not recommended. According to new American Heart Association (AHA) standards, a complete and careful personal and family history and physical examination designed to identify or raise the suspicion of cardiovascular lesions is the best available and most practical approach.

Symptomatic individuals and those athletes with significant familial medical history should be re-evaluated and scheduled for specific diagnostic tests. Individual symptoms and overall health should indicate to the physician whether or not clearance should be denied during the waiting period. In general, the athlete is allowed to continue participating.

Medical history

The most crucial portion of the PPE is the medical history. A complete history will identify approximately 75% of problems affecting athletes.

It is important to remember that frequently a medical history completed by the athlete does not reveal the same results as one completed by the athlete's parent or guardian. Ideally, the athlete and parent will complete the form together prior to the exam. There are many history forms available. Essential information should be obtained in the areas of cardiac history, medications and medical conditions, allergies, and family history.

Physical examination

The standard components of the preparticipation physical examination are listed below. This screening tool should be used to focus specifically on areas of concern in the particular athletic activity and areas identified as problems in the history. Males and females should be dressed in shorts, tank tops, and athletic shoes.

Height and weight

Height and weight should be recorded and reviewed yearly. Athletes who are extremely thin or obese should be questioned about sudden weight change, eating habits, and body image. Body composition determination is an optional station.

Head, eyes, ear, nose, throat (HEENT)

Visual acuity should be 20/40 or better in each eye. Protective eyewear should be recommended for use with corrective eyewear, history of serious trauma, or absence of an eye. Protective eyewear should always be checked prior to play. Pupils should be checked for anisocoria. If found, this baseline information should be clearly recorded in the medical record and communicated to members of the athlete's medical team. This is a significant point of reference in assessing for head trauma.

The general health of the remaining components of this exam should be assessed. In assessment of the ears, specifically check for scarring of the auditory canal, which may indicate the need for a hearing evaluation, and perforated tympanic membranes in athletes competing in water sports, which indicate the need for earplugs.

The oral cavity should be checked for ulcers and decreased enamel seen with bulimia; braces, which may indicate the need for a mouthguard; and a high-arched palate seen in those with Marfan syndrome. Nasal polyps, deviated septum, and repeated trauma to the nose should be assessed for referral.

Finally, any adenopathy should be assessed for infection or malignancy.

Cardiovascular

The AHA recently issued a new medical/scientific statement from the Sudden Death Committee and the Congenital Cardiac Defects Committee in which they believe that the standard preparticipation screening process for athletes appeared to be limited in its ability to identify cardiovascular lesions responsible for sudden death in young athletes.

As a consequence of this belief, the AHA statement recommends the development of a national standard for PPEs and strongly recommends that athletic screening be performed by health-care workers who possess the requisite training, skill, and background to reliably obtain a detailed cardiovascular history, perform a related physical examination, and recognize heart disease. The specific recommendation for a brachial artery blood pressure measurement was included in the statement.

The new AHA statement should be reviewed for further recommendations by all sports medicine providers to insure their professional liability. Blood pressure that is initially high should be repeated a few minutes after the initial check. If the condition continues, the athlete should be questioned about stimulants such as caffeine, ephedrine, or nicotine.

A radial and femoral pulse should be palpated for rate and rhythm. Auscultation of the heart should be performed with the athlete in supine and standing positions. A murmur of hypertrophic cardiomyopathy is best heard when the athlete is standing. Murmurs and the timing of murmurs should be assessed. Any detected murmur should be further clarified by instructing the athlete to perform deep inspiration, squat-to-stand, and Valsalva maneuver.

In detecting aortic stenosis, the systolic murmur will decrease with Valsalva and increase with squatting. Conversely, with hypertrophic cardiomyopathy, squatting will decrease the intensity of the murmur, and Valsalva maneuver will increase the intensity.

Benign systolic murmurs are common in young athletes. Innocent murmurs will also increase with squatting and decrease with Valsalva but can be differentiated from aortic stenosis by volume, location, radiation, and duration.

Arrhythmias may require electrocardiographic evaluation. Any further cardiac evaluation should be referred to a cardiologist.

Lungs

Clear breath sounds should be revealed during the pulmonary exam.

Abdomen

The athlete should be supine during assessment for masses, tenderness, and hepatosplenomegaly.

Genitourinary (GU)

The male should be assessed for singular or undescended testicles, testicular masses, and herniation. The female's GU exam should be deferred to a private primary care physician.

Musculoskeletal

The musculoskeletal system can be assessed with three different types of screening exams. The type and extent of musculoskeletal examination appropriate for the PPE is a widely debated topic.

Asymptomatic athletes with no history of injury rarely reveal a musculoskeletal injury. In fact, history alone has been shown to be 92% sensitive in detection of significant musculoskeletal injuries. A general screening examination is appropriate for asymptomatic athletes with no history of injury.

If an athlete is currently symptomatic of an injury or has a history of previous injury, weakness, or instability, the physician should perform a relevant joint-specific examination. If time is allowed, a joint-specific exam should be performed instead of a general screening; a sport-specific exam may be performed if time does not allow for a joint-specific exam.

General screening examination

A general screen will quickly assess range of motion, gross muscle strength, and muscle asymmetry along with identifying significant injuries. The general screening exam will not allow for specific diagnosis or severity of injury.

Joint-specific testing

Joint-specific testing assesses individual joints by inspection, palpation, and maneuvers. It is much more thorough than the general screening exam but also significantly more time consuming. A description of each joint-specific test is beyond the scope of this chapter but can be found in its entirety in Hoppenfeld's *Physical Examination of the Spine and Extremities*.

Sports-specific testing

Sports-specific examinations include endurance, strength, and flexibility testing in addition to an orthopedic examination. The focus is indicated by the particular sport and the area of greatest stress. For instance, runners would be assessed for knee and ankle stability, strength, and flexibility by use of specific orthopedic maneuvers.

The sports-specific exam is time consuming and requires greater knowledge of particular sports than does the joint-specific testing. Generally, sports-specific examinations can be saved for highly competitive and professional athletes.

Neurological

In general, a normal musculoskeletal examination denotes normal neurological function. However, for athletes who have suffered severe or multiple concussions, an exam of cranial nerves along with cerebellar and cognitive function tests may be indicated.

An athlete who has experienced recurrent nerve root or brachial plexus injuries ("stingers") should be assessed for deep tendon reflexes and upper extremity strength. Referral may be appropriate for any impairments noted.

Clearance

The culmination of the detailed medical history and lengthy physical examination in the PPE is the determination of clearance.

Clearance can be divided into three categories: 1) unrestricted clearance for contact, limited contact, or noncontact play; 2) clearance upon further evaluation or rehabilitation; and 3) clearance deferred for a specific or all sports. If a condition is detected, the following questions should guide the physician in determining clearance for an athlete:

1. Does the problem place the athlete at increased risk of injury?
2. Does the problem place any other participant at increased risk of injury?
3. Can the athlete safely participate with treatment?
4. Can limited participation be allowed while treatment is initiated?
5. If clearance is denied for specific sports, can other athletic activities be substituted?

Medicolegal considerations

Two very important medicolegal issues related to the PPE have been debated and should be reviewed. The primary legal issue is the athlete's right to participate. The right to make a final decision on whether to engage in athletics has been repeatedly recognized by the courts as resting with the athlete or with his or her parents.

A physician who disqualifies an athlete from play should consult with expert physicians. Both the examining and the consulting physician should clearly review all reasons why the athlete should not participate with the athlete and his or her parents.

Should the athlete choose to participate against medical advice, an exculpatory waiver stating that the physician(s) has clearly informed the family of all risks accompanying the participation of play should be signed. An exculpatory waiver is a written form stating that the family recognizes and assumes the risk of injury and releases the physician(s) and the school from liability. The validity of these waivers is not nationally recognized, and legal counsel is recommended for the physician on an individual-case basis.

The other major legal issue is professional liability for physicians performing PPEs as volunteers. Until recently, Good Samaritan laws did not cover preparticipation evaluations even if performed without charge. Some states have now instituted protection for examiners for athletic programs under Good Samaritan statutes. The physician should become familiar with his or her own state's statutes.

Physicians providing preparticipation evaluations should be familiar with standards set forth by significant medical committees such as those discussed throughout this chapter. After all, none of us can be protected from our own lack of knowledge.

Welcome meeting

The medical component of a generic welcome meeting or team gathering with your athletes and support staff should cover the following:

- Introduce yourself if not known to all
- Your contact details including emergency telephone number
- Arranging routine medical consultation
- Arranging emergency medical consultation
- What to do in the event of an emergency, e.g., road accident
- Drug-testing procedure
- Medical review and preparticipation exam
- "What-if" scenarios (e.g., what to do if a team member develops a contagious illness)
- Advice on avoiding problems, e.g., hydration, sun protection, insect problems, fluid and nutrition hygiene
- Questions. Make it clear that you will try to accommodate your team's individual needs as much as is possible

Drug testing

Your athletes will be required to have in- or out-of-competition drug testing. Establish a procedure in the event of a request for a drugs test.

As part of this you should identify the following:

- Appropriate drug-testing room (within limits imposed by available facilities)
- Who should be informed upon arrival of drug-testing officials
- Your role? Will you always be available as an athlete representative? If not, who will stand in should the athlete request a representative?
- What to do in the event of a positive test

Before competition has started

Visit the competition or athlete village medical center. Introduce yourself to reception staff and the lead physician if possible. Find out what facilities are on site and how to organize those tests that are not immediately available, e.g., MRI.

Where possible, visit the venues you are likely to be using and assess their facilities.

Establish where the nearest bank, telephone card sales, supermarket, opticians, dentist, and pharmacist are located. You'll be amazed how much athletes rely on the doctor and athletic trainer for day-to-day information.

Medical management

Whether you are a single-handed medical officer or the chief medical officer (CMO) of a team of medics, you will have management meetings to attend. These meetings are valuable opportunities for receiving or communicating information.

- Team leader meetings, meetings with leaders within your squad or team, e.g., team physicians, individual team leaders (at games there will be leaders for a number of areas, e.g., transport, nutrition, competition, media, security, etc), performance director, senior coaching staff, chief athletic trainer
- Team meetings, meetings with all members of your team
- Medical meetings. As CMO you should arrange to meet with the rest of your medical team on a regular basis. This should include meetings with the head or lead athletic trainer and athletic training colleagues
- Competition medical meetings. At major competitions there will usually be an opportunity for the games or competition medical committee to meet with medical representatives from competing teams or nations. This is a valuable opportunity to receive information on host medical protocols but more importantly to focus on areas that require attention, e.g., fluid and nutrition issues, drug-testing procedure, access to investigations.

Multi-sport events

The role of a medical officer is very different if you are responsible for a team at a multi-event competition.

As a medical officer to a team at a single sport competition, your focus is only on one sport, albeit with the different individual demands of those athletes under your care. This might vary from a group of football players all playing the same sport at the same time to an athletics squad with very different athletic disciplines, training and competing at different times.

Prioritizing

If working at a multi-sport event, you will have to balance the requirements of individual athletes (and their support staff) and different sports.

The key to successful games is communication and prioritizing. Most performance directors and coaches will appreciate that you have competing demands on your time.

Ask individual teams what medical support they would like and ask them to prioritize the training and competition elements of their program. Once you have an appreciation of each sport's requirements, go through the same exercise sport by sport from a medical viewpoint. This will reflect the following:

- Risk of serious injury of that sport, e.g., gymnastics vs. tennis
- Availability of medical support
- Athletic training support. It is vital that you discuss your plans with athletic training colleagues as there will be the option of a certain amount of cross-cover.
- Training vs. competition. Usually competition support is prioritized, however, there may be local medical services supporting competition that are not available for training, e.g., gymnastics training.
- Local medical services, e.g., venue medical provision (as above), athletes village medical center
- Requirement to provide medical consultations for those athletes not competing or training. In a games situation you will have to provide coverage at the athlete's village or equivalent.
- Logistical issues, e.g., ability to communicate with the team, access to transport. You may be able to cover adjacent venues if traveling times are short and communication via cell phone is easy. A distant venue may require that you travel with that squad, however, being conscious that this removes one member of the medical team from any cross-cover.
- This process should be flexible enough to accommodate sudden changes in circumstances, e.g., medical emergency, athletes progressing to final stages of competition.

The holding camp

There is an increasing tendency for athletes to go to a holding camp prior to major competition. This is valuable for a number of reasons:
- Environmental acclimatization (time zone, heat, humidity)
- Opportunity to fine-tune technical aspects
- Team building
- Tapering, focus, rest, and relaxation

You may travel with the team onward to competition or, alternatively, you may be employed solely to work at the holding camp. Working at a holding camp provides a unique opportunity to contribute to the preparation of elite athletes in a slightly more relaxed environment than what you will find at a games or championship.

Your medical management has to be tailored to the situation and the proximity to competition. This means that the time frames in which to work are very tight, and your practice may be modified accordingly.

The games

While caring for athletes at a championship event is a privilege, it is also the most demanding aspect of medical care because of the importance of the timing of any health issue. You may be faced with an athlete whose sole focus for the last 4 years has been Olympic competition and who may only have this one opportunity. Even simple problems may assume mammoth proportions in the athlete's mind.

Maintaining your focus

The pressure cooker environment of athletic competition puts an additional strain on relationships.

- Ensure you are working as a team
- Maintain composure and do not lose sight of why you are there. Do not become a "sideline fan"
- Communicate a concern before it becomes a problem; don't bottle things up
- Take adequate down time
- Be supportive of others taking their down time
- A hasty word can do irreparable harm. If tensions rise, walk away and figuratively count to 10
- Appreciate the stress of the situation and give colleagues some slack.
- A simple "thank you," a smile, or a hug (whichever is appropriate) costs nothing but makes a world of difference

Rest and relaxation (down time)

You will work long and unsociable hours, so it is vital that you take down time when you can. Establish a rotation so that you can cross-cover. If you are single-handed, ensure that you and your athletic trainer colleagues cover each other, leaving emergency contact details.

The return home

The evening after competition is usually celebrated by any closing ceremonies and time with your team. This is an important opportunity for everyone to unwind, but may have medical implications.

The journey home

You are still responsible for the medical care of those in your team so ensure that you have access to appropriate equipment for all stages of the journey home.

Compile a short medical report even if you are not required to do so as part of your medical officer responsibilities. It may help improve future trips and prove useful for successors.

Your arrival at home can be quite challenging for yourself and your partner and family. There is usually a feeling of deflation when your trip comes to an end. You will almost certainly be physically and, more importantly, mentally tired in addition to any jet lag.

You may be making the rapid transition from an exciting period of work in a new environment back to "the day job" with all the mundane roles and responsibilities that that involves (and, all too often, a backlog of work that has accumulated in your absence).

Be appreciative and balance recounting exciting moments from your travels with showing an interest in what others have been up to.

Allow yourself adequate time to recover from jet lag before returning to work.

Professional and ethical considerations

Medical work within sport is governed by exactly the same considerations and responsibilities that govern any other form of medical work. You have a duty of care to those that you are looking after and you must execute that duty of care within the framework of good medical practice. This encompasses all aspects of your work as a team doctor but has particular relevance to respecting patient confidentiality.

In addition to the medical work you carry out while away with a team, you have to comply with requirements for appraisal, revalidation, clinical governance, and your own continuing professional development.

Chief medical officer (CMO) role

If you are the CMO, you will have additional responsibilities as a medical team leader. It is your responsibility to ensure that all in your team are medically qualified and appropriately trained. If you were not involved with the interview process, ensure that you have seen proof of licensure and board certification.

Establish a code of conduct for all members of the medical team. There may well be a generic team code of conduct, which the medical team code of conduct has to incorporate.

Issues to consider as CMO are the following:

- Medical duties. Ensure that everyone has the same team philosophy
- Line management. As CMO you are responsible for all aspects of medical care and you need to ensure that your colleagues report any problems to you before they get out of hand. You will probably be responsible to a nonmedical colleague, e.g., coach, athletic director, parent, or camp director, and you should keep them equally informed without breaching confidentiality
- On-call arrangements. You have a duty to provide 24-hour emergency medical coverage or make clear what alternative arrangements are in place
- Rest and relaxation. You should ensure that all members of your team are taking adequate down time
- Alcohol consumption. Squads and teams may have their own generic views on alcohol consumption, and you must abide by the team code of conduct if a dry philosophy is adopted
- Wearing of team kit
- Medical representation at governing body, competition, games, and delegation management meetings
- Clinical governance issues of your team
- Mentoring and professional development. Be mindful that you may have considerably more experience than some of your colleagues. Particularly if this is their first competitive event, be supportive to ensure that their experience is a positive one

Patient confidentiality

Athletes deserve the same right to confidentiality as any other patient.

Medical indemnity

Ensure that your medical insurance and indemnity covers your scope.

Organizing a major sporting event

A major sporting event is a place of employment, entertainment, and competition and hence entails an unusually large and diverse number of potential areas of risk. It is vital to be able to deal with these crowds in a safe and efficient manner.

Accidents at sporting events have precipitated the development of guidelines to ensure crowd safety. The Mass Participation Event Management for the Team Physician: A Consensus Statement outlines such guidelines from the major sports medicine organizations in the United States.

First-aid minimum requirements

- No event should have fewer than two first-aiders.
- If there are seated and standing spectators, there should be 1 first-aider per 1000.
- If all are seated, there should be 1 first-aider per 1000 up to 20,000, then 1 per 2000.
- If there are more than anticipated, consult the local ambulance service.
- A first-aider holds a standard certificate of first aid issued by voluntary aid societies.
- First-aiders should be 16 years or older with no other duties at the event.
- First-aiders should be at the event prior to spectators arriving and remain until all spectators have left the grounds.
- They have a responsibility to provide room(s) for spectators in addition to other medical facilities.
- They should compliment the facilities provided by ambulance services.
- Consult with ambulance, local authorities, the crowd doctor, and appropriate voluntary aid services.
- A nonsmoking treatment area must be provided.
- Treatment area should be nonsmoking and minimum size 15 m^2, increased to 25 m^2, if >15000 spectators.
- To hold an exam table or stretcher(s), area for sitting casualties, extra table if necessary.
- Sufficient room for equipment and materials
- Blankets, pillows, stretchers, buckets, bowls, trolleys, and screens
- Suitable disposal facilities for sharps and waste
- Defibrillator (AED) if >5000 spectators expected. This can be provided by another agency if required.
- The first aid station should have an appropriate location allowing for access and egress, fittings and facilities.
- Crowd doctor. For >2000 spectators, a crowd doctor is needed who is trained in immediate care with appropriate qualifications, skills, experience, and support.

Knowledge of CPR, airway maintenance, spinal fracture immobilization, and treatment of anaphylaxis is required. Training should be in advanced life support and pediatric life support. Governing body rules will give recommendations regarding the level of qualification.

Important considerations for a crowd doctor are as follows:
- The first duty of the crowd doctor is to the spectators.
- The doctor's location should be known to first-aid, ambulance, and control point personnel and the doctor must be contactable
- Equipment levels and clinical protocols used should conform to guidelines published by the relevant sporting body.
- The crowd doctor should be in position before spectators arrive and remain until all spectators have left the premises.
- For <2000 spectators, there should be arrangements to summon a suitably trained and experienced crowd doctor.
- Be aware of the location and staffing arrangements of the first aid room and of ambulance and emergency plans for major incidents.

Ambulance provision
- One fully equipped ambulance if >5000 spectators and sourced from an approved group
- The relationship of an ambulance to access facilities should be known to management.
- Access for ambulance personnel to control point
- An ambulance must be present before and after spectators access and leave the premises.
- With 5000–25,000 spectators, there should be 1 accident and emergency ambulance with a paramedic crew. One ambulance officer, paramedic holds a certificate of proficiency in ambulance paramedic skills and has access to equipment, including drugs.
- With 25,000–45,000 spectators, there must be 1 accident and emergency ambulance with a paramedic crew, 1 ambulance officer, 1 major-incident equipment vehicle and a paramedic crew, and 1 control unit.
- With >45,000 spectators there must be 2 accident and emergency ambulances with paramedic crews; otherwise, as above.

Major incident plan
- Plans should be compatible with the local emergency services' major incident plan.
- Identify areas for dealing with casualties in multiple situations. This may include fire, accident, crowd disturbance, bomb scare, and adverse and inclement weather.
- Identify access and egress routes and rendezvous point for vehicles.
- Have an agreed-upon plan of action by all interested parties.
- All first-aid and medical staff must be briefed on their role in the major incident plan per event. A copy of this is kept in the first aid room.
- Risk assessments should be performed.

International governing body checklists
- Includes review of all medical arrangements
- Includes safety measures outside stadium
- Defines high-risk event
- Assesses size of stadium and provision of safety and medical coverage
- Reviews risks of trouble, including ticket forgery

- Fire brigade, ambulance, and security measures
- Practical issues regarding floodlights, etc.
- General rules regarding access of medical staff and stabilization of injuries on the field of play

Media issues

One of the biggest challenges of a major tournament is dealing with the media. Think very carefully before discussing any issues pertaining to the health of an athlete or group of athletes. Ideally, your team will be supported by a media representative who will guide you. Leave it to the experts, who will release well-scribed press statements that have been cleared with all concerned, most importantly, the athlete.

Issues to consider are as follows:
- Beware the quiet news day. Schedules still need filling.
- Requests for interviews are made to make news, not to find out what life as a doctor is like. Ideally, you should say nothing in saying something.
- Recorded interviews will be edited!
- Live interviews are less likely to be misrepresented at the time (they can be edited later for recorded news) but are extremely dangerous—interviewers are trained to produce a result.
- The media will work covertly and may pretend to be an interested fan.

Additional resources

American Academy of Family Physicians
American Academy of Orthopaedic Surgeons
American College of Sports Medicine
American Medical Society for Sports Medicine
American Orthopaedic Society for Sports Medicine
American Osteopathic Academy of Sports Medicine
Preparticipation Physical Evaluation, 3rd Edition (AAFP, AAP, ACSM, AMSSM, AOSSIM, AOASM) McGraw Hill, 2005, 1997, 1992
Mass Participation Event Management for the Team Physician: A Consensus Statement (ACSM), Medicine & Science in Sports & Exercise, 2003
Team Physician Consensus Statement (AAFP, AAOS, ACSM, AMSSM, AOASM, AOSSM) 2000

Further reading

Ades PA (1992). Preventing sudden death: cardiovascular screening of young athletes. *Phys Sports Med* **20**:75–89.

American Academy of Family Physicians (AAFP), American Academy of Pediatrics (AAP), American Medical Society for Sports Medicine (AMSSM), American Osteopathic Association of Sports Medicine (AOASM). *Preparticipation Physical Evaluation*, 2nd ed. Minneapolis, MN: Phys Sportsmed; 1997.

American Heart Association (1996). Cardiovascular preparticipation screening of competitive athletes. *Circulation* **94**:850–856.

26th Bethesda Conference: Recommendations for determining eligibility for competition in athletes with cardiovascular abnormalities. January 6–7, 1994. *Med Sci Sports Exerc* **26**(10 Suppl):S223–S283 [published erratum appears in *Med Sci Sports Exerc* 1994;**26**(12): following table of contents]; also in *J Am Coll Cardiol* 1994;**24**:845–899.

Committee on Sports Medicine (1983). *Sports Medicine: Health Care for Young Athletes.* Evanston, IL, American Academy of Pediatrics.

Feinstein RA, Colvin E, Oh MK. (1993) Echocardiographic screening as part of a preparticipation examination. *Clin J Sports Med* **3**:149–152.

Feinstein RA, Soileau EJ, Daniel WA Jr (1988). A national survey of preparticipation physical examination requirements. *Phys Sports Med* **16**:51.

Gallup EM (1995). *Law and the Team Physician*. Champaign, IL: Human Kinetic.

Gomez JE, Landry GL, Bernhardt DT (1993). Critical evaluation of the 2-minute orthopedic screening examintion. *Am J Dis Child* **147**:1109–1113.

Herbert D (1996). Pre-participation screening: competitive athletes and sudden death. *Sports Med Prim Care* **2**:90.

Hoppenfeld S (1976). *Physical Examination of the Spine and Extremities*. Appleton-Century-Crofts.

Johnson RJ. The sports qualifying screening evaluation.

Lombardo J (1991). Preparticipation examination. In Cantu R, Micheli L (eds.). *ACSM's Guidelines for the Team Physician*, 1st ed, Malvern, Lea & Febiger.

Lombardo JA, Robinson JB, Smith DM, et al. (1992). *Preparticipation Physical Evaluation*, ed. 1. Kansas City: American Academy of Family Practice, American Academy of Pediatrics, American Medical Society for Sports Medicine, American Orthopaedic Association for Sports Medicine, and American Osteopathic Association for Sports Medicine.

Sallis R (1997). The preparticipation examination. In Sallis R, Massimino F (eds.). *ACSMs Essentials of Sports Medicine*, 1st ed. St. Louis: Mosby, pp. 151–160.

Snoddy RO (1995). The preparticipation screening examination. In Baker CL (ed.). *The Hughston Clinic Sports Medicine Book*, 1st ed. Philadelphia: Williams & Wilkins, pp. 31–34.

Snoddy RO (1995). The preparticipation screening Examination. In Baker CL (ed.). *The Hughston Clinic Sports Medicine Book*, 1st ed. Philadelphia: Williams & Wilkins, pp. 31–34.

Taylor WC III, Lombardo JA (1990). Preparticipation screening of college athletes: value of the complete blood cell count. *Phys Sports Med* **18**:106–118.

Procedures

Joint injection overview

Indications

- Suppress inflammatory response
- Diminish pain
- Aid in therapeutic diagnosis

Conditions improved with local corticosteroid injection:

- Osteoarthritis
- Crystal-induced arthritis (gout, pseudogout)
- Rheumatoid arthritis
- Seronegative spondyloarthropathies (ankylosing spondylitis, psoriasis, Reiter's syndrome, arthritis associated with inflammatory bowel disease)
- Bursitis (subacromial, olecranon, trochanteric, pes anserine, pre-patellar, retrocalcaneal)
- Periarthritis (adhesive capsulitis)
- Tenosynovitis or tendonitis (De Quervain's, trigger finger, bicipital tendonitis, medial or lateral epicondylitis, plantar fasciitis)
- Neuritis (carpal tunnel, tarsal tunnel, Tietze's, costochondritis)

Contraindications

- Cellulitis over injection site
- Severe primary coagulopathy
- Uncontrolled anticoagulant therapy
- Septic effusion
- Suspected bacteremia with joint not being source
- More than three previous injections in same weight-bearing joint in preceding 12-month period
- Lack of response to two or three prior injections
- Inaccessible joints
- Joint prosthesis

Supplies needed

- Sterile or nonsterile gloves
- Povidone-iodine or alcohol wipes
- Sterile drapes (optional and usually not necessary)
- Ballpoint pen or other skin marker (optional)
- 1 mL to 10 mL syringe
- 18- to 20-gauge needle
- 22- to 25-gauge (use 25-gauge for smaller joints) 1.5-inch needle
- Ethyl chloride spray
- Local anesthetic or favorite corticosteroid preparation
- 4 × 4 gauze made wet with sterile saline or alcohol
- Dry 4 × 4 gauze
- Band-Aid

Procedure

- Draw up proper amounts of local anesthetic and then steroid into a single 1 mL to 10 mL syringe using 18- to 20-gauge needle. Remove needle used to draw up preparation and replace with 22- to 25-gauge needle
- Identify site of entry and mark with ballpoint pen, skin marker, or needle with cap in place
- Prep the area with a povidone-iodine or alcohol wipe.
- Sterilely drape area if desired
- Mix preparation by tipping the syringe forward and backward.
- Spray site of entry with ethyl chloride until skin begins to whiten to locally anesthetize skin
- Insert needle into site. Pull back on plunger to ensure that the needle is not in a blood vessel. If blood returns, reposition needle. If not, inject local anesthetic or corticosteroid preparation into joint. Little resistance should be felt if in the joint space. If resistance is met, attempt to reposition slightly. Be sure to pull back on the plunger with each needle repositioning
- Remove needle; clean area with wet gauze pad and then dry gauze
- Place Band-Aid over puncture wound

Aftercare and return to play

Leave the Band-Aid on for 6–12 hours. It is essential to rest the affected area after injection for 24–48 hours to keep medication within the joint space. The patient should immediately report fevers, chills, or local signs of infection or allergic reaction.

The joint should be re-examined if discomfort is not improved within 72 hours post-injection. The patient may bathe normally after injection and return to normal activity after 48–72 hours.

Inform patients that pain diminished within the first hour are due to the local anesthetic and symptoms may return after the medication wears off. The corticosteroid effects may take 48–72 hours to reach maximal benefit.

Adverse effects and complications

- Post-injection steroid flare
- Steroid arthropathy
- Tendon rupture or injury
- Infection
- Injection into blood vessel or blood vessel injury
- Nerve injury
- Subcutaneous fatty atrophy
- Skin depigmentation
- Adverse drug or hypersensitivity reaction
- Osteoporosis and cartilage damage
- Facial flushing
- Transient paresis of injected extremity
- Asymptomatic pericapsular calcification

Shoulder

Glenohumeral joint (see Fig. 23.1)

Technique
- The patient sits supported with the arm resting comfortably by their side.
- Palpate and identify the head of the humerus, the coracoid process, and the acromion. Mark on the skin if necessary

Anterior approach
- Have the shoulder slightly externally rotated to open up joint space. Insertion site is approximately 1 cm lateral to the coracoid process and medial to head of the humerus
- Direct needle posteriorly and slightly superiorly and laterally into joint.
- The needle should not contact bone. If it does, pull back and redirect at a slightly different angle

Posterior approach
- Have the arm held in medial rotation across the waist. Insertion site is 2–3 cm inferior and medial to the posterolateral corner of acromion. Place thumb of the non-injecting hand at the angle of acromion and index finger anteriorly on the coracoid process.
- Direct needle anteriorly in the direction of the coracoid process.
- Suggested preparation: 6 mL 0.25% bupivicaine, 1 mL (4 mg) dexamethasone, and 1 mL (40 mg) kenalog in a 10 mL syringe. Inject with a 22-gauge needle.

For a picture of the anterior approach, see Joint aspiration, Figure 23.28.

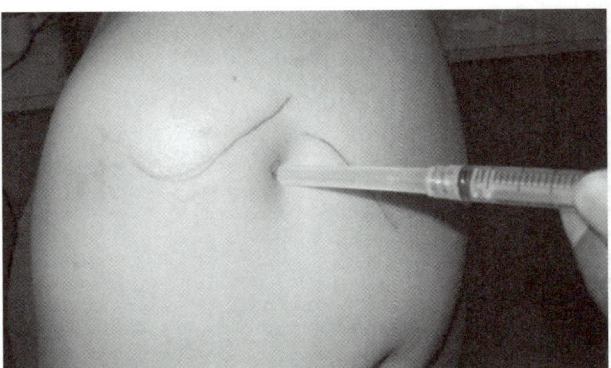

Figure 23.1 Glenohumeral posterior.

Acromioclavicular joint (see Fig. 23.2)

Technique

- The patient sits supported with the arm hanging by their side to slightly separate the joint surfaces
- Identify joint by palpating laterally along the clavicle until its termination. At this point, a slight depression will be noted. This is site of the joint line, lateral edge of acromion, and entry site
- Insert needle angling medially about 30° and pass through capsule
- Suggested preparation: 1 mL of 0.25% bupivicaine with 0.25 mL (10 mg) kenalog in 3 mL to 5 mL syringe. Inject with a 25-gauge needle

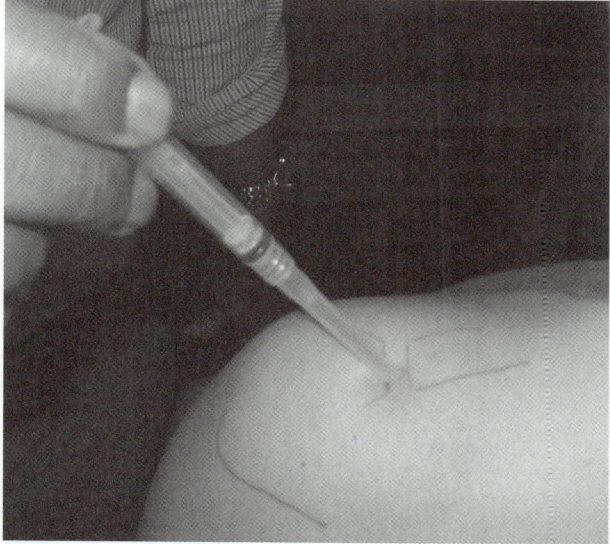

Figure 23.2 Acromioclavicular joint injection.

Subacromial bursitis (see Fig. 23.3)

Common indications
- Subdeltoid bursitis
- Rotator cuff impingement
- Rotator cuff tendinosis
- Adhesive capsulitis

Technique
- The patient sits supported with arm resting comfortably by their side.
- Palpate laterally along the clavicle until its termination. At this point, a slight depression will be noted. This is the lateral edge of the acromion. Just inferior to that is a soft spot that is the subacromial space.
- Insertion site is 2–3 cm inferior and medial to the posterolateral corner of acromion.
- Direct needle at a 45° angle superiorly into the bursa. There should be no resistance or discomfort to the patient.
- Suggested preparation: 6 mL of 0.25% bupivicaire, 1 mL (4 mg) dexamethasone, 1 mL (40 mg) kenalog in a 10 mL syringe. Inject with a 25-gauge needle.

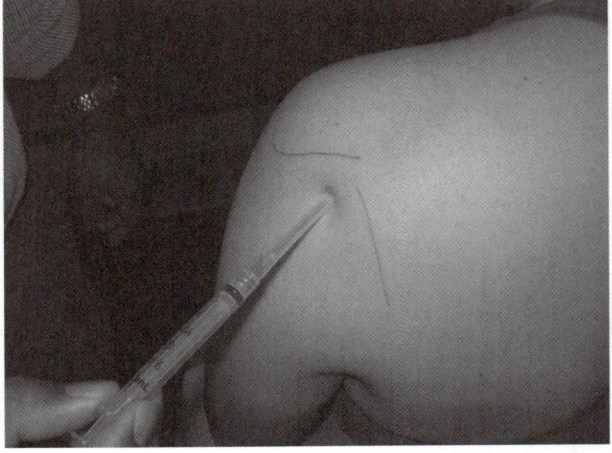

Figure 23.3 Subacromial bursitis injection.

Biceps tendonitis (see Fig. 23.4)

Technique
- The patient sits supported with arm resting comfortably by their side.
- Do not inject into the tendon.

Short head
- The short head of the biceps attaches to the coracoid process. If this area is tender, insert needle directly into the point of maximal tenderness until it reaches bone. Withdraw the needle 1–2 mm and inject.

Long head
- Identify the biceps tendon by rotating the patient's arm and shoulder outward. The bicipital groove is palpable anteriorly and tendon rotation can be palpated. Identify the most tender area (usually in bicipital groove).
- Insert needle at 30° and direct it parallel to the groove. The objective is to infiltrate the area in and around the groove and not into the tendon.
- Redirect if resistance is felt, as it is likely within the tendon. You may use a fanlike pattern to bathe more of the tendon if the patient has continued pain.
- Suggested preparation: 1 mL of 0.25% bupivicaine with 0.25 mL (10 mg) kenalog in 3–5 mL syringe. Inject with a 25-gauge needle.

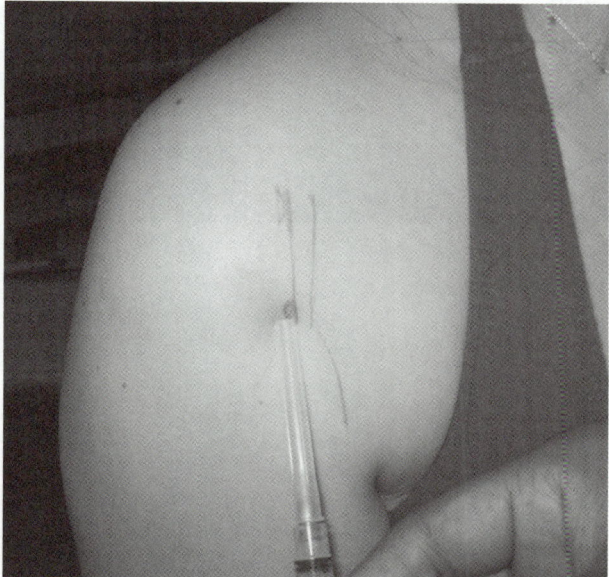

Figure 23.4 Biceps tendonitis injection.

Elbow

Elbow joint (see Fig. 23.5)

Technique
- The patient sits with the elbow supported and flexed at 90°.
- Identify joint by palpating soft tissue within triangle formed by the lateral epicondyle, radial head, and olecranon process. This is the entry site.
- Insert needle aiming for the medial epicondyle. If the needle hits bone, it should be pulled back and redirected at a different angle.
- Suggested preparation: 3–5 mL of 0.25% bupivicaine with 1–2 mL (40–80 mg) methylprednisolone in a 5 mL to 10 mL syringe. Inject with a 25-gauge needle.

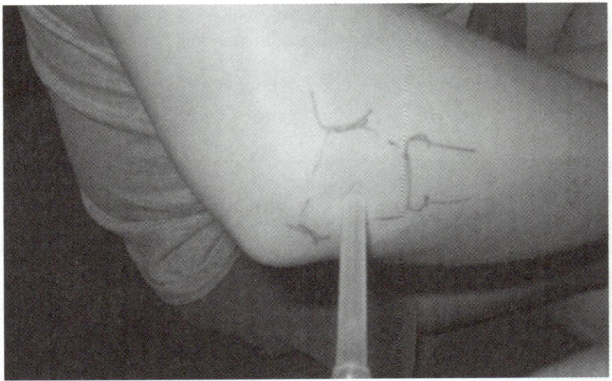

Figure 23.5 Elbow joint injection.

Lateral epicondylitis (see Fig. 23.6)

Technique

- The patient sits with the elbow supported and flexed at 45° and forearm pronated.
- Identify the most tender point of lateral epicondyle by gentle palpation. This is entry site.
- Insert needle at 90° down to the level of bone. Then pull back 1–2 mm and inject preparation slowly.
- Suggested preparation: 3 mL of 0.25% bupivicaine with 1 mL (4 mg) dexamethasone in a 5 mL syringe. Inject with a 25-gauge needle.

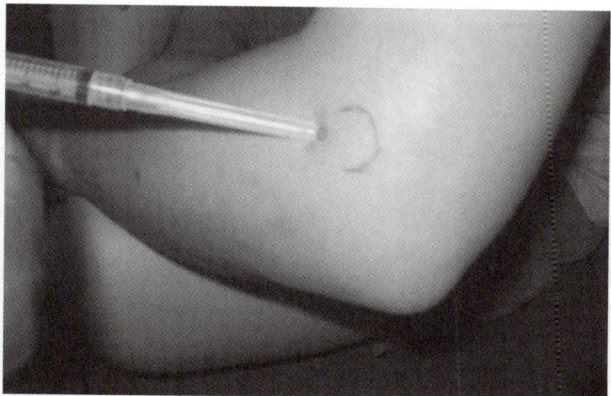

Figure 23.6 Lateral epicondylitis injection.

Medial epicondylitis (see Fig. 23.7)

Technique

- The patient sits with the elbow supported, flexed at 45°, and abducted and forearm supinated.
- Identify the most tender point of medial epicondyle by gentle palpation. This is entry site.
- Insert needle at 90° down to the level of bone. Then pull back 1–2 mm and inject preparation slowly.
- Suggested preparation: 3 mL of 0.25% bupivicaire with 1 mL (4 mg) dexamethasone in a 5 mL syringe. Inject with a 25-gauge needle.

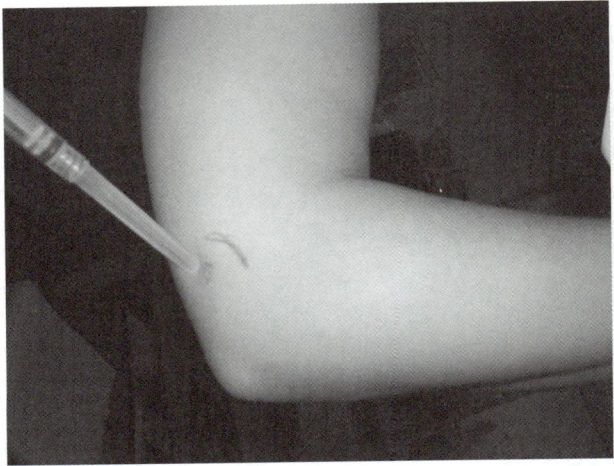

Figure 23.7 Medial epicondylitis injection.

Olecranon bursitis (see Fig. 23.8)

Technique

- The patient sits with the elbow supported and maximally flexed and forearm pronated. The patient may also lie supine with the elbow maximally flexed over their chest.
- Identify olecranon process and fluctuance noted above it.
- Insert needle directly into the bursa.
- Injection usually follows aspiration of bursa.
- Suggested preparation: 3 mL of 0.25% bupivicaine with 1 mL (40 mg) methylprednisolone in a 5 mL syringe. Inject with a 25-gauge needle.

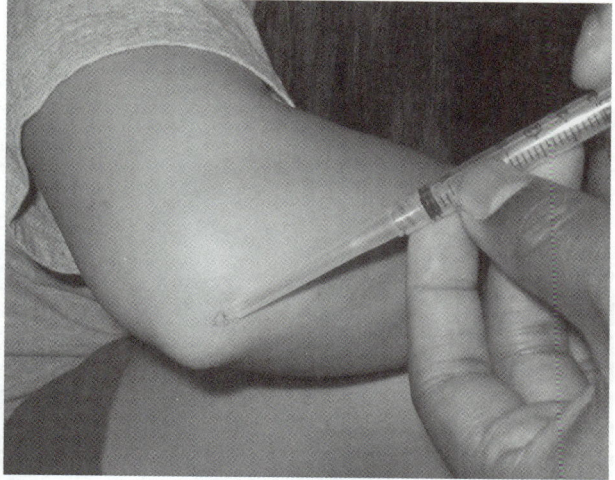

Figure 23.8 Olecranon bursitis injection.

Hand/wrist

First carpometacarpal joint (see Fig. 23.9)

Technique

- The patient sits with the hand supported on a flat surface with the ulnar side down and thumb opposed.
- Identify the joint space between the trapezium and first metacarpal. Traction may be used on thumb to open the joint space more.
- Insert needle just proximal to the first metacarpal on the extensor surface, toward the ulnar side of the extensor pollicis brevis tendon (to avoid radial artery).
- This is best if done under fluoroscopy.
- Suggested preparation: 0.5 mL of 1% lidocaine with 0.5 mL (20 mg) methylprednisolone in a 3 mL syringe. Inject with a 25-gauge needle.

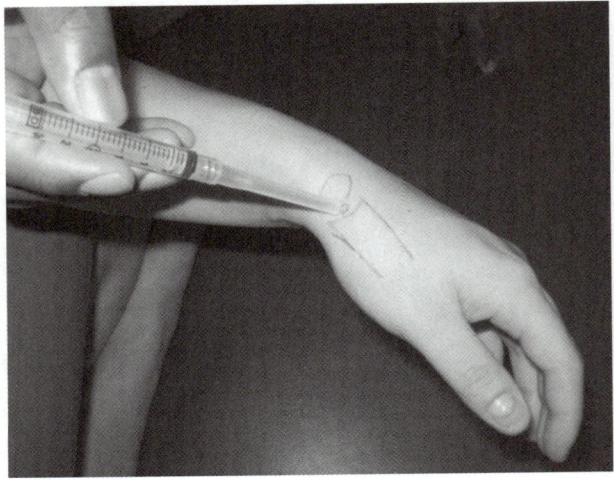

Figure 23.9 First carpometacarpal joint injection.

Carpal tunnel (see Fig. 23.10)

Technique

- The patient sits with wrist dorsiflexed at 30° and rested on a rolled towel with the palmar side upward.
- Identify proximal palmar crease by having the patient flex their wrist.
- Identify palmaris longus tendon by having the patient flex the third finger against resistance with flexed wrist. Site of needle insertion is just medial to the palmaris longus tendon at proximal palmar crease.
- Insert needle at 30° aiming distally toward the ring finger. If the patient has discomfort or experiences paresthesias, withdraw and reposition needle more toward the ulnar side. Advance needle 1–2 cm until there is no resistance, and inject medication.
- Suggested preparation: 2–3 mL of 1% lidocaine with 1 mL (40 mg) methylprednisolone in a 5 mL syringe. Inject with a 25-gauge needle.

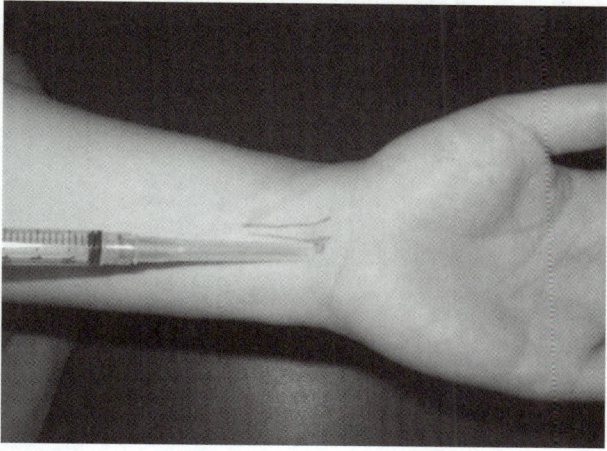

Figure 23.10 Carpal tunnel injection.

Trigger finger (see Fig. 23.11)

Technique
- The patient sits with the hand supported and palmar side upward.
- Identify the flexor tendon involved. There is often a palpable nodule or thickening of sheath.
- Insert needle distally at a 30° angle and aim proximally, almost parallel to the skin, toward the nodule. Inject into the nodule.
- Suggested preparation: 0.5 mL of 1% lidocaine with 0.5 mL (20 mg) methylprednisolone in a 3 mL syringe. Inject with a 25-gauge needle.

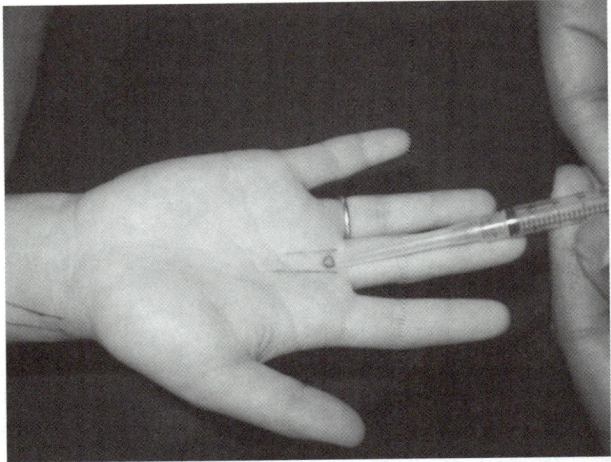

Figure 23.11 Trigger finger injection.

De Quervain's tenosynovitis (see Fig. 23.12)

Technique
- The patient sits with the hand supported on a flat surface with the ulnar side down and thumb maximally abducted.
- Identify radial styloid, extensor pollicis brevis, and abductor pollicis longus by having the patient fully extend and abduct the thumb.
- Insert needle parallel to the tendons (but not into the tendon) aiming toward the radial styloid. The patient should be comfortable throughout the procedure.
- Suggested preparation: 2 mL of 1% lidocaine with 1 mL (4 mg) dexamethasone in a 5 mL syringe. Inject with a 25-gauge needle.

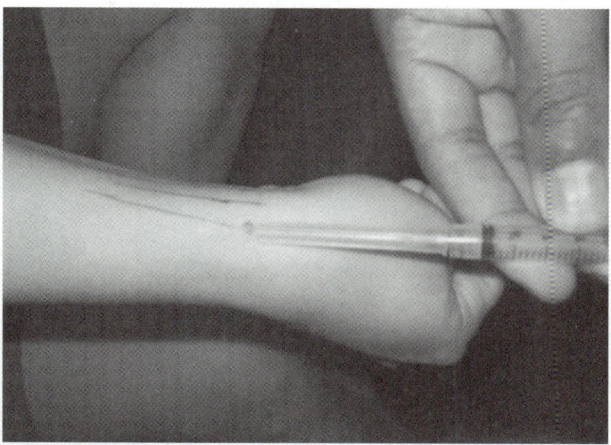

Figure 23.12 De Quervain's tenosynovitis injection.

Hip

Trochanteric bursitis (see Fig. 23.13)

Technique

- The patient lies in lateral decubits position with the affected hip upward and a pillow between the knees to relax the iliotibial band. The patient's hip is flexed 30°–50° with knee flexed 60°–90° for comfort and stabilization.
- Identify the point of maximal tenderness along the greater trochanter. This is the entry site.
- Insert needle perpendicular to the skin until bone is contacted. Withdraw 1–2 mm and inject into bursa.
- Suggested preparation: 6 mL 0.25% bupivicaine, 1 mL (4 mg) dexamethasone, and 1 mL (40 mg) kenalog in 10 mL syringe. Inject with a 22-gauge needle.

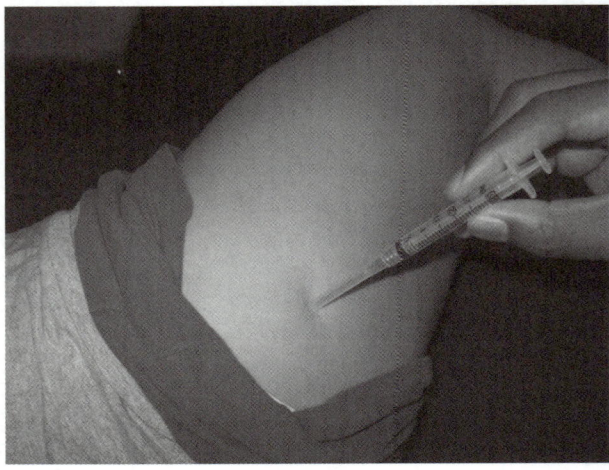

Figure 23.13 Trochanteric bursitis injection.

Hip pointer (see Fig. 23.14)

Technique

- The patient stands or may lie in lateral decubits position with the affected hip upward and a pillow between the knees.
- Identify the point of maximal tenderness along the iliac crest. This is the entry site.
- Insert needle perpendicular to the area until it contacts bone. Withdraw 1–2 mm and inject.
- Occasionally there may be a hematoma over this area that can be drained prior to injection.
- Suggested preparation: 5 mL 0.25% bupivicaine and 1 mL (4 mg) dexamethasone in a 10 mL syringe. Inject with 22-gauge needle.

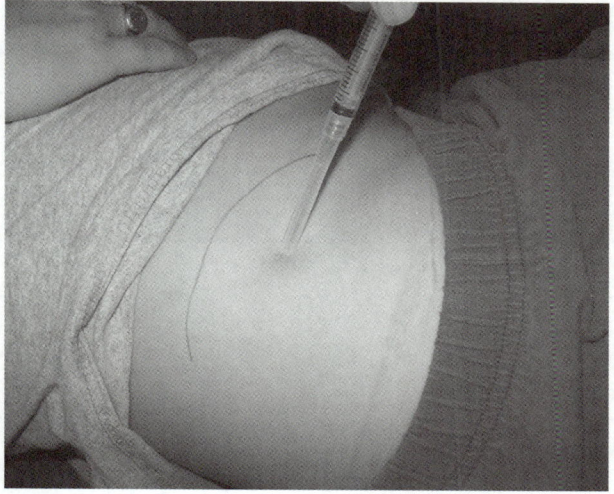

Figure 23.14 Hip pointer injection.

Proximal iliotibial band (see Fig. 23.15)

Technique
- The patient lies in lateral decubitus position with the affected side upward and knees flexed 20°–30°. Palpate the iliotibial band along the lateral thigh to its origin on the greater trochanter.
- Identify the point of maximal tenderness at the origin and insert needle into this site.
- Suggested preparation: 5 mL 0.25% bupivicaine and 1 mL (4 mg) dexamethasone in a 10 mL syringe. Inject with 22-gauge needle.

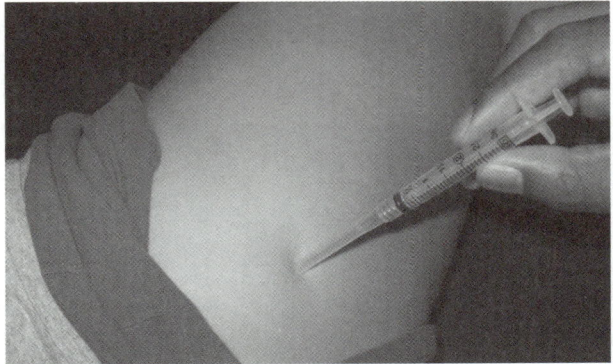

Figure 23.15 Proximal iliotibial injection.

Knee

Intra-articular joint—supine lateral (see Fig. 23.16)

Technique

- The patient lies supine with knee slightly flexed with a pillow or rolled-up towel in the popliteal space.
- Identify the lateral and superior borders of the patella. Mark if necessary. Site of entry is 1 cm superior and 1 cm lateral to superior-lateral corner of the patella.
- Direct the needle under the superior-lateral corner of the patella. No resistance should be met if in the joint space.
- Suggested preparation: 6 mL 0.25% bupivicaine, 1 mL (4 mg) dexamethasone, and 1 mL (40 mg) kenalog in 10 mL syringe. Inject with a 22-gauge needle.

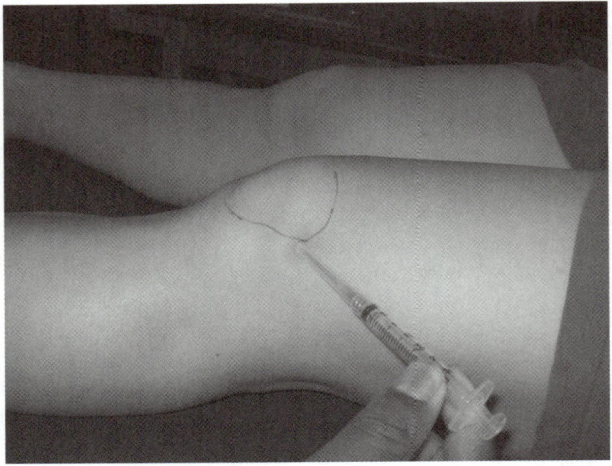

Figure 23.16 Knee supine lateral injection.

Intra-articular joint—seated lateral (see Fig. 23.17)

Technique

- The patient sits with legs hanging comfortably off the table with knees flexed at 90°.
- Identify lateral and inferior borders of the patella. Draw lines outlining each border (either imagined or on skin). The entry site is at the intersection of these two lines.
- Insert needle at a 45° angle, aiming into the joint space. No resistance should be met if in the joint space.
- Suggested preparation: 6 mL 0.25% bupivicaine, 1 mL (4 mg) dexamethasone, and 1 mL (40 mg) kenalog in 10 mL syringe. Inject with a 22-gauge needle.

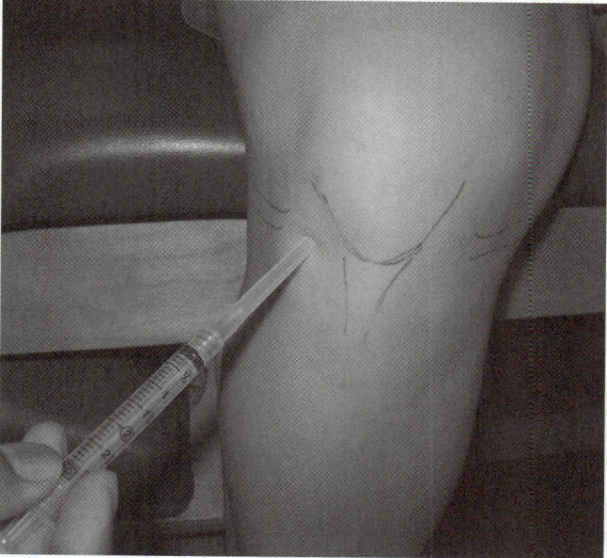

Figure 23.17 Knee seated lateral injection.

Intra-articular joint—medial (see Fig. 23.18)

Technique

- The patient sits with legs hanging comfortably off the table with knees flexed at 90°.
- Identify medial and inferior borders of the patella. Draw lines outlining each border (either imagined or on skin). The entry site is at the intersection of these two lines.
- Insert needle at a 45° angle, aiming into the joint space. No resistance should be met if in the joint space.
- Suggested preparation: 6 mL 0.25% bupivicaine, 1 mL (4 mg) dexamethasone, and 1 mL (40 mg) kenalog in 10 mL syringe. Inject with a 22-gauge needle.

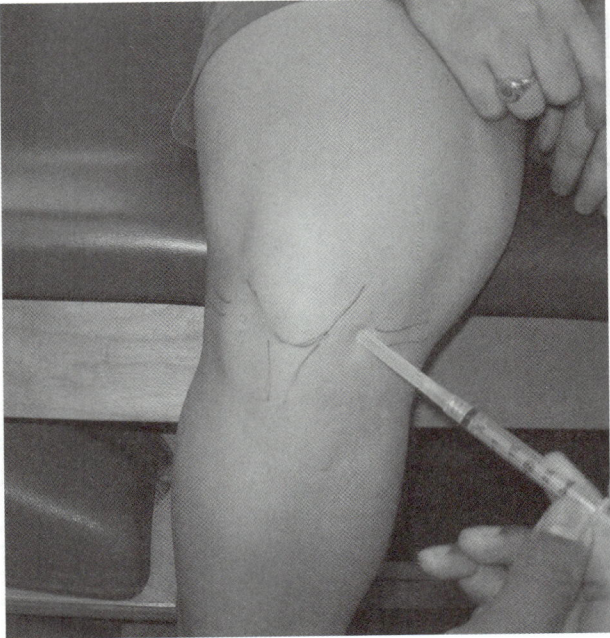

Figure 23.18 Knee medial injection.

Pes anserine bursitis (see Fig. 23.19)

Technique

- The patient lies supine with knee slightly flexed with a pillow or rolled-up towel in the popliteal space.
- Identify the tendinous border of medial thigh muscles and follow them across the joint line to their insertion at the pes anserine. The point of maximal tenderness is the entry site.
- Insert needle perpendicular to the tibia until contacting bone. Withdraw 2–3 mm and inject.
- Suggested preparation: 4 mL 0.25% bupivicaine, 1 mL (4 mg) dexamethasone in 10 mL syringe. Inject with a 22-gauge needle.

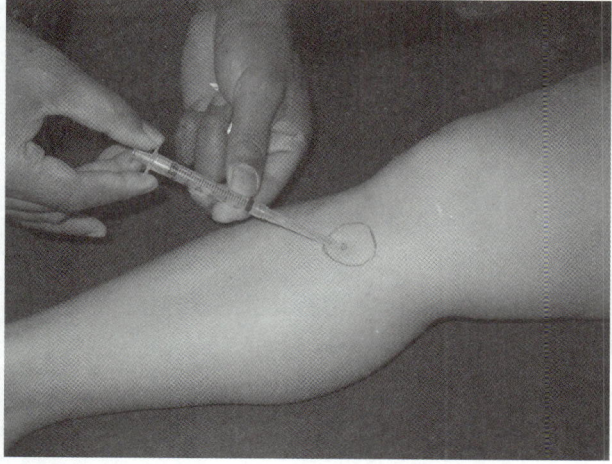

Figure 23.19 Pes anserine bursitis injection.

Prepatellar bursitis (see Fig. 23.20)

Technique

- The patient lies supine with knee slightly flexed with a pillow or rolled-up towel in the popliteal space.
- Palpate over the patella for fluctuance anterior to the patella.
- Insert needle directly into the fluid pocket from either the medial or lateral side.
- May need to aspirate fluid from bursa prior to injection. Aspiration is recommended only if infected fluid is suspected.
- Suggested preparation: 3 mL 0.25% bupivicaine and 1 mL (4 mg) dexamethasone in 3–5 mL syringe. Inject with a 25-gauge needle.

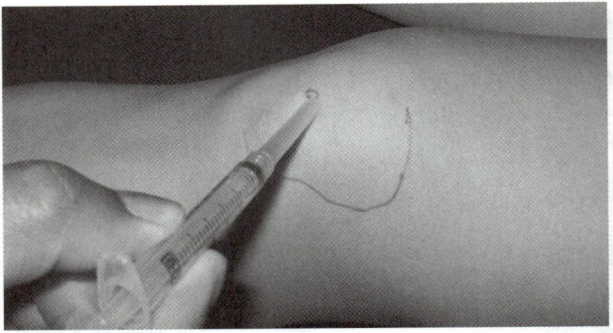

Figure 23.20 Prepatellar bursitis injection.

Distal iliotibial band (see Fig. 23.21)

Technique

- The patient lies in lateral decubitus position with the affected side upward and knees flexed 20°–30° to relax the iliotibial band.
- Palpate the iliotibial band along the lateral thigh, across the lateral femoral condyle to its insertion at Gerdy's tubercle. Identify the point of maximal tenderness near Gerdy's tubercle. This is the entry site.
- Insert needle into this site and inject.
- Suggested preparation: 5 mL 0.25% bupivicaine and 1 mL (4 mg) dexamethasone in 10 mL syringe. Inject with 22-gauge needle.

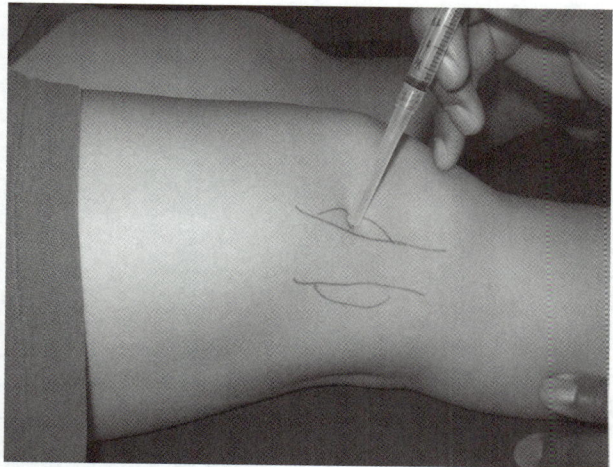

Figure 23.21 Distal iliotibial injection.

Ankle/foot

Ankle joint (see Fig. 23.22)

Technique

- The patient lies supine with knee in flexion and foot firmly supported on the table. The patient may also be seated with the foot supported.
- Identify the space between the anterior border of the medial malleolus and the medial border of the tibialis anterior tendon for articulation of the talus and tibia.
- Insert needle, angling posterolaterally into the joint. No resistance should be met.
- Suggested preparation: 3–5 mL 0.25% bupivicaire and 1 mL (4 mg) dexamethasone in 10 mL syringe. Inject with 25-gauge needle.

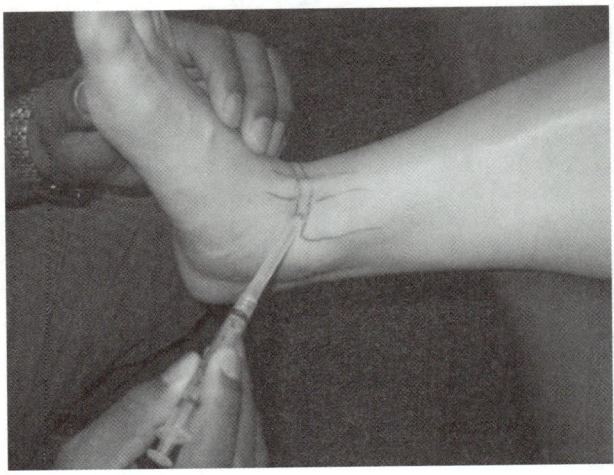

Figure 23.22 Ankle joint injection.

Sinus tarsi (see Fig. 23.23)

Technique

- The patient lies supine with knee in flexion and foot firmly supported on the table. The patient may also be seated with the foot supported.
- Identify the sinus tarsi, or talocalcaneal sulcus, by palpating between the talus and superior aspect of distal calcaneus. This space is inferior and posterior to the anterior talofibular ligament.
- Insert needle into this space for injection.
- Suggested preparation: 2 mL 0.25% bupivicaine and 1 mL (4 mg) dexamethasone in 10 mL syringe. Inject with 25-gauge needle.

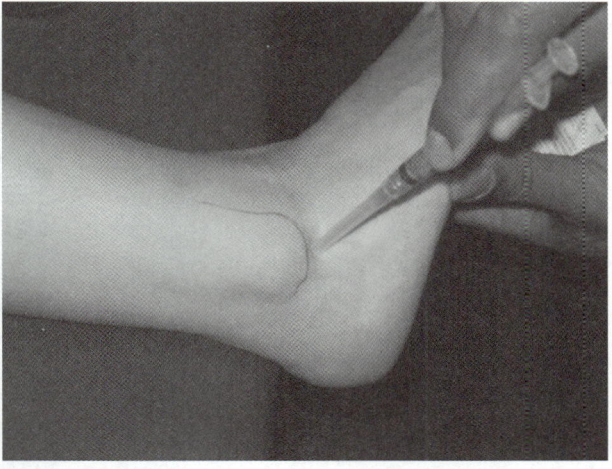

Figure 23.23 Sinus tarsi injection.

Tarsal tunnel (see Fig. 23.24)

Technique

- The patient lies in lateral decubitus position with the affected foot down.
- Identify the posterior tibial nerve behind the medial malleolus by having the patient actively invert the foot against resistance and first identifying the posterior tibial tendon. The nerve lies posterior to the tendon. The entry site is 2 cm proximal to the nerve.
- Insert needle at a 30° angle and direct distally. Inject slowly.
- Suggested preparation: 1 mL 0.25% bupivicaine and 0.5 mL (2 mg) dexamethasone in 3 mL syringe. Inject with 25-gauge needle.

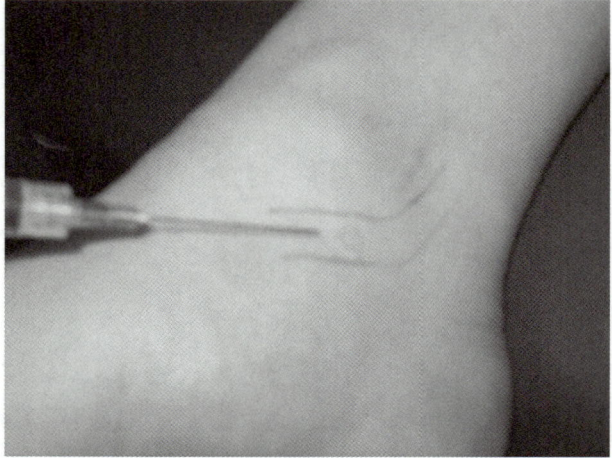

Figure 23.24 Tarsal tunnel injection.

Plantar fasciitis (see Fig. 23.25)

Technique

- The patient lies in lateral decubitus position with the affected foot down and medial aspect of the affected heel upward.
- Identify area on the medial calcaneus where it curves upward. This is the entry site.
- Insert needle directly down, perpendicular to the skin, past the midline of the width of the foot. Inject slowly and evenly through the middle one-third width of the foot while the needle is slowly withdrawn.
- Avoid injecting through the base of the foot at the fat pad.
- Suggested preparation: 2 mL 0.25% bupivicaine and 1 mL (4 mg) dexamethasone in 3 mL syringe. Inject with 25-gauge needle.

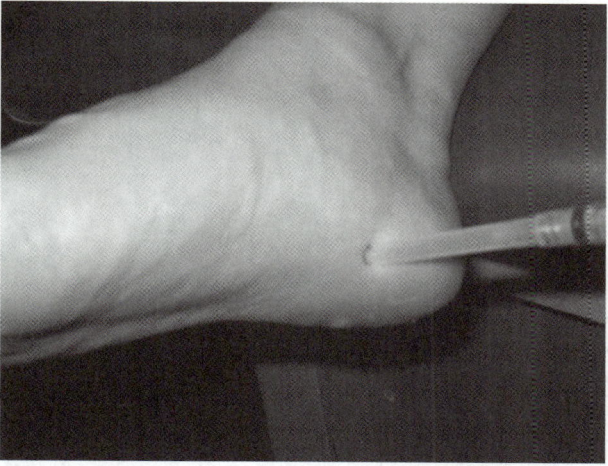

Figure 23.25 Plantar fasciitis injection.

First metatarsophalangeal joint (see Fig. 23.26)

Technique
- The patient lies in supine position with the knee in flexion and foot firmly supported on the table.
- Identify the MTP joint line on dorsum of the foot by passively flexing and extending the first toe. Distal traction may be applied to the first toe to open the joint space.
- Insert needle either on the dorsomedial or dorsclateral aspect at a 60°–70° angle to plane of the foot distally to match the slope of the joint. Inject slowly. No resistance should be met.
- Suggested preparation: 1 mL 0.25% bupivicaine ard 0.5 mL (2 mg) dexamethasone in 3 mL syringe. Inject with 25-gauge needle.

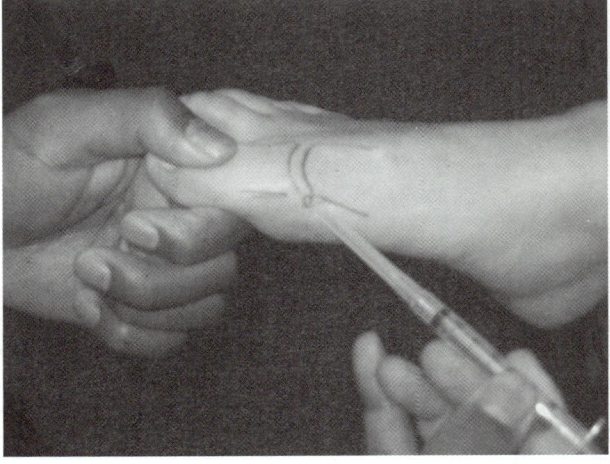

Figure 23.26 First metatarsal joint injection.

Morton's neuroma (see Fig. 23.27)

Technique
- The patient lies in supine position with the knee in flexion and foot firmly supported on the table.
- Palpate the area of tenderness and fullness on the dorsum of the foot between the affected metatarsal heads. This is the entry site.
- Insert needle at a 45° angle distally to proximally on dorsal foot surface down to the area of fullness.
- Avoid injecting into the plantar fat pad.
- Suggested preparation: 2 mL 0.25% bupivicaine and 0.5 mL (2 mg) dexamethasone in 3 mL syringe. Inject with 25-gauge needle.

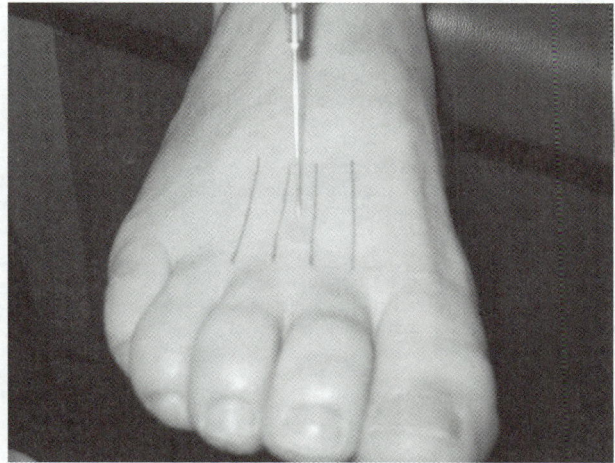

Figure 23.27 Morton's neuroma injection.

Joint aspiration

Indications
- Evaluate synovial fluid and determine cause of effusion
- Diminish pain or intra-articular pressure
- Remove exudative fluid from a septic joint
- Injection of medications

Contraindications
- Cellulitis over injection site
- Severe primary coagulopathy
- Uncontrolled anticoagulant therapy
- Suspected bacteremia with joint not being source
- Inaccessible joints
- Joint prosthesis

Supplies needed
- Sterile or nonsterile gloves
- Povidone-iodine or alcohol wipes
- Sterile drapes (optional and usually not necessary)
- Ballpoint pen or other skin marker (optional)
- 1 mL to 10 mL syringe (one or two)
- 10 mL to 60 mL syringe
- 18- to 20-gauge needle (two or three)
- 22- to 25-gauge (use 25-gauge for smaller joints) 1.5-inch needle
- Hemostat (if also injecting)
- Ethyl chloride spray
- Local anesthetic
- Tubes for culture or other laboratory studies
- Corticosteroid preparation (if also injecting)
- 4 × 4 gauze wet with sterile saline or alcohol
- 4 × 4 dry gauze
- Band-Aid
- Compression dressing (optional)

Procedure
- Draw up sufficient amount of local anesthetic into a 1 mL to 10 mL syringe using an 18- to 20-gauge needle.
- Remove needle used to draw up local anesthetic and place a 22- to 25-gauge needle on syringe with local anesthetic only.
- If planning to also inject corticosteroid preparation, draw up proper amounts of local anesthetic then steroid into a 1 mL to 10 mL syringe using an 18- to 20-gauge needle. Mix well by tipping the syringe forward and backward.
- Identify the site of entry and mark with a ballpoint pen, skin marker, or needle with cap in place.

- Prep the area with a povidone-iodine or alcohol wipe.
- Sterilely drape area if desired.
- Spray site of entry with ethyl chloride until skin begins to whiten to locally anesthetize the skin.
- Inject local anesthetic, creating a wheal at skin surface. Allow a few minutes for the skin to properly anesthetize.
- Insert 18- to 20-gauge needle attached to a 10 mL to 60 mL syringe into the site previously identified. Pull back on the plunger to aspirate joint fluid. Milking fluid toward the injection site may be beneficial. Fluid needed for laboratory studies should be transferred to tubes.
- If also injecting corticosteroid into the joint, keep the needle in place using hemostat. Remove aspiration syringe and replace it with a syringe containing corticosteroid preparation. Mix injection well by tipping syringe backward and forward. Inject medication slowly. There should be no resistance.
- Remove needle and clean the area with a wet gauze pad and then dry gauze pad.
- Place a Band-Aid over the puncture wound. Compression dressing may be needed.

Aftercare and return to play

Leave the Band-Aid or dressing on for 6–12 hours. The patient should immediately report fevers, chills, or local signs of infection if they occur. The patient may bathe normally and return to play immediately after aspiration.

If injected, please refer to Joint injection overview section (p. 768) for aftercare and return-to-play guidelines.

If laboratory studies are being sent, inform patients of the time frame anticipated to provide them with results.

Adverse effects and complications

- Infection
- Inability to aspirate fluid
- Post-injection steroid flare
- Steroid arthropathy
- Tendon rupture or injury
- Injection into blood vessel or blood vessel injury
- Nerve injury
- Subcutaneous fatty atrophy
- Skin depigmentation
- Adverse drug or hypersensitivity reaction
- Osteoporosis and cartilage damage
- Facial flushing
- Transient paresis of injected extremity
- Asymptomatic pericapsular calcification

Shoulder

Technique

- The patient sits supported with arm resting comfortably by their side.
- Identify and palpate the head of the humerus, the coracoid process, and the acromion.

Anterior approach (see Fig. 23.28)

Have shoulder slightly externally rotated to open up joint space. The insertion site is approximately 1 cm lateral to the coracoid process and medial to the head of the humerus. Direct the needle posteriorly and slightly superiorly and laterally into the joint for aspiration. The needle should not contact bone. If it does, pull back and redirect needle at a slightly different angle.

Posterior approach

Have the arm held in medial rotation across the waist. The insertion site is 2–3 cm inferior and medial to the posterolateral corner of acromion. Place thumb of the non-injecting hand at the angle of acromion and index finger anteriorly on the coracoid process. Direct needle anteriorly in the direction of the coracoid process for aspiration.

For a picture of the posterior approach, please see Figure 23.1.

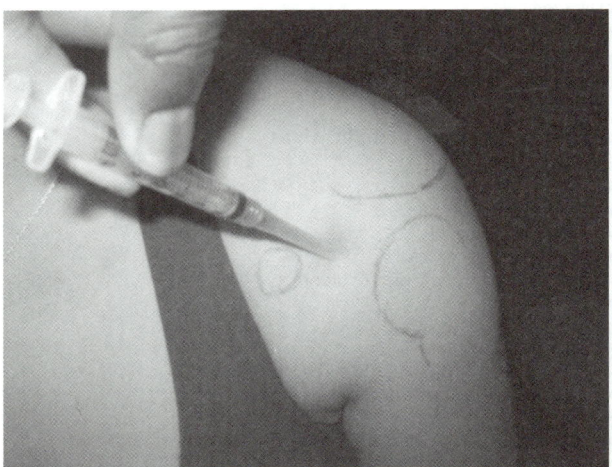

Figure 23.28 Glenohumeral anterior.

Elbow (see Fig. 23.29)

Technique

- The patient sits with the elbow supported and flexed at 90°.
- Identify the joint by palpating soft tissue within the triangle formed by the lateral epicondyle, radial head, and olecranon process.
- Insert needle aiming for the medial epicondyle for aspiration. If the needle hits bone, it should be pulled back and redirected at a different angle.

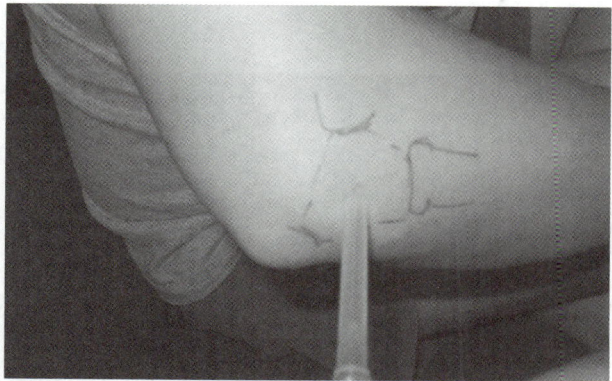

Figure 23.29 Elbow aspiration.

Knee (see Fig. 23.30)

Technique

- The patient lies supine with legs extended and relaxed. A pillow or a rolled towel may be placed under the popliteal space to slightly flex the knee.
- Identify the most superior and lateral aspect of the patella.
- Insert needle 1 cm superior and 1 cm lateral to this point for aspiration. Apply gentle pressure to the contralateral side of the knee to encourage fluid to pool in the area of aspiration. Direct needle at a 45° angle under the patella to the midjoint area.

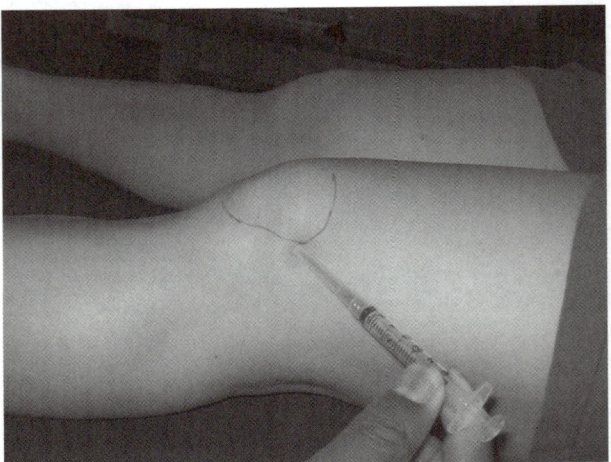

Figure 23.30 Knee aspiration.

Ganglion cyst aspiration, injection

Indications
- Relieve pain and/or paresthesias caused by cyst
- Cosmetics

Contraindications
- Cellulitis over injection site
- Severe primary coagulopathy
- Uncontrolled anticoagulant therapy
- Proximity to radial artery
- Continued recurrence may require surgical removal.

Supplies needed
- Sterile or nonsterile gloves
- Povidone-iodine or alcohol wipes
- Sterile drapes (optional and usually not necessary)
- 1 mL to 10 mL syringe
- 2–1 mL to 3 mL syringe
- 3–18- to 20-gauge needle
- 22- to 25-gauge (use 25-gauge for smaller joints) 1.5-inch needle
- Ethyl chloride spray (optional)
- Local anesthetic (i.e., 1% lidocaine)
- Hemostat (optional)
- Corticosteroid of choice (i.e., 1 mL/40 mg methylprednisolone), optional
- 4 × 4 gauze wet with sterile saline or alcohol
- 4 × 4 dry gauze pad
- Band-Aid
- Compression dressing (optional)

Procedure
- Draw up local anesthetic into one 1 mL to 3 mL syringe using an 18- to 20-gauge needle; use another same-size syringe and needle to draw up 1 mL of corticosteroid if desired to inject as well.
- Remove the needle used to draw up local anesthetic and replace it with a 22- to 25-gauge needle. Remove needle used to draw up corticosteroid.
- Identify ganglion site.
- Prep the area with a povidone-iodine or alcohol wipe.
- Sterilely drape area if desired.
- Spray site of entry with ethyl chloride until the skin begins to whiten to locally anesthetize skin.
- Insert needle with local anesthetic just beneath the skin and inject, making a wheal. Allow several minutes for anesthetic to take effect.
- Attach an 18- to 20-gauge needle to 1 mL to 10 mL syringe.

- Insert needle into the site previously anesthetized. Pull back on plunger to aspirate contents of cyst. The contents are often thick and gel-like.
- If you wish to inject corticosteroid, apply hemostat to an 18- to 20-gauge needle already in the skin and remove the syringe from the needle. Attach the syringe of corticosteroid to the needle and nject it slowly into the cyst.
- Remove needle and clean area with wet gauze pad and then dry gauze pad.
- Place a Band-Aid over the puncture wound.
- Apply a compression dressing if desired.

Aftercare and return to play

Leave the Band-Aid on for 6–12 hours. Return to play is immediate. Inform the patient that ganglion cyst may recur with or without corticosteroid injection. Definitive treatment for continued recurrence is surgical removal.

Adverse effects and complications

- High recurrence rate
- Inability to aspirate cyst
- Infection
- Post-injection steroid flare

Trigger point injection

Indications
- Trigger point: a focal, hyperirritable, knot-like area within a band of skeletal muscle

Contraindications
- Anticoagulation therapy or bleeding diathesis
- Local or systemic infection
- Allergy to medications to be injected
- Acute muscle trauma

Supplies
- Gloves
- Alcohol pads
- Gauze sponges
- Bupivicane 0.25% without epinephrine or an alternative anesthetic, 3–5 mL (one can add a corticosteroid as well)
- 3 mL or 5 mL syringe
- 25-gauge needle of various lengths depending on injection site
- Adhesive bandage

Procedure
- With gloved hands locate the trigger point.
- Squeeze it with the index finger and thumb.
- Clean the skin with an alcohol pad.
- Slowly direct the needle into the muscle toward the trigger point.
- Aspirate to confirm that the needle is not in a vessel.
- Inject a small amount of anesthetic.
- Withdraw the needle to the level of subcutaneous tissue, redirect superiorly, inferiorly, medially, and laterally, injecting the remainder of the anesthetic.
- Withdraw the needle completely and maintain firm pressure for 2 minutes.
- Apply adhesive bandage.

Aftercare and return to play
The patient should remain active but avoid strenuous activity for 2–3 days after injection.

Adverse effects and complications
- Post-injection soreness
- Hematoma formation
- Medication reaction if steroids used
- Skin infection
- Pneumothorax, depending on injection site location

Peripheral intravenous access

Indications
- Significant volume depletion or dehydration
- Unable to restore volume losses through oral intake
- Severe muscle cramping
- Profuse vomiting and/or diarrhea

Contraindications
- Area with overlying infection
- An extremity with shunts or fistulas
- Extremity on the side of radical mastectomy

Supplies
- Gloves
- Alcohol pads
- Tourniquet
- Gauze sponges
- Tape
- Tegaderm
- Angiocatheters 16, 18, 20, and/or 22 gauge
- Saline lock tubing

Procedure
- Position patient comfortably and apply tourniquet around the upper arm or forearm.
- With gloved hands, clean the site with an alcohol pad.
- Use your thumb to stabilize the vein inferiorly with light traction downward.
- Use the index finger on the more proximal area with upward pressure.
- Hold the angiocatheter between the thumb and index finger on the dominant hand.
- With the bevel up, puncture vein at an angle of 10°–30° to the skin.
- After flash is seen, advance several more millimeters to ensure being completely in the vein.
- Advance only the angiocatheter.
- Remove the needle, making sure to place pressure on the vessel to decrease blood loss.
- Connect the saline lock or IV tubing.
- Cover the IV site with Tegaderm and use tape on the tubing to prevent accidental dislodgement.

Aftercare and return to play
If running fluid, turn it off. Pull out the angiocatheter and hold firm pressure with a gauze sponge for 2 minutes. Tape the gauze sponge down.

Adverse effects and complications
- Phlebitis
- Infiltration
- Infection
- Nerve damage
- Bruising

Compartment testing (exertional)

Indications
- When there is concern for exertional compartment syndrome

Contraindications
- Overlying skin infection
- Bleeding dyscrasia

Supplies
- Gloves
- Povidone-iodine (Betadine) swabs
- Lidocaine 1% without epinephrine or alternative anesthetic
- Handheld compartment pressure monitor (see Fig. 23.31)
- Gauze sponges
- Adhesive bandages

Procedure

General procedure overview
- Position the patient supine.
- Assemble the handheld device per manufacturer instructions.
- With gloved hands, prep the skin with Betadine swabs.
- Make a skin wheal with the anesthetic, making sure not to infiltrate the compartment.
- Calibrate or "zero" device before use.
- Avoid neurovascular structures while inserting the device needle into the compartment.
- Keeping device parallel to the table, slowly inject a small amount of saline (<0.3 mL) into compartment.
- Record the number after it equilibrates.
- Withdraw needle and apply an adhesive bandage.
- Have the patient perform enough exercise to provoke symptoms.
- Repeat the above steps for measuring at 1 and 5 minutes after exercise.

Compartment testing in lower leg
- Perform measurements 4 to 5 finger-widths below tibial tuberosity.
- Palpate lateral leg for the septum dividing the anterior (above septum) and lateral (below septum) compartments (see Fig. 23.32).
- Measure pressures above and below septum with 2 separate injections.
- On the medial aspect, the superficial posterior and deep posterior compartments can be measured with one injection (see Fig. 23.33).
- Only one injection site is needed if close enough to the septum.
- Insert pressure needle a finger-width below the septum, only a couple of centimeters to get superficial posterior pressure (see Fig. 23.34).
- Along the same trajectory continue inserting the needle deeper to measure deep posterior compartment pressure.

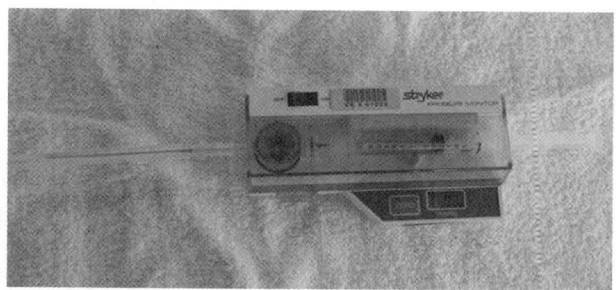

Figure 23.31 Compartment testing device.

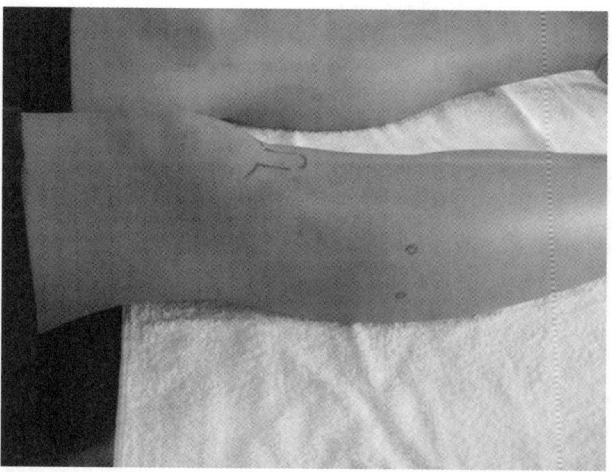

Figure 23.32 Lateral landmarks for compartment testing.

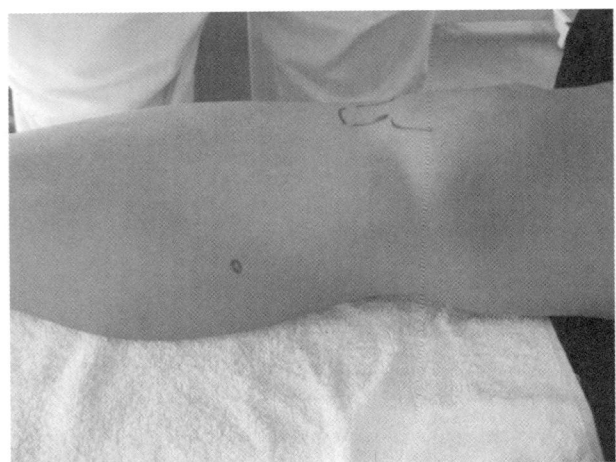

Figure 23.33 Medial landmark for compartment testing.

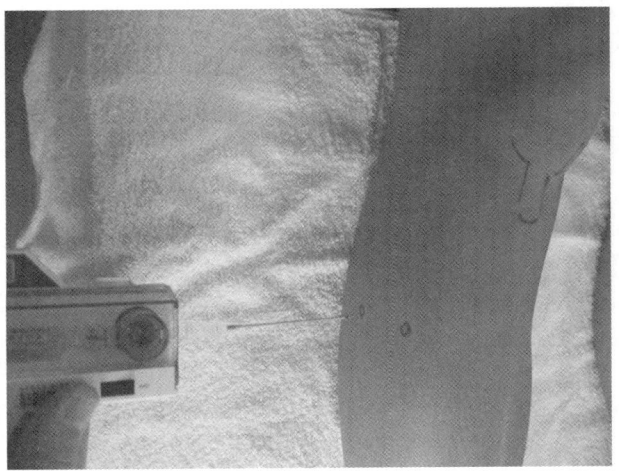

Figure 23.34 Correct position in which to hold device.

Aftercare and return to play

One should consider a surgical referral or evaluation for possible fasciotomy or fasciectomy if the following occur:

- Resting compartment pressures are >15 mmHg
- Exertional pressures at 1 minute are >30 mmHg
- Pressures are >20 mmHg at 5 minutes

Adverse effects and complications

- Can be painful
- Infection
- Bleeding
- Nerve and/or vascular damage

Laceration repair

Indications
- Laceration is too wide to heal well without re-approximation

Contraindications
- Grossly contaminated wounds
- Animal bites

Supplies
- Gloves
- Eye protection
- Suture material (€4.0 for large mobile areas; 5.0 for smaller areas; 6.0 for face).
- Laceration repair kit (or at least needle drivers and tissue forceps)
- Lidocaine 1% or alternative anesthetic with or without epinephrine, depending on area
- Saline 100 mL to 300 mL (minimum) for average-sized wounds
- 5 mL syringe
- 20 mL or larger syringe
- 19-gauge angiocatheter
- 25- or 27-gauge needle
- Tetanus prophylaxis, if patient is not up to date
- Dermabond*

Procedure
- Document a thorough physical and neurovascular exam.
- Locally anesthetize the wound with the 25- or 27-gauge needle.
- Perform a nerve block in areas with little subcutaneous tissue (e.g., fingers) to prevent tissue distortion.
- Use 19-gauge angiocatheter and larger syringe for high-pressure irrigation with saline.
- Debride devitalized tissue.
- Follow standard wound closure technique and principles.
- With delayed or grossly contaminated wounds, clinical judgment is imperative with regard to wound closure and management.
- Protect the wound from external contaminants during the vulnerable 24- to 48-hour period. Give tetanus prophylaxis if appropriate.
- Clean the wound as detailed earlier.
- Approximate the wound (see Figs. 23.35 and 23.36).
- For dermaband use, apply the substance in four to five layers. Allow each layer to dry between applications. Avoid eyes and hair.

Aftercare and return to play
Reinforce wound coverage if the patient is practicing or competing. Frequently check the area for signs of infection. Prophylactic antibiotic use can be considered. Sutures should be removed at 5–14 days, depending on location.

*Dermabond should only be used in low-tension areas (e.g., face) and when the likelihood of wound contaminants is extremely low.

Adverse effects and complications

- Infection
- Wound dehiscence
- Hypertrophic scarring

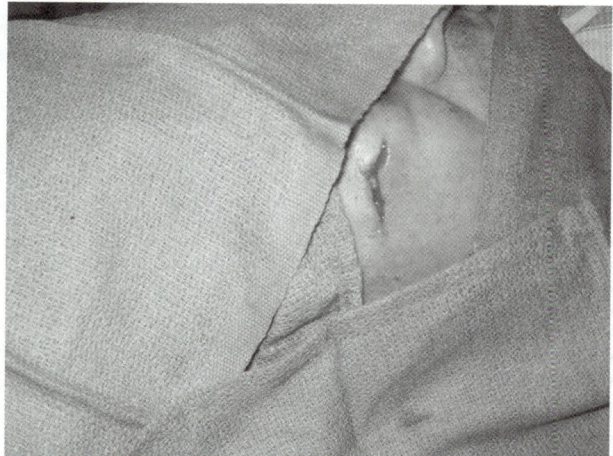

Figure 23.35 Laceration under right eye.

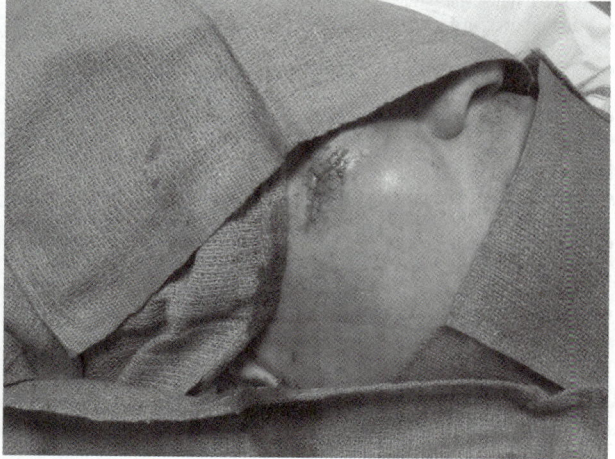

Figure 23.36 Repaired laceration with wound edges well approximated.

Auricular hematoma aspiration/incision ("cauliflower ear")

Indications
Hematoma formation within the ear

Contraindications
Overlying skin infection

Supplies
- Gloves
- Gauze sponges
- Elastic gauze roll
- Lidocaine 1% without epinephrine
- Povidone-iodine (Betadine) swabs
- 19-gauge needle
- 10 mL syringe
- Antibiotic ointment
- Dental rolls
- 4–0 nylon suture
- Collodoin
- Cotton balls

Procedure
- Use gloved hands to clean the ear with Betadine swabs.
- Give either a local anesthetic or perform auricular nerve block (see Fig. 23.37).
- Insert needle into the most fluctuant portion of hematoma.
- Aspirate fluid while "milking" the hematoma (see Fig. 23.38).
- Maintain pressure for 3 minutes after withdrawing needle (see Fig. 23.39).
- For incision, make the incision along the pinna and posterior edge of the hematoma.
- Evacuate the hematoma and irrigate the area.
- Apply antibiotic ointment over the area.

Pressure dressing
- Suture anterior and posterior dental rolls through the ear, compressing the pinna.
- Alternatively, soak cotton balls in collodoin. Before the cotton hardens, mold it to the ear at the site of aspiration or incision. Place gauze behind the ear and fluffed gauze anterior to it.
- Wrap elastic gauze around the head.

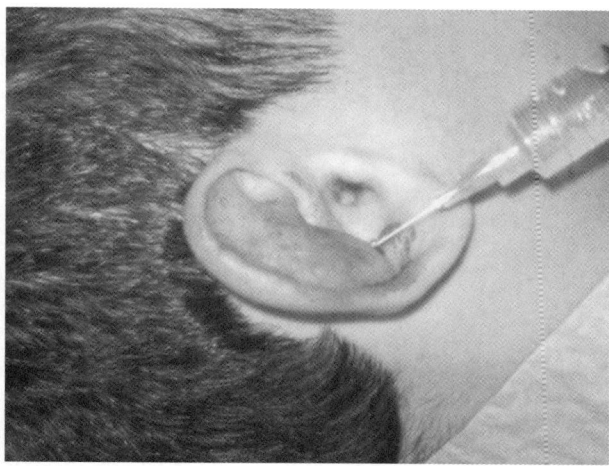

Figure 23.37 Anesthetizing well-clean cauliflower ear.

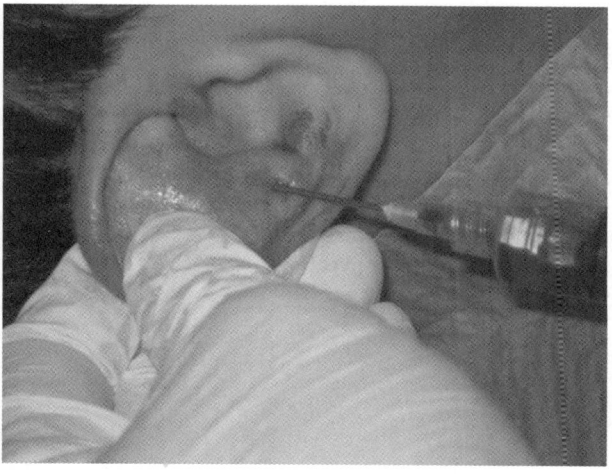

Figure 23.38 Aspiration of serosanguinous fluid.

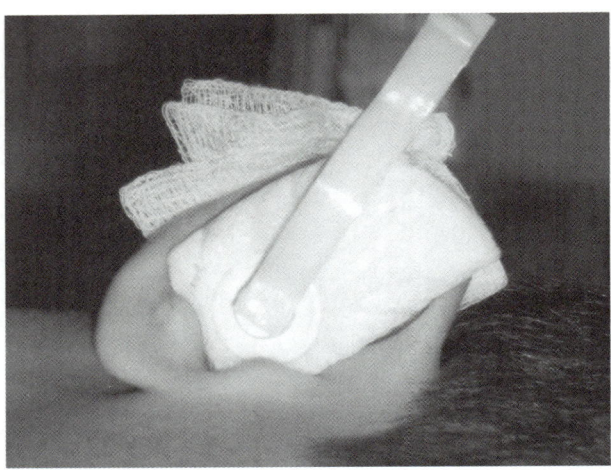

Figure 23.39 Clamp on ear after aspiration to maintain pressure.

Aftercare and return to play

- Prescribe an antistaphylococcal antibiotic.
- Examine the ear after 24 hours for hematoma reaccumulation.
- Reaspiration may be necessary.
- Closely monitor the area for signs of infection.
- Remove the dressing in 1 week.
- Consider an ear, nose, throat (ENT) follow-up.
- If there is an infection, surgical drainage is necessary along with IV antibiotics.

Adverse effects and complications

- Infection
- Hematoma reaccumulation
- Auricular deformation, permanent "cauliflower ear"

Abscess incision and drainage

Indications
- Abscess formation with detectable area of fluctuance

Contraindications
- Early abscess without localization of pus

Supplies
- Gloves
- Lidocaine 1% or alternative anesthetic
- 5 mL syringe
- 25- or 27-gauge needle
- Gauze sponges
- Incision and drainage kit, including scalpel and hemostat
- Wound culture swab
- Cotton-tipped applicator
- Packing gauze
- Tape
- Elastic gauze
- Antibiotics*

Procedure
- Use gloved hands to make a skin wheal with anesthetic.
- Use scalpel to incise over the area of maximal fluctuance about 1–3 cm.
- Incise in the direction that conforms to the natural skin creases.
- Make a smaller incision in special areas (e.g., face).
- Culture a sample of purulent material with swab to check for community-acquired methicillin-resistant *Staphylococcus aureus* (CA-MRSA).
- Break up loculations inside the abscess with a hemostat.
- Use a cotton-tipped applicator for smaller areas.
- Pack the abscess loosely with gauze packing.
- Secure edges of nonadherent dressing with tape or circumferentially with elastic gauze.

Aftercare and return to play
- Reassess the wound in 48 hours.
- Repacking may be required.

Adverse effects and complications
- Vascular and/or nerve injury
- Bleeding
- Hypertrophic scarring

* Antibiotic choice requires clinical judgment and knowledge of bacterial resistance patterns.

Ingrown toenail removal

Indications
- Ingrown toenail

Contraindications
- None

Supplies
- Gloves
- English nail anvil or suture scissors or #11 scalpel blade
- Hemostat
- Lidocaine 1% or alternative anesthetic
- 25- or 27-gauge needle
- 5 mL syringe
- Saline
- Alcohol wipes
- Phenol 70% to 90% or silver nitrate sticks
- Cotton-tipped applicator
- Toe tourniquet
- Antibiotic ointment

Procedure
- Clean toe gently with gloved hands.
- Perform a digital block after cleaning areas to be injected with alcohol (see Fig. 23.40).
- Squeeze the toe to exsanguinate and apply toe tourniquet (see Fig. 23.41).
- Use English anvil nail splitter or scissors to make a longitudinal cut along the lateral one-fourth of the nail.
- If using the nail splitter, go one-half to two-thirds back, then switch to scissors or scalpel.
- If using only scissors, maintain upward pressure to prevent from cutting nail bed.
- Divide nail several millimeters past the proximal nail fold until resistance is no longer felt.
- Grasp the end of the nail with the hemostat and pull in the plane of the nail while twisting toward the remaining nail.
- Ensure that there is no remaining nail.

If there is recurrence, one can consider using the following additional technique:
- Make sure the nail bed is completely dry and apply the phenol only under the proximal nail fold in three 30-second intervals.
- Do not get the phenol on the healthy nail bed.
- Alternatively, use silver nitrate on the nail bed to dry it out.
- Use a gloved finger to remove traces of dried phenol.
- To finish the procedure in general, remove the tourniquet, apply antibiotic ointment, and cover with a nonadherent dressing.

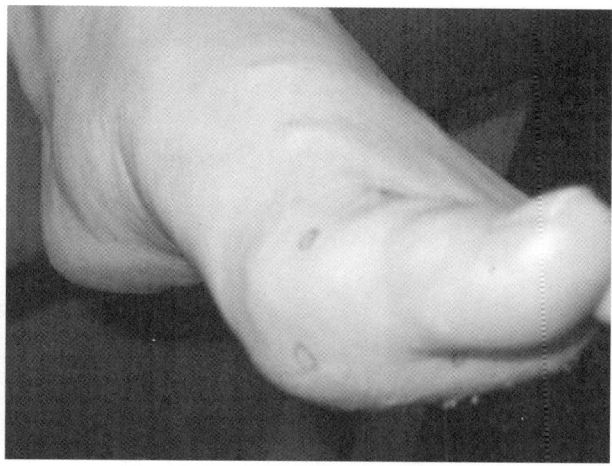

Figure 23.40 Injection landmarks for great toe digital block.

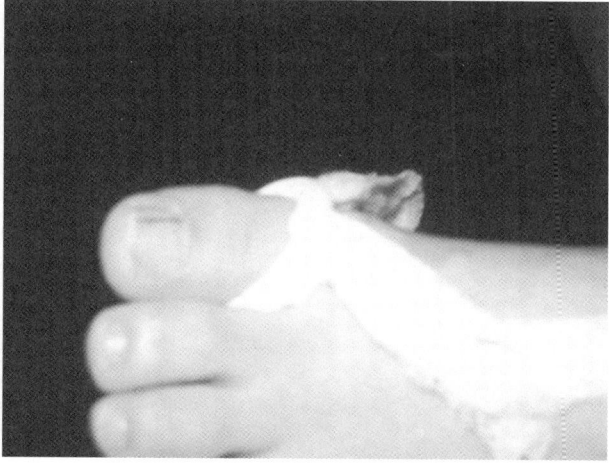

Figure 23.41 Tourniquet on toe and marker on toenail representing portion to cut along and remove.

Aftercare and return to play
- Wash the wound twice a day with fresh dressing changes.
- Look for signs of infection.
- Wrap the wound well, but can continue to play and practice.

Adverse effects and complications
- Regrowth of nail
- Infection
- Inclusion cyst growth
- Delayed healing

Subungal hematoma drainage

Indications
- Painful subungal hematoma greater than one-third nail

Contraindications
- >36 hours, because blood has likely coagulated

Supplies
- Gloves
- Alcohol wipes
- Electrocautery device or
- Paperclip or
- 18-gauge needle
- Gauze sponges
- Tape

Procedure
Multiple devices can be used to achieve the same goal. There may be slight discomfort with the procedure, but anesthesia is not necessary.
- With gloved hands, clean the nail with alcohol wipes.
- If using the cautery device, touch the nail, creating either multiple small holes or one large one to facilitate blood drainage.
- If using a paperclip, heat until red hot and use it in the same manner.
- If using the 18-gauge needle, spin needle until the nail is penetrated and stop before the sensitive nail bed is reached.
- Squeeze as much blood out as possible and dress the wound.

Aftercare and return to play
Warn the patient that the nail could be lost and when it grows back there could be a permanent nail deformity.

Adverse effects and complications
- Infection
- Permanent nail deformity

Epistaxis control

Indications
- Epistaxis

Contraindications
- Massive facial trauma

Supplies
- Gloves
- Face shield
- Gauze sponges
- Topical anesthetic
- Topical vasoconstrictor
- Afrin nasal spray (tetracaine 1% and 0.05% oxymetazoline), an anesthetic and vasoconstrictor
- Nasal speculum
- Dental rolls or cotton
- Bayonet forceps
- Silver nitrate sticks

Procedure
- Wear mask and gloves.
- Use a nasal speculum to locate the source of bleeding.
- Soak dental rolls or cotton in Afrin.
- Wring out soaked material and place it in the affected naris with a forceps for 5 minutes.
- In addition, have the patient firmly pinch the nostrils.
- Once hemostasis is achieved, cauterize the area with silver nitrate sticks by gently touching area for 4–5 seconds.

This technique should be sufficient for most nosebleeds. For more complicated nosebleeds, persistent cases, or bleeds with a posterior bleeding, seek additional care at an emergency department.

Aftercare and return to play
- Prescribe antibiotics (amoxicillin, trimethoprim/sulfamethoxazole, etc.) if leaving in the packing.
- Profuse bleeds should be re-evaluated in 48 hours and removal of the nasal packing should be considered.

Adverse effects and complications
- Septum perforation with the silver nitrate
- Infection of sinuses
- Toxic shock syndrome; exceedingly rare

Tooth avulsion management

Indications
- Avulsed tooth

Contraindications
- If it is a primary tooth do not reimplant. This can interfere with secondary tooth eruption.
- If tooth is fractured
- If significant maxillofacial trauma

Supplies
- Gloves
- Transport media (e.g. Hank's balanced salt solution, Save-A-Tooth, milk, water)
- Periodontal paste or composite
- Saline
- Gauze sponges
- Tetanus if not up to date

Procedure
Time is more critical if a liquid medium is not available. Anything over 60 minutes is unlikely to be successful. Some commercial agents can extend this time window up to 12 hours.
- Only handle the tooth by the crown with gloved hands.
- Gently clean off any debris with saline.
- Remove any clot in the socket with irrigation.
- Place the tooth in the socket.
- Have the patient bite on the gauze to help realign it.
- Use the composite to form a splint using neighboring teeth.

Aftercare and return to play
The patient should have close dental follow-up within 24 hours. The American Association of Endodontics does not recommend routine antibiotic use. However, some clinicians do and if given, antibiotics should cover oral flora (e.g., penicillin, clindamycin, etc.).

Patients should be on a soft diet until they follow up with a dentist.

Adverse effects and complications
- Infection
- Reimplantation failure

Common joint reductions

Indications
- Joint dislocation

Contraindications
- None

Supplies
- Specific joint immobilization devices
- For upper extremity can use a sling

Procedure
- General principles include documenting a physical and neurovascular exam before reduction attempts and after the reductions are achieved.
- Exaggerate the direction of the deformity before reducing the joint (especially true with fingers)
- Reducing quickly if a fracture is not obvious is easier before spasm sets in.
- Several reduction methods should be known for large joints because more than one technique may be necessary.
- If a field reduction is not done and there is no neurovascular compromise, prereduction radiographs should be obtained.
- Postreduction films are strongly encouraged except in certain cases (e.g., radial head dislocation).

Anterior shoulder dislocation
The *traction counter-traction* method stabilizes the torso while gently pulling on the arm at a 45° angle.

The *external rotation method* gently and slowly externally rotates the arm with the elbow at 90°, using the forearm as a lever.

In the *Spaso technique*, the patient is supine with the affected arm fully extended toward ceiling. Vertical traction is applied and the arm externally rotated at the forearm or wrist.

In the *scapular manipulation technique*, the patient lies in a prone position with a portion of the body off the edge. The affected arm hangs perpendicularly toward the floor. Weights (10 kg) are attached at the wrist or an assistant can create traction by pulling downward. With thumbs together, the operator places one hand on the superior aspect of the scapula and the other on the inferior aspect. The technique stabilizes the superior part while pushing the lateral edge of the scapula medially and dorsally with the thumbs.

Posterior elbow dislocation
In the *traction method* the patient lies prone and an assistant applies countertraction on the humerus toward the patient. The operator applies opposite traction on the forearm while flexing the elbow with a hand stabilizing the distal humerus and correcting any olecranon lateral displacement.

Another method has the patient lying prone. An assistant pulls on the forearm while the operator encircles the distal humerus and uses both thumbs to apply olecranon pressure. The arm is in slight flexion, which relaxes the triceps. There should be no mechanical block with full range of motion, as well as stability in the joint.

Finger dislocation
Exaggerate the injury with slight traction and hyperextension before bringing it back in a reduced position. The joint should be checked after reduction for stability.

Lateral patella dislocation
Extend the knee and apply gentle medially directed patella pressure.

Aftercare and return to play

Anterior shoulder dislocation
Immobilize the shoulder with a commercial device. Alternatively, one can use a sling and swath to immobilize the arm. Follow up with orthopedics in 1–2 weeks.

Posterior elbow dislocation
Immobilize at 90° with a long arm posterior splint. Make sure there is no neurovascular compromise or injury. Follow up with orthopedics in 1 week.

Finger dislocation
If stable, splint the finger in 20°–30° of flexion for 3 weeks. One can also "buddy-tape" the finger for 3–6 weeks. Refer to orthopedics in 1–2 weeks.

Lateral patella dislocation
Use commercial knee immobilizer device with the knee in full extension. Follow up with orthopedics in 1–2 weeks.

Adverse effects and complications
- Vascular injury
- Nerve injury
- Residual joint instability

Casting, splinting, and taping

See Figures 23.42 and 23.43.

Indications
- Fracture, dislocation, ligament, or tendon injury

Contraindications
- If injury is significant, swelling casts should be avoided.

Supplies
- Gloves
- Eye protection
- Stockinette
- Plaster of Paris (POP) or
- Fiberglass cast material
- Prefabricated splint rolls
- Padding, such as Webril
- Elastic bandages
- Adhesive tape
- Utility knife or scissors
- Bucket of water

Procedure

General principles include close examination of skin before applying any material. The skin should be clean. Bony prominences should have extra padding. The joint should be immobilized in neutral or functional positions (e.g. "wine glass" position for wrist). If applying a cast, make sure swelling is minimal and more swelling is unlikely. Inattention to this can lead to either ischemic injury or improper immobilization.

- Place on the stockinette and apply 2–4 layers of padding.
- Place extra padding at the ends; the stockinette should be long at the ends.
- With gloved hands, dip the fiberglass in water for 1–2 minutes.
- Gently wring and wrap circumferentially from proximal to distal.
- Overlap material by one-half.
- Strategic cuts may be necessary to wrap with minimal wrinkles and to go around digits.
- Fold the extra stockinette and the edge of the padding over the fiberglass to create a smooth edge.
- Use the second wrapping to secure the folded edges down.
- Wet gloves frequently and smooth down the entire cast.
- The position of immobilization needs to be maintained until the material adequately hardens.
- Pay close attention that no skin is in contact with the sharp edges of dried fiberglass.
- Use a utility knife or scissors to remove exposed sharp edges.
- Recheck neurovascular status and reassess pain.

Use of splinting is better in the acute setting because of the increased likelihood of swelling.

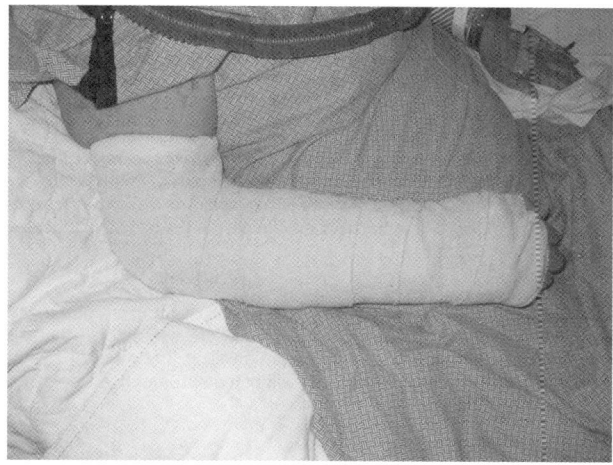

Figure 23.42 Upper extremity cast for distal radius or ulna fracture.

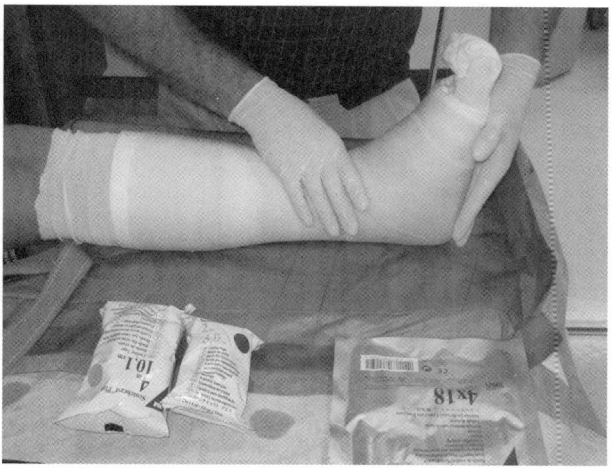

Figure 23.43 Lower extremity cast for distal leg fractures.

- Apply padding in a similar fashion to cast application.
- Use either 6 to 8 layers of plaster or prefabricated splint material.
- The material needs to be wet to initiate the hardening process.
- Use elastic wrap to cover the splint while maintaining the ideal immobilization position.
- Recheck neurovascular status and reassess pain.

Specific finger injuries (e.g., mallet finger) require special splints, but taping is ideal for some mild collateral ligament finger injuries. "Buddy taping" or taping a finger to the neighboring one is convenient and allows early motion. Improper immobilization can cause stiffness in the hand and lead to a significant loss of function.

Aftercare and return to play
The length of time differs for specific injuries and their degree of severity. Frequent periodic checks and close follow-up are necessary if there is concern for wound infection or significant swelling. The material cannot get wet. At the very least, its integrity will be compromised if it does not fall completely apart.

Adverse effects and complications
- Thermal injury
- Ischemic injury, including pressure sores or compartment syndrome
- Nerve damage
- Infection
- Joint stiffness
- Muscle atrophy

Office spirometry

Indications
- Detecting pulmonary disease
- Exertional dyspnea
- Wheezing

In addition to these indications, there are myriad others, ranging from neuromuscular dysfunction (e.g. myasthenia gravis) to evaluating disability status.

Contraindications
Acute disorders that would affect performance (e.g., nausea, vomiting) are contraindications. The following most likely do not pertain to the athlete, but are included for completeness:
- Recent eye surgery
- Hemoptysis of unknown origin
- Pneumothorax
- Recent abdominal or thoracic operation
- Recent myocardial infarction or unstable angina
- Thoracic aneurysm (risk of rupture)

Supplies
- Spirometer

Procedure
There can be a great deal of patient variability in spirometry testing. One of the most important factors affecting the results is patient effort.
- Have patient fully inspire so the lungs are at capacity.
- The patient should tightly seal lips around mouthpiece.
- The patient should immediately blow the air out as fast and as long as possible until the lungs are empty.
- Validate the test with at least three reproducible trials.

Reproducible in this regard means that each FEV_1 (forced expiratory volume in 1 second) measurement is within 200 mL of each other. This should hold true for each FVC (forced vital capacity) measurement as well.

If trials are not reproducible, eight is the maximum number performed. The highest FEV_1 and FVC are recorded even if they are measured in separate trials.

The volume–time curve is helpful with validating the results. Expiration should occur for at least 6 seconds. After validation, the flow–volume curve should be closely analyzed and interpreted (see Figs. 23.44 and 23.45).

The pulmonary process can be normal, restrictive, or obstructive. If an abnormality is discovered, more specialized testing or care may be necessary.

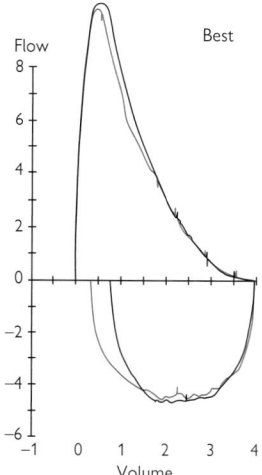

Figure 23.44 Example of a normal flow–volume loop.

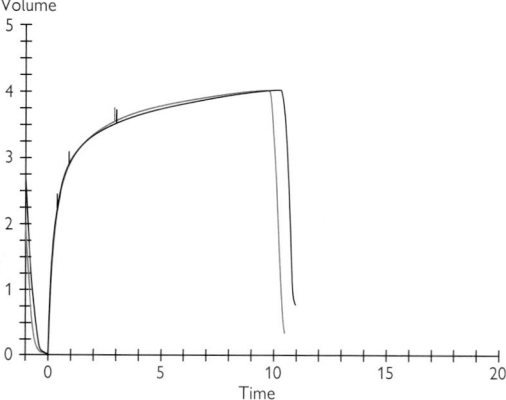

Figure 23.45 Example of a normal volume–time curve.

Aftercare and return to play

Clinical knowledge of how to interpret the data is critical. Normal ranges of values are dependent on height, weight, age, and gender. The FEV_1 and FVC are decreased in both restrictive and obstructive processes.

When the absolute FEV_1/FVC ratio is normal or increased, a restrictive process is possible. Static lung volume measurements are necessary to make the diagnosis.

If the TLC (total lung capacity) is <80%, it is strongly suggestive of a restrictive process. The FRC (functional residual capacity) measurements make the diagnosis definitive.

A decreased FEV_1/FVC ratio is consistent with an obstructive process. The patient can be retested after a bronchodilator challenge to judge reversibility.

The American Thoracic Society has developed a scale using FEV_1 and TLC to grade severity. Clinical judgment is crucial for deciding on the athlete's return to play.

Adverse effects and complications

Symptoms consistent with any of the above contraindications can be exacerbated.

Treadmill testing

Indications
- Evaluation of patients with chest pain
- Prognosis and severity of disease
- Evaluation of arrhythmias
- Screening for coronary artery disease
- Evaluation of patients with congestive heart failure (CHF)
- Evaluation of functional capacity
- Sports medicine

Treadmill testing is recommended by the American College of Sports Medicine (ACSM) for males older than 40 years and females older than 50 years who are planning on participating in vigorous exercise.

Contraindications
Absolute
- Acute myocardial infarction (MI)
- Acute myocarditis or pericarditis
- Severe symptomatic aortic stenosis
- Acutely ill patients (severe anemia, hyperthyroidism, and infections)
- Rapid arrhythmias
- Patients with problems walking
- Unstable angina

Relative
- Aortic stenosis that is not severe (no symptoms)
- Severe left main disease (>70%)
- Severe hypertension (240/130)
- CHF
- ST-segment depression at rest
- Hypertrophic cardiomyopathy (use caution because of risk of sudden death after exercise)

Supplies
- Treadmill
- Cardiac monitoring equipment
- Crash cart
- Defibrillator

Procedure
Termination of the test
- Premature ventricular complexes (PVCs) that develop in pairs or with increasing regularity
- Atrial tachycardia, fibrillation, or flutter
- Onset of second- or third-degree heart block
- Chest pain
- ST-segment depression >3 mm
- Heart rate or blood pressure that drops with exercise
- Extreme elevations in blood pressure with dizziness or changes in vision

- Patient reached maximal heart rate
- ST elevation 2 mm or more in precordial or inferior leads that do not have a resting Q wave
- Patient is unable to continue because of dyspnea, fatigue, or faintness
- ST-segment depression present at rest and progressive with exercise

Stress-test protocol

Many protocols exist, some of which are listed below. For the purposes of this chapter we will focus on the Bruce protocol, which is most widely used.

- Balke protocol
- Bruce protocol
- Ellestad protocol
- Modified astrand protocol

Bruce protocol

Increase in both speed and grade of the treadmill is used to produce a positive test.

A. Get consent from the patient.
B. Attach ECG leads and blood pressure (BP) cuff (see Fig. 23.46).
C. Take baseline vitals and obtain ECG.
D. Start treadmill test (see Table 23.1)
E. Exercise usually lasts 10 minutes unless the patient is in excellent condition.
F. Recovery period
   a. It is very important to monitor for ECG in the initial moments after the test.
   b. The BP and ECG are monitored at 1-minute intervals for 6 minutes.

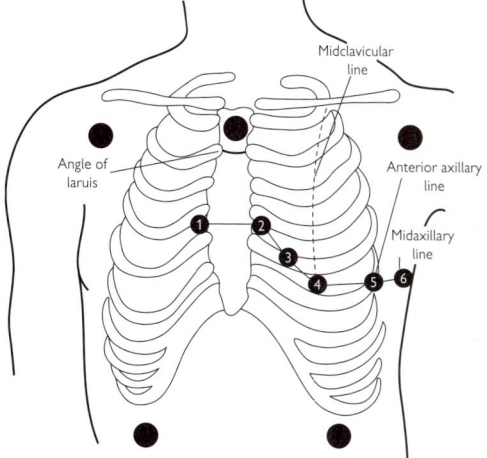

Figure 23.46 Locations of ECG leads for treadmill testing.

Table 23.1 Treadmill test values

Stage	Speed	Grade	Time	Cumulative time
1	1.7	10%	3 min	3 min
2	2.5	12%	3 min	6 min
3	3.4	14%	3 min	9 min
4	4.2	16%	3 min	12 min
5	5.0	18%	3 min	15 min
Recovery	0	Supine	6 min	21 min

Treadmill criteria definitions

Negative adequate (no diagnostic ST-segment changes with peak exercise heart rate = 85% of target heart rate): target heart rate (HR) = 220 − age × .85

Negative inadequate (no diagnostic ST-segment changes with peak exercise heart rate <85% of target heart rate)

Uninterpretable because of the following:
- Exercise-induced conduction disturbance (not right bundle branch block [RBBB])
- Rest and exercise-induced conduction disturbance (not RBBB)
- Rest and exercise-paced ventricular rhythm
- Lead fell off
- Patient fell
- Artifact
- All patients with left bundle branch block (LB3B)
- Patients with RBBB, V1–V3, and AVR are considered to have uninterpretable results, but the remainder of the ECG should be read according to the rules below.
- ECG with unstable baselines

Positive ST-segment changes (see Fig. 23.47)

Treadmill interpretation
- Isoelectric line: flat portion of the PR interval

Positive treadmill test
- 0.1 mV deviation of the ST segment from the isoelectric line at 60 msec, unless there is J-point depression with an up-sloping ST segment. The ST segment must be horizontal or moving away from the isoelectric line to be considered positive.

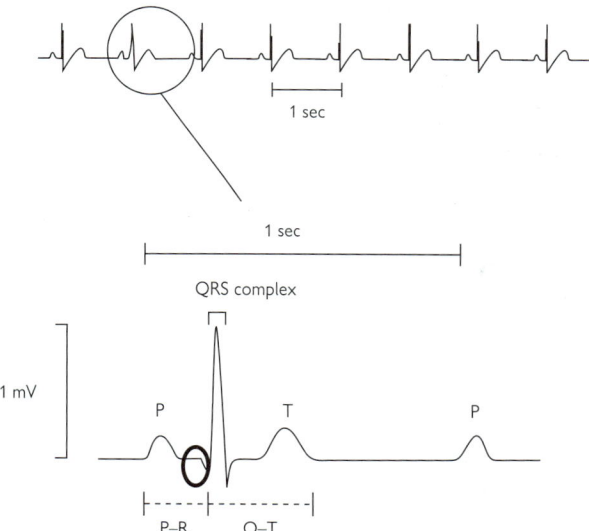

Figure 23.47 Positive ST-segment changes.

Resting ECG abnormal
- *ST segment elevation:* The J point must move an additional 0.1 mV away from the isoelectric line in combination with a ST segment that is either horizontal or moving away from the baseline in order to fulfill the criteria for a positive test.
- *ST segment depression:* If depression is ≤.05 mV at rest, an additional .1 mV of ST depression must be present to be called positive. If resting depression is >.05 mV, then an additional 0.2 mV of ST depression must be present in combination with an ST segment that is either horizontal or moving away from the baseline in order to fulfill the criteria for a positive test.

Treadmill report
- Dates and patient-identifying information
- Percent of maximal heart rate
- Blood pressure and pulse at each stage
- Physicians diagnosis

Aftercare and return to play
If the test is positive, refer to cardiology for follow-up. Please see reference in Further reading for more information on stress testing.

Further reading
Ellestad M (2003). *Stress Testing Principles and Practice*, 5th ed. New York: Oxford University Press.

Index

Shoulder (glenohumeral) joint: movements, principal muscles, and their innervation

Movement	Principal muscles	Peripheral nerve	Spinal root origin
Flexion	Pectoralis major (clavicular part)	Pectoral nerve (medial and lateral)	C 5, 6
	Deltoid (clavicular part)	Axillary nerve	C 5, 6
Extension	Latissimus dorsi	Nerve to latissimus dorsi (thoracodorsal nerve)	C 6, 7, 8
Abduction	Supraspinatus (initial 20°)	Suprascapular nerve	C 5, 6
	Deltoid	Axillary nerve	C 5, 6
Adduction	Pectoralis major	Pectoral nerves (medial and lateral)	C 5, 6
	Latissimus dorsi	Nerve to latissimus dorsi	C 6, 7, 8
Medial (internal) rotation	Pectoralis major	Pectoral nerves (medial and lateral)	C 5, 6
	Latissimuss dorsi	Nerve to latissimuss dorsi	C 6, 7, 8
	Subscapularis	Subscapular nerves (upper and lower)	C 5, 6
	Teres major	Lower subscapular nerve	C 5, 6
Lateral (external) rotation	Infraspinatus	Suprascapular nerve	C 5, 6
	Teres minor	Axillary nerve	C 5, 6
	Deltoid (posterior fibers)	Axillary nerve	C 5, 6
Circumduction	Combinations of the above		

Reproduced with permission from MacKinnon P, Morris J (2005). *Oxford Textbook of Functional Anatomy*, Vol 1. Oxford, UK: Oxford University Press. ©2005.

Radioulnar and wrist joint: movements, principal muscles, and their innervation[1]

Movement	Principal muscles	Peripheral nerve	Spinal root origin
Supination	Biceps	Musculocutaneous nerve	C 5, 6
	Supinator	Radial nerve (deep branch)	C 5, 6, 7
Pronation	Pronator teres	Median nerve	C 5, 6, 7
	Pronator quadratus	Median nerve	C 5, 6, 7, 8
Flexion	*Common flexor origin muscles*		
	Flexor carpi radialis	Median nerve	C 5, 6, 7
	Flexor carpi ulnaris	Ulnar nerve	C 5, 6, 7, 8
	(Palmaris longus)	Median nerve	C 5, 6, 7
	Long digital flexors	Median and ulnar nerves	C 5, 6, 7
Extension	*Common extensor origin muscles*		
	Extensor carpi radialis longus and brevis	Radial nerve (trunk and deep branch*)	C 5, 6, 7
	Extensor carpi ulnaris	Radial nerve (deep branch*)	C 5, 6, 7, 8
	Long digital extensors		
Abduction	Flexor carpi radialis	Median nerve	C 5, 6, 7
	Extensor carpi radialis longus and brevis	Radial nerve	C 5, 6, 7
	Abductor pollicis longus and brevis	Radial nerve (deep branch*)	C 5, 6, 7, 8
Adduction	Flexor carpi ulnaris	Ulnar nerve	C 5, 6, 7, 8
	Extensor carpi ulnaris	Radial nerve (deep branch*)	C 5, 6, 7, 8

* The deep branch of the radial nerve is also called the posterior interosseous nerve from its position in the extensor compartment posterior to the interosseous membrane.

1 Reproduced with permission from MacKinnon P, Morris J (2005). *Oxford Textbook of Functional Anatomy*, Vol 1. Oxford: Oxford University Press. © 2005.

About the Oxford American Handbooks in Medicine

The Oxford American Handbooks are flexi-covered pocket clinical books, providing practical guidance in quick reference, note form. Titles cover major medical specialties or cross-specialty topics and are aimed at students, residents, internists, family physicians, and practicing physicians within specific disciplines.

Their reputation is built on including the best clinical information, complemented by hints, tips, and advice from the authors. Each one is carefully reviewed by senior subject experts, residents, and students to ensure that content reflects the reality of day-to-day medical practice.

Key series features

- Written in short chunks, each topic is covered in a two-page spread to enable readers to find information quickly. They are also perfect for test preparation and gaining a quick overview of a subject without scanning through unnecessary pages.
- Content is evidence based and complemented by the expertise and judgment of experienced authors.
- The Handbooks provide a humanistic approach to medicine—it's more than just treatment by numbers.
- A "friend in your pocket," the Handbooks offer honest, reliable guidance about the difficulties of practicing medicine and provide coverage of both the practice and art of medicine.
- For quick reference, useful "everyday" information is included on the inside covers.
- Made with hard-wearing plastic covers, tough paper, and built-in ribbon bookmarks, the Handbooks stand up to heavy usage.